Ocular Trauma in Armed Conflicts

Shrikant Waikar
Editor

Ocular Trauma in Armed Conflicts

Springer

Editor
Shrikant Waikar
Department of Ophthalmology
Institute of Naval Medicine, INHS Asvini
Mumbai, Maharashtra, India

ISBN 978-981-19-4020-0 ISBN 978-981-19-4021-7 (eBook)
https://doi.org/10.1007/978-981-19-4021-7

This Springer imprint is published by the registered company Springer Nature Singapore Pte Ltd.
The registered company address is: 152 Beach Road, #21-01/04 Gateway East, Singapore 189721, Singapore

Dedicated to all my patients
who have always reposed unstinted faith in me and have been
my source of
inspiration and motivation.

Foreword

Trauma is as old as the human civilization and ocular trauma is no exception. Even cave men fought with each other over food and prey. Armed conflicts have been raging across the globe in the form of conventional or unconventional warfare. The worst sufferers of these conflicts are young men. There is not only loss of young lives but also mutilation of body parts and visual morbidity. Having experience of 1965 and 1971 Indo-Pak and Sri Lanka operations I can vouch for the fact that ocular trauma in armed conflicts requires a highly specialised approach to its management. Ocular trauma is mostly a part of poly trauma in such cases. There is always a time lag in these cases reaching specialised centres of treatment due to evacuation difficulties. The foremost priority is saving of life/limb and preserving the visual function. Loss of vision has a devastating effect and rehabilitation post-treatment is very important. It involves both visual and cosmetic rehabilitation. There is thus a need for an exclusive book on management of ocular trauma sustained in armed conflicts. This book is an attempt in that direction.

Trauma in a conflict situation can be of varying nature. It could be mechanical trauma which can be direct or indirect in the form of missiles or blast injuries. It can be chemical, biological, radiological or nuclear trauma. This textbook covers every aspect of ocular trauma sustained in armed conflicts. Each contributing author has a vast experience of tackling such injuries.

Time is of utmost importance in any case of ocular trauma. In a conflict situation a lot of time is lost before the casualty can reach a tertiary facility. Hence the book covers trauma care right from its inception till the tertiary care level. **Lifesaving** takes **precedence** but an appropriate timely management at the onset of trauma and early introduction of antibiotics and prevention of further aggravation can go a long way in the final outcome. Battle scenario is very different from a civil setup. The book starts with a chapter on the changing nature of ocular trauma and battlefield trauma presentation and prehospital care followed by a chapter on **the forward surgeons'** perspective on the management of battlefield polytrauma. Due to the peculiar constraints of a battle situation such as terrain, time, weather or intensity of conflict, it is only infrequently that a casualty can be air lifted directly to a tertiary care centre. In most cases the care at this level is provided by fellow soldiers, paramedics and medical officer. The next level of care is provided by the forward general surgeon. An appropriate timely management goes a long way in **not only saving the life** but also by stabilising the casualty so that further management can be taken over by the concerned specialists. These chapters have been enriched **by real-life experiences of the authors in battle scenarios**. Chemical, biological, radiological and nuclear (CBRN) warfare injuries and management are well covered. Detailed initial evaluation by first contact ophthalmologist and meticulous primary repair of open globe injury is the most important step which will determine future course of the injured eye. A separate chapter is devoted towards this step. There have been a number of advances in imaging and ophthalmic investigative procedures, and these have been covered in detail as also the classification of ocular trauma. War injuries are often associated with orbital and craniofacial injuries, and they have been **covered in detail by** a maxillofacial and reconstructive surgeon. Renowned subspecialists in cornea, cataract and refractive surgery, glaucoma, uvea, vitreo-retina and oculoplasty have come together to elaborately cover every aspect of globe injury in various chapters. Head injury has a number of neuro-ophthalmological manifestations and that has also been covered in detail. **Finally, a chapter** on low visual aids, prevention of trauma and rehabilitation of ocular trauma cases is also included.

This textbook comprehensively **covers the complete spectrum** of ocular trauma in armed conflicts right from its occurrence to primary, secondary and tertiary management. There is a smooth flow of information. The text is easy to understand and is well supported by diagrams and colour photographs. **It is an ideal reference book for** all trauma care personnel, viz. paramedics, medical officers and **general surgeons** located in forward areas in war. It will also be of immense benefit not only for postgraduate students and general ophthalmologists but also those practicing sub-specialities.

Ocular Trauma Society of India
New Delhi, India
Armed Forces Medical College
PuneIndia

M. S. Boparai

Preface

The thought process for this textbook on *Ocular Trauma in Armed Conflicts* originated when I took upon the task of organising a continuing medical education programme on ocular trauma. I realised that even two full days of the CME were insufficient to cover such trauma in toto. The vast, diverse and complex nature of ocular injuries in armed conflicts coupled with scanty and scattered literature available led me to the conceptualisation of this textbook. A complete manual on ocular trauma in armed conflicts which would cover management strategies right at the occurrence of injury and continued at every step along the chain of evacuation was essential. The aim was to provide an ideal reference manual for trauma care personnel, medical officers and general surgeons in war zone and a complete textbook for ophthalmology practitioners. Appropriate management has to be instituted right at the time of injury and continued further at primary, secondary and tertiary level. Having served in the armed forces for over 30 years, first as a medical officer with troops in forward locations in conflict zone and then as an ophthalmologist in peripheral hospitals and later as a senior specialist in the tertiary care centres, I experienced at first hand difficulties and constraints in management of ocular trauma at each level. Substantial difficulties are faced at the grassroots level in managing a casualty in the middle of a conflict. There are peculiar constraints of such a situation. The medical officer has to provide medical care in a hostile environment. The evacuation is difficult and the resources are limited. The focus is on saving life. Also due to limited training in management of ocular trauma at medical school level, the eyes are often neglected. If an evacuation gets delayed there may be irreversible damage by the time the casualty reaches an Ophthalmologist. The first contact ophthalmologist has a very important role to play. An appropriate management at this level and a meticulous primary repair would form the base for future interventions by various sub-specialists. This aspect has been covered in detail and would be of immense benefit not only to the residents but also to all ophthalmology practitioners. Various investigative modalities available in the armamentarium have been covered in detail. An attempt has been made to elaborately cover the management strategies at each level and also the specialised management of trauma to various ocular structures. Basic and advanced management of orbital and adnexal trauma, anterior and posterior segment injuries have been covered in detail. Ocular trauma in an armed conflict in a young individual not only leads to structural and functional ocular damage but also leads to cosmetic disfigurement and immense psychological impact.

Prevention of trauma, management of low vision and rehabilitation have also been covered. Experienced specialists in the respective domains have come together to contribute towards this book with the aim of advancing the knowledge in this field. I truly hope this effort will enhance the skills of all trauma care personnel in managing ocular injuries and create a positive impact on the lives of the injured.

Mumbai, Maharashtra, India Shrikant Waikar

Acknowledgements

As I ventured upon the path of writing this textbook the enormity of the mammoth task overwhelmed me. I thank my parents for their blessings which provided me the guiding light along the difficult path. It made the seemingly impossible task achievable.

I thank Dr. Sandeep Saxena whose unconditional support and encouragement made me embark upon the path of writing this book and turned this book from a concept into a reality. I thank my wife Meenakshi who stood by me and was the pillar of support throughout the journey of writing this book. I am thankful to my children Pooja and Aashish for bearing with my busy schedule and helping me to complete the commitment.

The specialised management of complex ocular trauma required the experts in various specialities to contribute to this task. I am thankful to all the authors for having come forward and contribute towards this text despite their heavy commitments. I am thankful to my colleagues who contributed with inputs from their experience of managing ocular injuries in forward hospitals. I thank Suvendu Panda who helped me with the drafting and organising the text. I thank my organisation for granting me the permission to write this book. I thank all those whose names I may have missed but their contribution was invaluable. I finally thank the publishers for having agreed to publish this textbook on the vital issue of ocular trauma in armed conflicts.

As I ventured upon the path of writing this textbook the enormity of the mammoth task overwhelmed me. I thank my parents for their blessings which provided me the guiding light along the difficult path. It made the seemingly impossible task achievable.

Disclaimer

Views expressed in this book are those of the Authors and do not represent views or position of Indian Armed Forces.

Contents

About the Editor

Shrikant Waikar is presently Professor and Head of the Department of Ophthalmology at Institute of Naval Medicine, INHS Asvini, Colaba, Mumbai, India, and is a Senior Adviser to 16 armed forces hospitals across India. He graduated from Armed Forces Medical College (AFMC), Pune, India, in 1989. After graduation, he actively participated as a medical officer with the fighting forces in various counter-terror operations. He has seen active armed operations at close quarters and managed multiple forms of trauma for 3 years before specialising in the field of Ophthalmology from AFMC Pune (MS) followed by a Diplomate of National Board (DNB) and fellowship from Sankara Nethralaya, Chennai (FMRF). He is also a member of the National Academy of Medical Sciences (MNAMS). He has served as an ophthalmologist and anterior segment microsurgeon in various armed forces hospitals in India. He has vast experience in managing all forms of ocular trauma, both military and civil. He has been taking lectures on ocular trauma in various forums and organised a national level CME at Lucknow, India, for armed forces and civil ophthalmologists. He has several publications and has delivered numerous national and international conference presentations.

1 Changing Nature of Oculofacial Trauma in Armed Conflicts

Meenakshi Sharma

The history of mankind goes hand in hand with the history of conflicts. Starting his journey from the Paleolithic age as a hunter gatherer, conflicts started between man and animals. Weapons made of stones and wood were devised to aid in hunting. As human population increased also increased the mutual intolerance. The desire for dominance, supremacy, and control over the limited resources led to conflicts between human communities. Bands of armed men raided adjoining settlements frequently, leading to violent conflicts. Humans, sitting at the top of the pyramid of the animal kingdom, rapidly advanced in every field. The gap between humans and animals increased, but the basic animal trait of violence and intolerance never went away. Through the Neolithic Age and the Metal Age more and more lethal weapons were devised for offense and defense. They were used not only for hunting but also against fellow humans. Human settlements progressed from small groups and tribes to larger civilizations and kingdoms, and eventually to the nations of today. History is witness to large scale conflicts and wars over the ages, with the loss of millions of lives and injuries. Wars led to the downfall of thriving civilizations. Weapons have continued to evolve from the prehistoric era to the present, changing the nature of trauma over the ages.

1.1 Evolution of Weapons Leading to Changing Nature of Ocular Trauma

1.1.1 Prehistoric Era: The Era Before the Origin of Script

Paleolithic age (2.5 million years BCE to 10,000 BCE): Weapons were made of stone, bones, and wood. Crude stone axes were also used. These earliest weapons, made of stones and sticks, caused blunt injuries, while heavier stones would lead to crush injuries.

Mesolithic age (10,000 BCE to 8000 BCE): Polished small stones were attached to wood, bones, or antlers for use as spears or arrows. These were devised for hunting to cut through the thick hide of animals. The sharp, polished stones along with the wooden spears caused deeper injuries.

Neolithic Age (8000 BCE to 3000 BCE): Man settled down from a nomadic lifestyle. Used tools for agriculture. Stone weapons, bows and arrows and spears were used for offense or defense [1]. Civilizations flourished in Mesopotamia, Egypt, Greece, Rome,the Indus Valley, and China from the neolithic age onwards, going into the ancient history era. This was an era of wars and inva-

M. Sharma (✉)
Ex Army Dental Corps, India, Delhi, India

S. Waikar (ed.), *Ocular Trauma in Armed Conflicts*, https://doi.org/10.1007/978-981-19-4021-7_1

sions. The rulers tried to expand their kingdoms, leading to violent conflicts.

Chalcolithic (Bronze) Age (3000 BCE to 1300 BCE): Bronze, an alloy of copper and tin, was discovered. Civilizations now used bronze for sharper and pointed weapons and also blunt heavy maces. The Sumerians in Mesopotamia were the first to use metals in weapons. The pointed metal weapons caused deep penetrating injuries, while the heavy maces caused blunt injuries.

Protohistory: The transition period from oral to written records started in the late Neolithic to early Chalcolithic ages.

1.1.2 Ancient History Era: The Era of Written History

Ancient history consisted of the period from the onset of written history up until 500 CE, around the fall of the Roman Empire. This period included the Iron Age from 1300 BCE-900 BCE. Advances in weapons took place. Bronze could not hold its sharpness, so iron weapons were devised [2]. At this time, iron was considered even more precious than gold.

The discovery of metals allowed the development of metal spears, arrows, swords, and knives. These newer weapons were more dangerous and lethal causing severe lacerations and deeper penetrating injuries. Newer weapons were designed. Catapults were devised in ancient Greece around 400 BCE and further refined by the Romans [3]. They were used to launch large stones and multiple darts. At times poisonous snakes, containers of bees, and even dead bodies infected with plague were launched. This was probably the earliest instance of biological warfare.

Middle Ages—500–1500 CE: This period extended from the fall of the Roman Empire until the fall of Constantinople. A new weapon, fire in the form of flame throwers, was used by the Greeks to cause fires in the enemy ships and cause a large number of casualties by thermal burns. This incendiary substance was invented in 672 CE and was called Greek fire. The nature of this substance still remains unknown. It was probably a mixture of naphthalene, pine resin, quick lime, sulphur ,and calcium phosphide. It would cling to skin and cause extensive burns, and it even burned in water.

Around 1000 CE, gunpowder was invented in China from saltpeter (potassium nitrate), sulfur and carbon. Europeans called salt peter as snow from China or Chinese salt. This was used to improve the existing weapons. Crude hand grenades and canons started being used by the Chinese around 1200 CE. They also used early forms of rockets. Around 1440 CE in the later part of a 100-years war, the French used gunpowder in artillery guns against the English army. The use of gun powder laden weapons caused a large number of casualties due to secondary missiles and splinters [4].

Modern age—1500–1800 CE: This period included the age of discovery. Sea expeditions and discovery of new lands of America, Africa and India led to wars between the colonialists and the natives and also the violence related to slave trade.

For centuries, wars were fought with weapons made of metal and wood, like swords, bows and arrows and spears, until gunpowder was invented. This led to the invention of guns and canons. Armed with this newer and superior weaponry, colonialists easily conquered large areas, defeating native armies with primitive weapons. Mysorean rockets were pioneered by Tipu Sultan, ruler of Mysore in India, who used them against the British Army in the 1780s. This rocket technology was later adopted by Napoleon Bonaparte in France.

Contemporary age, 1800 CE to present day: In this era, over a period of time, there was a shift in the mode of warfare from close hand-to-hand combat to the increasing use of projectile weaponry. With these weapons came new forms of injury caused by higher-velocity bullets or splinters. Secondary missiles in the form of high-speed stones and pebbles as a result of cannon balls also caused ocular injuries. In 1803, the British used shrapnel. Shrapnel would burst close to the target releasing multiple pellets or shrapnels and were much more devastating than earlier weapons. Rifles though invented in 1498 became practical for use in warfare around 1850s when they were used effectively by Prussians against Austria. Soon machine guns were invented causing multiple high velocity bullet wounds. The pace of inventions increased in twentieth century.

The advances in arms and ammunition and in modern weaponry brought about more destruction and injuries. Newer explosive devices, besides direct trauma from fragments and splinters, also generated shock waves due to blast, which were extremely damaging to hollow organs and also the eye. The transmission of shock waves into the eye caused damage to all intraocular structures, even in a closed globe injury.

Chemical weapons were used in the First World War, causing mass blindness. They were again used in gas chambers during the Holocaust in the 1930s. The nuclear bombs were dropped for the first and fortunately the last time on the Japanese cities of Hiroshima and Nagasaki in 1945, towards the end of the Second World War.

These weapons of mass destruction, like chemical, biological, and nuclear weapons used in the first and second world war, led to large-scale destruction and death.

All these weapons resulted in a wide spectrum of injuries due to direct blunt or penetrating trauma, foreign bodies, thermal, chemical, and radiation injuries, as well as damage due to shock waves due to blasts. Contamination and infection further compounded the problems. Newer developments in laser weapons have further made the eyes vulnerable.

The human race has entered the third decade of the twenty-first century. But still, there is no end to armed conflicts. The twentieth century saw two world wars and many large scale wars. There has been no respite in the twenty-first century either. The major wars starting with World War I are enumerated below.

1.1.3 Wars in the Contemporary Age

World War I (1914–1918)
World War II (1939–1945)
Cold War (Soviet Union and United States, and their allies, 1945–1991)
Korean War (1950–1953)
Vietnam War (1955–1975)
India-China War 1962
Indo Pak War 1965 and 1971
Bosnian War (1992–1995)
Kargil War 1999
War on Terrorism (2001–present)
War in Afghanistan (2001–2021)
War in Iraq (2003–2011)
Syrian Civil War (2011–present)
Libyan Civil War (2014–2020)
War in Donbass (2014–present)
War between Armenia and Azarbaijang 2020
Russia–Ukraine war 2022

Besides these, numerous low-intensity conflicts and anti-militancy operations are continuing across the world. The concept of war has changed over the years. Instead of causing death, the aim in today's warfare is to maim the soldier, which would occupy the fellow soldiers in attending to and evacuating the injured, thus reducing the number of fighting troops. As a result, the weapons of today cause multiple injuries to incapacitate the soldiers.

1.2 Protective Gear

The evolution of weapons has been coupled with the evolution of protective gear. The discovery of metals allowed not only the development of weapons but also of protective gear. Shields were devised to protect against swords and spears. The primitive warfare made the upper torso more susceptible. The head and neck were particularly susceptible. The eyes being unprotected and exposed, were especially vulnerable to trauma. Body armour of metal was made which was worn by warriors going into war [5]. Protective head gear was also devised. The earliest helmets were made of bronze. Later, iron helmets were made and used for protection. Protective metal face masks were also devised. The early helmets were heavy and impaired the field of vision. Newer helmets were devised, improving visibility while protecting the head. While the whole body could be protected by body armour, the eyes remained exposed and susceptible to trauma. Sight being vital to warriors, any ocular trauma would incapacitate them and make them susceptible to further injury. History is replete with instances of such trauma. There is a mention in history of an arrow injury to Philip II,father of Alexander the Great in the year 354 BCE, leading to the loss of his right eye [6]. King Antigonos I Monophthalmus, the successor of Alexander, had a similar injury to his eye, hence the suffix to his name meaning one eyed [7]. Much later in history, another reference is the tapestry of Bayeux, preserved in a museum in France. This depicts the arrow injury to the right eye of King Harold of England in the Battle of Hastings in the year 1066, leading to his death. Several soldiers with eye injuries are also depicted in this tapestry. There are other recorded instances in history of such trauma among various warriors.

To protect the eyes visors were designed for helmets. There were thin slits for vision. Even these were not foolproof. Slivers of lances could pass through these slits and cause injuries that were at times fatal.

The invention of gunpowder and firearms required new kinds of eye protection. Visors were not sufficient protection against bullets. Splinters could go through the slits and injure the eyes. Chemical warfare and the use of poisonous gases in the first and second world wars made the use of gas masks with eye protection essential. Mobile armored vehicles and tanks required the use of protective glasses for protection against mud, stones, and dust. Thick shock resistant polycarbonate glasses are being devised for eye protection. But still ,protective measures are not universal and foolproof. Till foolproof protective gear is designed, eyes will continue to remain vulnerable.

1.3 Changes in Medical Care Over the Years

No proper system of medical care or evacuation was there in olden times. As huge armies indulged in hand-to-hand combat, heaps of bodies would pile up in the battle field.

With no proper system of evacuation and medical care, they were left to fend for themselves and many would succomb to their injuries.

The kings had their royal physicians available to treat him. Philip's eye injury was successfully treated by his physician Critobulos, who excelled in the removal of arrows using a special instrument called the "spoon of Diocles' [6]. Much later, in 1403 CE, King Henry V had a similar arrow injury to his eye, which was saved by London surgeon John Bradmore [8]. However, such successful outcomes were rare. Others were not so fortunate. In most cases, the injured died for lack of proper medical care. Such was the state right from ancient days until modern times.

Even in modern times, injured people were kept in inadequately staffed wards under unhygienic conditions, where many would die of diseases. Baron Dominique Larrey was the first military surgeon to organize battlefield trauma care during the Napoleonic Wars in France. He utilized horse-drawn ambulances called 'Flying Ambulances' and prioritized evacuating more serious casualties first [9]. The British trauma care system was much less organized, and it was during the Crimean War that Florence Nightingale was first sent to provide the healing touch to injured soldiers. This led to further improvements in the care of the injured. The International Red Cross then stepped in to provide medical care to the injured. Over the years, a lot of advances have taken place in tactical battlefield trauma care and evacuation, leading to much better outcomes. Early evacuation has not only allowed more lives to be saved but also ensured access to advanced tertiary care.

In ancient times, the care of the injured consisted of the removal of the embedded arrow and the application of herbs to the wound. Careful observations and innovations over the years have led to advancements in medical care. Knowledge has grown progressively since ancient times. Refinement in surgical techniques, antibiotics, and surgical asepsis have all improved the outcomes of war injuries. War wounds have even led to newer inventions. The invention of the intraocular lens (IOL) is attributed to one such observation. Prof. Harold Ridley observed during the Second World War that the intraocular foreign body consisting of tiny splinters of the transparent canopy of fighter aircraft in RAF pilots did not cause any reaction. This observation and the resultant invention of the IOL has revolutionized cataract surgery today [10]. The advancements in ophthalmic, maxillofacial, and oculofacial surgical techniques has enabled visual and cosmetic rehabilitation in most cases of ocular trauma.

Due to increased awareness of the futility of war and the destruction and deprivation caused by war, large scale wars have decreased, but there is unrest across the world. Violent conflicts continue in the form of conventional wars or unconventional warfare, terror attacks and counter terror operations, territorial wars, mob violence, etc. New weapons continue to be devised to find a ready market. Medical care has to keep pace so as to remain one step ahead to provide succour to the needy and injured.

References

1. McEwen E, Bergman R, Miller C. Early bow design and construction. Sci Am. 1991;264:76–82.
2. Kanz F, Grossschmidt K. Head injuries of Roman gladiators. Forensic Sci Int. 2006;160(2–3):207–16.
3. Rossi C, Russo F. A reconstruction of the Greek–Roman repeating catapult. Mech Mach Theory. 2010;45(1):36–45.
4. Hall B. Weapons and warfare in renaissance Europe: gunpowder, technology, and tactics. Baltimore: The Johns Hopkins University Press; 2001. p. 320.
5. Clements J. Medieval armor: plated perfection. Mil Hist. 2005;22(4):38–41.
6. Lascaratos J, Lascaratos G, Kalantzis G. The ophthalmic wound of Philip II of Macedonia (360–336 BCE). Surv Ophthalmol. 2004;49(2):256–61.
7. Lascaratos J. "Eyes" on the thrones: imperial ophthalmologic nicknames. Surv Ophthalmol. 1999;44:73–8.
8. Sadun AA. The eye injury that changed history. San Francisco: AAO, Scope, Senior Ophthalmologists; 2017.
9. Katoch R, Rajagopalan S. Warfare injuries: history, triage, transport and field hospital setup in the armed forces. MJAFI. 2010;66:304–8.
10. Apple DJ, Sims J, et al. Harold Ridley and the invention of the intraocular lens. Surv Ophthalmol. 1995;40:279–92.

2 Battlefield Trauma Care: Prehospital Management

Ashwani Shukla

Since the earliest days of civilisation, it has been recognised that a fit army is an effective army. The assurance that they will be efficiently attended to in the event of any injury is a big morale booster for the fighting soldier and also acts as a force multiplier for the commander on the battlefield. Hence, protocols for triage and surgery were developed as early as Hammurabi's Babylon, - documented in the Edwin Smith papyrus (1500 BC.) [1]. The Greeks required physicians to be present during the battle, and the Romans established hospitals close to the battlefield. Indian mythology and historical texts also recount the close association of 'vaids' and healers with the battling armies.

The modern concepts of military surgery and trauma care were established by Dominique Larry (1776–1842), the chief surgeon of Napoleon's army, who developed concepts of sanitation, epidemiology, triage, evacuation, and training of medical personnel. He organised a system of prehospital transportation to carry the wounded from the battlefield to a central location by a horse drawn wagon called the 'Flying Ambulance' [2]. These concepts continue to shape military medicine to this day. The British Indian Army soon incorporated these principles and established the first corps of stretcher bearers ,followed by the Royal Bengal Medical Corps, which was a full-fledged organisation specifically for the care of the sick and wounded in the army. The father of our nation, Mahatma Gandhi, too, started his journey in public service by organising a St. John's Ambulance Corps during the Boer War in South Africa.

Broadly, the medical setup in all armies across the world is top down and bottom-up, where the organisation and protocols are standardised from above and implementation is left to the practitioners below, who improvise the delivery as per the fluid situation on the ground. At the level of a fighting unit, i.e., a regiment, there is a doctor, called the Regimental Medical Officer (RMO), generally a GP, who has a few trained medical personnel (medics or nursing assistants), under him or her and also a special group of combatant soldiers (BFNAs, or Battle Field Nursing Assistants) who are specially trained in basic life support. BFNAs are embedded in small groups of a platoon or less at the site of action to carry out first aid and evacuation, for the doctor cannot be everywhere. Additionally, it is one of the duties of the RMO to constantly train all soldiers in the best practices for avoiding and managing injuries sustained by them and to help their buddies in the heat of battle.

The most common wounding agent in modern warfare is artillery bombs, not bullets. Bombs cause blast injuries to those directly exposed and

A. Shukla (✉)
Ex Army Medical Corps, India, Delhi, India
Reliance Industries Ltd, Mumbai, India

S. Waikar (ed.), *Ocular Trauma in Armed Conflicts*, https://doi.org/10.1007/978-981-19-4021-7_2

multiple penetrating wounds on the bodies of survivors from multiple bomb fragments. This is a deliberate policy—to incapacitate, not to kill; so that the enemy is burdened by a large number of war-wounded—to be evacuated, treated, and then rehabilitated, mitigating the actual effort of an army, which is to fight and kill. Seeing a fellow soldier in pain and mortally wounded has a very bad effect on the morale of the fighter and lessens his will to fight. Pre-hospital trauma management therefore incorporates features of injury prevention, mitigation, and the development of standardised protocols that can be incorporated at scale throughout a fighting force.

The compulsions of pre-hospital care are dictated by epidemiological studies, which show that there is a three-fold increase in mortality for every 30-min period that passes without medical care [3]. An injured soldier can be given little more than basic first aid during the thick of the battle and needs to be brought to a medical facility for definitive treatment. The ability to be evacuated depends on the asymmetry of logistics available between the opposing sides. Here, an early evacuation to a surgical hospital by helicopter has been shown to significantly reduce mortality.

Conversely, another review has found out that 18% of trauma deaths were caused due to pre-hospital transportation and could have been prevented by on-site rapid management. This include cases like exsanguination, airway obstruction and ventilatory compromise [4]. However, this is easier said than done because trauma under active military conditions has several constraints. Slow and difficult evacuations, lack of diagnostic aids and peer help, poor resuscitative and operative conditions and an irregular supply of medicines and blood. Finally, a transient patient and doctor population requires the development of protocols that serve as guidelines for general injury management and to provide a continuum of care progressively towards definitive care and rehabilitation.

The Tactical Combat Casualty Care (TC3) project was initiated by the Naval Special Warfare Command in 1993 and later continued by the U.S. Special Operations Command (USSOCOM). As part of this concept, besides addressing a casualty's medical condition, responding medical personnel also addresses the tactical situation faced while providing casualty care in combat.

The kind of terrain where combat is taking place makes a huge difference in casualty care. Different terrains like mountains, deserts, jungles, and glaciers result in different kinds of physiological derangements in casualties. Also, the terrain determines the mode and speed of evacuation.

2.1 The Echelon Concept of Care

(Echelon: *Noun*—a level or rank in an organisation, profession or society. OED).

A concept of levels (Echelons) of care has evolved to plan battlefield medical support. Its broad framework is as below:

2.1.1 First Echelon of Care

This is the Regimental Aid Post (RAP), manned by the RMO and a couple of medics. This is just adjacent to the actual site of engagement but not in direct line of enemy small arms fire. Patient flow in and out happens depending on the ebb and flow of the battle. with more coming in during a lull in fighting. The goal at this level is rapid treatment along the lines of ATLS/BLS and triage, with the aim of evacuation from the field or return to duty if physically and mentally fit to fight.

2.1.2 Second Echelon of Care

At the second echelon, patients are brought in from multiple RAPs, so the flow is more continuous. This is away from the frontline but well within the enemy's artillery fire range. This is staffed by a doctor or sometimes by a limited surgical team. The aim is for more definitive resuscitation, including blood and some limited damage control, while holding patients for further evacuation after fresh triage.

2.1.3 Third Echelon of Care

At the next level are Base/General or Zonal hospitals. They are staffed with multiple surgical teams and major specialties. Here definitive management of life- and limb-threatening injuries, post-operative intensive care, and limited holding facilities are available. Ophthalmic injuries will get expert initial management at this level.

2.1.4 Fourth Echelon of Care

This is a fully equipped and staffed hospital where patients can receive definitive operative and non-operative long-term care and rehabilitation.

Not every casualty needs to pass through all four stages for full treatment. Depending on the injury and the evacuation facilities available, the patient can be triaged and decisions taken accordingly.

In this chapter, we shall limit ourselves to prehospital trauma care at levels I and II.

There may not be any combat medical personnel available when the casualty occurs. Initial care may have to be provided by the combatants. The first responder can be one's self, fellow combatants, or battle field nursing assistants (BFNA,) who are combatants trained in medical care.

Care under fire is the care rendered by the first responder or combatant at the scene of the injury while he and the casualty are still under effective hostile fire. Available medical equipment is limited to that carried by the individual or by the medical provider in his or her aid bag.

Self-care: The casualty should try to return fire to keep the enemy at bay. If unable to fight, should lie flat if there is no cover and move to nearby cover as soon as possible. If hemorrhage from a limb is present, a tourniquet available in the soldier's kit should be applied.

Buddy Care: Try to shift the casualty to nearby cover while returning fire. Should reassure the casualty. Attend to his wounds. Apply a tourniquet if required.

BFNA care: BFNA is a link between medical services and fighting arms. He is capable of carrying out resuscitation and providing first aid before casualties can be evacuated further. He has analgesic injections,dressings,a tourniquet, IV fluids, antibiotics, etc. in his kit. He also has antibiotic eye drops, eye ointment, and a sterile eye patch or shield.

2.2 Care at First Echelon

This is the medical aid given by the Army medic at the scene of the battle. The casualty may still be facing direct enemy fire or be protected by a natural or makeshift structure. The first objective is to prevent further injury. Shift the person to a place not in direct enemy fire, like a trench or behind a mound. Minor wounds are given first aid, and the soldier is sent back to battle if he is physically and mentally sound. Moderate or more severe wounds are examined here and treatment is initiated. The principles of care cater to all types of injuries seen on the battlefield. A resourceful doctor can mitigate much future suffering by following certain time-tested drills. However, there are two life-threatening conditions that should be addressed immediately and pay excellent dividends if treated in time.

- An obstructed airway or a large sucking chest wound compromising ventilation
- Haemorrhage

2.2.1 Airway

May be obstructed because of head injuries. Unconscious or semiconscious patient may have poor respiratory effort, collection of secretions in the pharynx, or the tongue may fall back. The decreased oxygenation in turn will cause acidosis and brain edema leading to secondary brain injury and further worsening of the patient.

Facial injuries cause loss of integrity of the facial bones or the mandible, causing the oral and pharyngeal soft tissue to collapse into the airway space. Besides, blood and mucus may trickle down the airway if the weak patient is unable to cough or spit.

Patients with head, abdominal, or severe traumatic injuries often have nausea and vomiting. Vomit can be aspirated by a semiconscious patient.

Airway obstruction is easy to identify. The person would have air hunger, tachypnoea, stridor, or there would be poor respiratory effort. A cyanotic pallor may be observed if the condition is severe.

2.2.2 Clear the Airway by

Turn the patient to one side. If the soldier is unconscious, clear the secretions, foreign bodies, broken teeth, etc., from the mouth and throat using a gauze or gloved finger after inserting a mouth gag.

Use an oral sucker with a secretion trap—part of the medic kit.

For multiple mandibular fractures, pass a strong silk stitch through the tongue and hitch it to the chin so that the tongue does not fall back during transport.

Transport the patient by laying him on his side without a pillow so that gravity ensures that the secretions fall down onto the stretcher.

Cricothyroidotomy may be resorted to in very dire circumstances, because ensuring all the conditions needed for its success —desperation, technical skill, security, and maintenance of the air passage—together is a rare possibility.

2.2.3 Treat Pneumothorax

This may be an open, sucking chest wound, often seen with a flailing chest or a tension pneumothorax.

A sucking chest wound is easily identified by the sucking sound and the vicarious movement of a segment of the chest during inspiration and expiration. There will be other telltale signs of a chest wall injury and severe pain due to multiple rib fractures. During inspiration, the intrapleural pressure is reduced. In normal circumstances, this automatically pulls in air through our glottis and trachea. In an open chest injury, the air from outside tries to rush into the pleura during inspiration. Since it does not contribute to the O_2-CO_2 exchange, the oxygenation of blood is compromised. Treat this injury with a Vaseline gauze & shell dressing with Elastoplast covering three sides of the dressing, permitting the fourth side to allow air to escape as the normal lung expansion takes place.

A tension pneumothorax is more common in the relatively uninjured-looking chest wall, which has suffered a point-source penetrating injury or an isolated rib fracture. The injured lung parenchyma allows for communication between the airway and the pleura(chest wall). However, since the chest wall is intact, the air that has leaked out from the bronchioles is trapped between the pleura and the lungs. This causes on increase in intrapleural pressure, causing the lung to collapse and later the mediastinum to be shifted to the opposite side. Very soon, the venous return to the heart starts to get compromised, and the patient suddenly collapses. A tension pneumothorax is recognised by a dyspnoeic patient with a tracheal shift, distant or absent breath sounds on the affected side, and a 'boxy' percussion note.

The immediate first aid of a tension pneumothorax is the insertion of a wide-bore needle in the second intercostal space in the mid-clavicular line of the affected side. This allows for the leak of some air and gives you a few precious minutes to arrange for a one-way valve chest tube or a water-sealed drainage tube. A more definitive and secure chest tube insertion can be done in the second-level station. Transfer the patient with chest trauma into a semi-recumbent state supported by a few pillows.

2.2.4 Control Haemorrhage

Controlling preventable exsanguination is important because a morbidity analysis of war wounds showed that of all cases of death, 5% could be primarily attributed to blood loss [5]. These are preventable deaths. Bleeding may be internal or external. Internal organ bleeding needs surgical attention. Here, the responsibility of the battlefield doctor is to recognise the injury and arrange for rapid evacuation of the casualty after securing an intravenous access. With modern body protective armor, those who sustain internal injuries despite it are usually those who sustain severe blast or close-quarter heavy fire and are potentially unsalvageable, but the majority of war injuries (60%) reaching the hospital are extremity injuries. These include a combination of soft-tissue and bony injuries. Pressure and elevation are the two golden principles for managing such injuries.

Apply pressure dressing with a liberal amount of gauze and firm wide bandaging. The bandage should be wide enough to dissipate the pressure along either end of the extremity wound so that a localised wet bandage does not become a tourniquet over time. A scalp wound would need a crepe bandage for better security. Trunk wounds should be strapped with Elastoplast. Elevation of the bleeding part reduces the venous loss considerably.

Extremities with bony injuries may lose a lot of blood into the muscle belly, which may not be obvious at first glance. Splinting of the limb reduces the mobility of the injured part, thus promoting stasis and clot formation and temporarily stopping bleeding.

If time and skill permit, superficial bleeding wounds may be addressed with a quick figure-eight suture. No attempt should be made to do a complete closure as war wounds are very contaminated and shall need a thorough surgical debridement before any permanent management.

Tourniquets should be used as a last resort and need to be applied correctly. They should be applied on the proximal part of the limb over a single bone, i.e., the humerus or femur, and be tight enough to block both the arterial and the venous flow. Once applied, they should be released every 30 min for 3 min to provide perfusion for the viable muscles and tissues. The patient with a tourniquet should not be left unattended, and information about it should be documented and transmitted, including to the receiving doctor at the next station, when handing over. A prominent mark, like a ‘T,” on the forehead should be made so that the receiving station is aware of the tourniquet. Once a patient reaches a surgical center, the wound is explored and the bleeding is controlled under anesthesia on a priority basis. Teaching why, when, and how to tie a tourniquet is also one of the tasks of the RMO [6]. A tourniquet assembly is present in the kit of every soldier.

In the absence of these immediately life-threatening conditions among the casualties at the regimental aid post level, the doctor should follow a quick drill of primary survey, initial resuscitation, secondary survey, and triaging followed by treatment.

2.2.5 Reassure Patients

A reassuring word from an authority figure helps a frightened and anxious patient a lot. Quiet efficiency in general demeanor is the best reassurance.

2.2.6 Combat Hypothermia

In chilly weather and at night (when most of the fighting takes place these days!), Hypothermia for an exposed patient is a real danger. A vasoconstricted patient feels even more cold. Moreover, it is one factor that you can control and thus break the (often fatal) triad of trauma: hypothermia coagulopathy, and metabolic Acidosis.

Cover the patient with blankets. Do not attempt to heat the patient or place a hot water bottle underneath the blankets. It is often forgotten in the heat of more pressing issues and goes on to produce burns on the already injured patient. If time permits, or at the second echelon, warmed intravenous fluids should be given.

2.2.7 Analgesia

The concepts for analgesia keep changing, as so does the availability of drugs to the RMO. Suffice it to say that alleviating pain reduces the parasympathetic drive, reduces anxiety, and improves peripheral circulation, allowing the doctor to assess the patient better and also giving time to formulate strategy. There is still a place for opioid analgesia in safe dosages.

2.2.8 Dress and Splint Limbs

Remove the torn and debris-laden clothing, clean the wounds as best as you can, and dress the wounds with sterile dressings held in position with adhesive bandages. Splinting reduces pain and blood loss by preventing the fractured bone from digging into the soft tissue and producing further trauma. Upper limbs are best splinted with a padded Kramer-wire splint supported by a triangular bandage, and the lower limb with a Thomas splint. The RMO must drill his or her team to apply a Thomas splint with expertise and explain the physics behind the effectiveness of the nineteenth-century 'relic'.

POP, when applied, should be well padded to permit for reactionary edema. Thus, instead of a complete cast, a POP back slab with padding and bandaging is a better alternative.

2.2.9 Intravenous Resuscitation

Unlike in ER of a hospital, starting an intravenous infusion is not an automatic response in a battlefield situation. Besides rationing it for those who truly require it, the other decision a medic in the field has to take is ensuring its sustenance and care till the patient reaches the next echelon of care and is handed over to a bigger setup. Traumatic shock is generally due to hypovolemia. Once the pain has been addressed with opioids and the injury splinted, if the patient is still in shock, an intravenous line with crystalloids should be started. The aim of perfusion is to sustain vital organs with relative hypotension (90–100 mmHg systolic BP) because, in the absence of adequate surgical control, raising the blood pressure will result in a increase in bleeding [7]. If delay in evacuation is anticipated, start a ringer lactate drip with a bolus of 250 mL, followed by the rest of the fluid over 30 min. If BP is sustained, fine, or else after 2–3 units, consider giving haemaccel and trying early evacuation. Blood is not available at the forward line.

2.2.10 Antibiotics

War wounds are grossly contaminated with polymicrobial flora representing dirt, vegetation, clothing particulate matter, and chemicals. Besides, these contaminants are buried deep into the wound due to the kinetic insult at the time of injury. The correct treatment for such wounds is proper surgical debridement under anesthesia with good lighting. If available and if delay is anticipated, a broad-spectrum antibiotic may be given as prophylaxis. The provisioning and administration policies for antibiotics and drugs are constantly under review depending on the theater concerned, and the RMOs should keep themselves updated regarding them.

2.2.11 Tetanus Toxoid

As a policy, soldiers are immunised against tetanus, but an additional dose is given to all open wounds.

2.2.12 Start Oral Feeds: A Hot Cup of Sweet Tea

A hot cup of tea is a great tonic for a tired, thirsty, and hungry soldier and an effective booster of morale. Exceptions should be made for those who are in shock, have abdominal or chest wounds, or are likely to undergo surgery, such as an open globe injury.

2.2.13 Care of Ocular Injuries

- Reassure the patient.
- No pressure bandage is to be applied if there is doubt about an open globe injury.
- Eye shields are better than eye patches for protecting injured eyes.

- A sterile saline wash may be given for chemical injury or the removal of an extraocular foreign body. It should be avoided if there is a suspicion of an open globe injury.
- Broad spectrum antibiotic drops may be applied; ointment is to be avoided in case of open globe injury. Systemic antibiotics are required in such a case or any other systemic injury. Oral or systemic analgesics may be administered to alleviate the pain.

2.2.14 Documentation

The importance of clarity, brevity, and consistency in documentation while describing war injury cannot be underestimated because the injured soldier may have to pass through different medical teams, who should all be able to understand the condition of the patient, before specific treatment can be initiated. Moreover, the initial documentation carries a lot of weight in the compensation claims for a war wounded. A standard field medical card goes a long way towards fulfilling this requirement.

Flowchart for Battlefield Trauma

Primary Survey

Airway

Patent—Yes/No. If NO apply suction, chin lift, jaw thrust, oral/nasopharyngeal airway as appropriate

If trauma is blunt, watch for C spine injury and protect it

Breathing

Look for—Equal chest movements, tracheal shift, wounds and cyanosis

Listen for—breath sounds, percussion

Feel for—crepitus, surgical emphysema, pain

Record respiratory rate

Decompress chest and bandage as per requirement

Circulation

Assume all hypotension is due to hypovolemia unless proved otherwise

Control external haemorrhage

Record pulse rate, blood pressure, capillary refill

If situation permits, establish intravenous access and perfuse crystalloids

Disability Assessment (Neurological)

Prevent secondary brain injury by ensuring **ABC**

Isolated head injury does not cause shock—give fluids

Record status by AVPU/GCS

Exposure

Beware of weapon/ordinance attached to clothing, especially grenades

Expose all patients before secondary survey. Cover with blankets as soon as possible to minimise hypothermia

Bag and label all clothing and personal effects

Don't forget the back. Log roll if suspecting spinal injury

Secondary Survey

Start secondary survey after completing primary survey and after the patient is haemodynamically stable

Document all findings

Head

Head and neck is relatively exposed in cases of shrapnel and blast injuries hence

Check for small wounds

Look for bruising, swelling and asymmetry

Identify any fractures, broken teeth or altered bite. If broken, can it compromise airway during transfer?

Look for CSF leak, otorrhoea, rhinorrhoea or hemotympanum.

Look for ocular injury, periorbital odema, haemorrhage, diplopia, gaze abnormality or globe injury – cover it with a well-padded secure bandage.

Gently palpate all skull wounds for fracture or fragments

Repeat GCS

Chest

Re evaluate breathing and palpate entire chest wall including clavicles and sternum

Abdomen

Any obvious abdominal injury. Entry/ exit wounds. Localised or generalised bruising/ guarding.

Examine pelvic integrity by compression by the sides and over symphysis pubis

Perform rectal examination to look for blood, integrity of rectal wall, anal tone bony fragments

Any scrotal haematoma, meatal blood

Limbs

Most commonly injured

Look for obvious wounds, deformity, swelling, abnormal movements, pain, absence of peripheral pulses, local neurological deficits.

Splint the limb in anatomical position and recheck for peripheral pulses

Drugs

Give Analgesia and antibiotics as per protocol [8]

2.2.15 Priority in Casualty Evacuation

Triage is a dynamic assessment that should be carried out repeatedly at every level. The broad principles for selecting the priority for casevac are as follow:

- First Priority
  - Wounds of the abdomen and lower chest requiring resuscitation and urgent surgery
  - Patients with respiratory difficulty needing further management surgically (including maxillofacial wounds)
  - Gross limb injuries needing tourniquets
  - Burns over 20% BSA
- Second Priority
  - Patients who need early surgery but are in good general condition
- Third Priority
  - Rest of the cases
- Fourth Priority
  - Patients with extensive injuries or who are obviously moribund (because they shall take away the resources which could be better utilised to save first and second priority patients without any significant improvement in the chances of the survival). Principle of greatest common good

Primary care of the wounded and their early evacuation to a specialist facility is the most important intervention in reducing the morbidity and mortality of soldiers injured on the battlefield. A smart application of protocols and their dynamic modification by an alert doctor is very often the difference between life and death for a soldier and win or defeat for the Army of the day.

Appendix

Distribution of injuries: Blast vs. Gunshot wounds

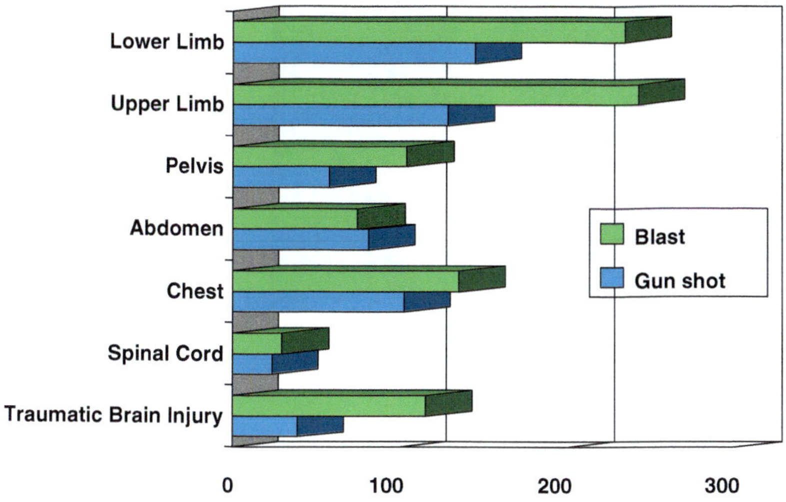

Pattern 1: Small amount of explosive

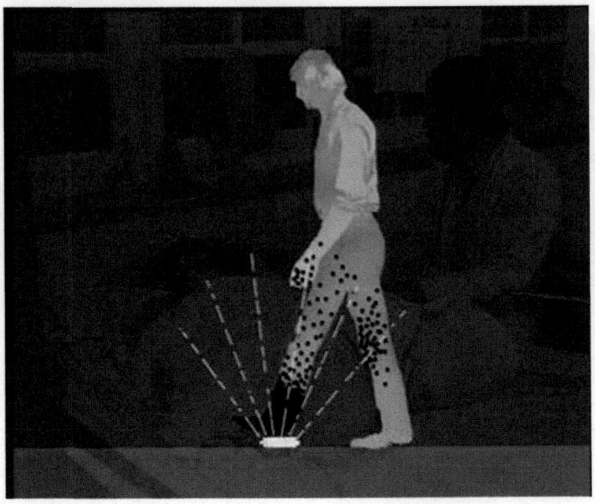

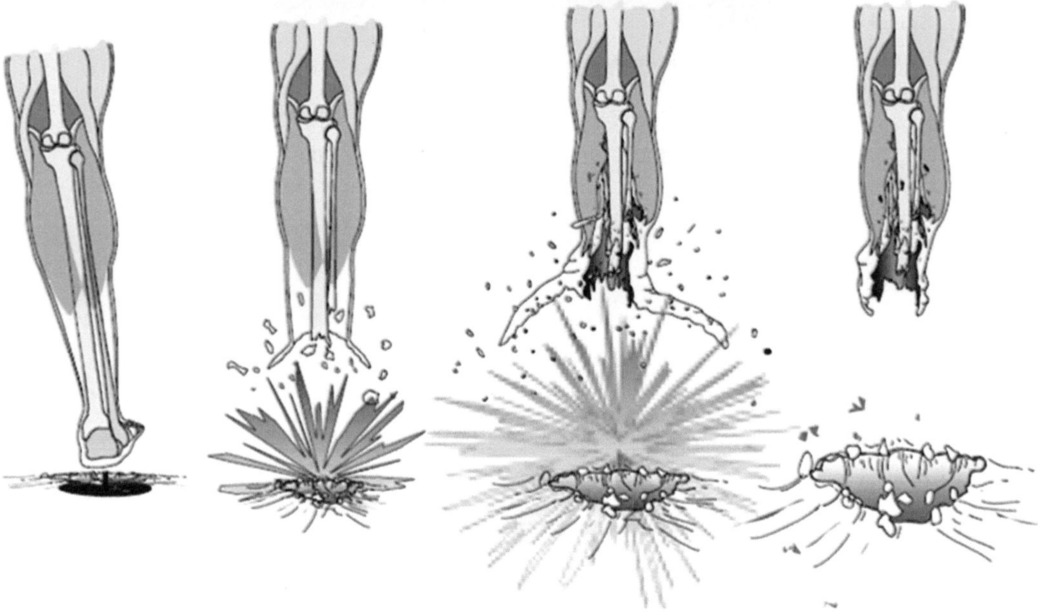

Pattern 2: Injury

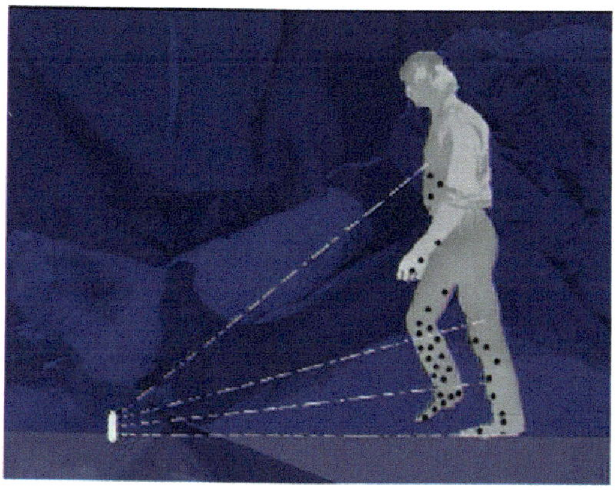

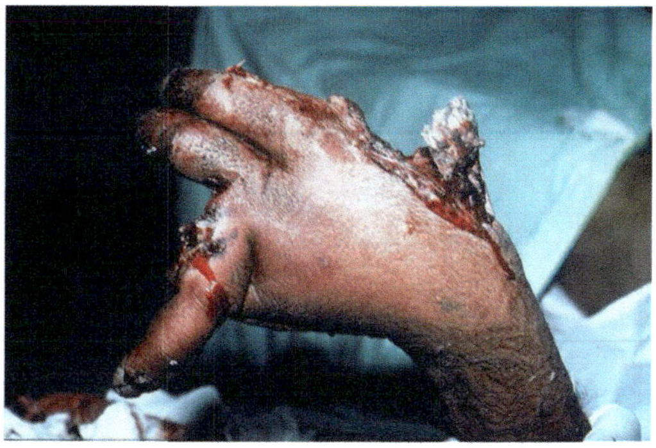

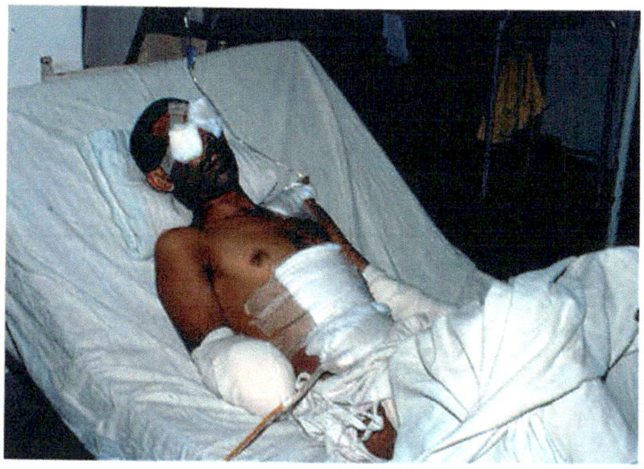

Pattern 3: Injury—manipulation of mine

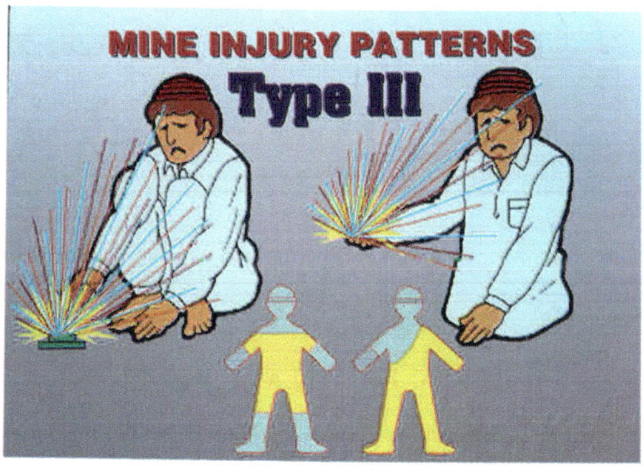

References

1. Anon. The Edwin Smith Papyrus, case 36. Classics of surgery Library. Birmingham, AL: Gryphon; 1984. p. 354–6.
2. Cushing J, Larry DJ. Memoirs of a Military Surgeon. Baltimore: Wilmont R; 1984.
3. Crowley RA, Hudson F, Scarlian E, et al. An economical and proved helicopter program for transporting the emergency critically ill and injured patient in Maryland. J Trauma. 1973;13:1029–38.
4. Frey CF, Huelke DF, Gikas PW. Resusitation and survival in motor vehicle accidents. J Trauma. 1969;9:292–310.
5. Maughen JS. An enquiry into nature of wounds resulting in killed in action in Vietnam. Mil Med. 1970;135:8–13.
6. Butler FK Jr, Hagaman J, Butler EG. Tactical combat casualty care in special operations. Mil Med. 1996;161:3–16.
7. Bickwell WH. Are victims of injury sometimes victimized by attempts at fluid resuscitation. Ann Emerg Med. 1993;22:225–6.
8. Kochar SK. Trauma care: echelon concept and relevance. Principles and practices of trauma care. New Delhi: Jaypee; 1998. p. 76–8.

3 Management of Battle Field Polytrauma: A Forward Surgeon's Perspective

Arup Ratan Basu

3.1 Introduction

Hippocrates (c. 460–377 BC) had said, "He who wishes to be a surgeon must go to war." Centuries have elapsed, but the principle of Hippocrates still holds good. Every war, conflict, or mass disaster has increased our knowledge regarding the treatment protocol for such casualties. War or battlefield surgery is somewhat different than civilian trauma or mass casualties in some manners, and these need to be understood for proper management of patients [1].

- A war scenario is highly unpredictable and yet quite basic. A few high-end tertiary centers may be present as base hospitals, but the majority of forward hospitals are likely to lack sophisticated diagnostic and therapeutic techniques.
- A war scenario is hostile and unsafe. The forward surgical team is often at personal risk from the dangers of war and often follows the "shoot and run" policy of the fighting arms of war. The safety of the surgical team must be ensured at all times.
- The casualty is transported from the forward-most areas to the surgical setup through various echelons of medical care. A well-coordinated, adequately trained team needs to be in place at the various echelons to ensure smooth transit of patients while ensuring lifesaving resuscitative measures.
- As the casualties are usually in huge numbers at any given time, the concept of mass casualty management and triage needs to be kept in mind. "Do the best you can for the time being, but not necessarily the maximum," is the policy to be followed.
- The pattern of injury in war surgery is different than civilian polytrauma and disaster. The modern weapons of war deliver high amounts of energy, which are directly transferred to the patient on contact, causing extreme polytrauma.
- Ethical and legal norms need to be practiced rigidly and differently than civilian polytrauma in cities and towns. Medical personnel at war are guided by International humanitarian law under the Geneva Convention, the ICJ at The Hague ,and the United Nations. Patients have to be treated on the basis of their needs and the severity of their injuries, without any bias toward their country, race, religion, etc. Equal and fair treatment needs to be accorded to the host and enemy nations' casualties. This might require changing the mindset of the treating surgeon and the entire team as they are in the thick of war, facing direct enemy action and its consequences. Anger management is of the utmost impor-

A. R. Basu (✉)
Department of Surgery, Manipal Tata Medical College, Jamshedpur, Jharkhand, India

S. Waikar (ed.), *Ocular Trauma in Armed Conflicts*, https://doi.org/10.1007/978-981-19-4021-7_3

tance, and a cool and balanced mind should be at the forefront. As the medical personnel face the problem of getting attacked by the enemy, adequate protection needs to be accorded to the entire medical team. This, however, is not always followed, as many times in guerilla warfare the medical team gets attacked in crossfires.

3.2 War Injuries

- The various injuries encountered in war are due to blunt injuries, penetrating wounds, anti-personnel landmines, explosive blasts, burns, and non-conventional weapons.
- Blunt trauma can be caused by road traffic accidents, collapsed buildings and falls from a military barrack, explosions and anti-tank mines, and beatings of prisoners or sympathisers.
- Penetrating trauma can be caused by fragment wounds from splinters, shrapnels,pieces of artillery shells, mortars, grenades, which travel at very high speeds and have an irregular penetrating trajectory near the site of impact. Bullet wounds are from machine guns, rifles, pistols, shotguns, etc. and may cause lethal wounds. Cut wounds, "*arme blanche,*" can be caused in close quarter battle with knives, bayonets, and machettes.
- Anti-personnel mine injuries are due to blast mines, fragmentation mines, butterfly mines, or IED (improvised explosive devices). They can cause extensive damage, like splinter injuries combined with the effect of blast injuries.
- Explosive blast injuries are due to the detonation of high-energy explosives that create a moving pressure blast wave in the air.
  - The primary blast injuries are caused by direct pressure effects with rupture of the tympanic membrane and rupturing of the alveoli and capillaries ("termed as blast lung").
  - The secondary injuries are caused by wounds caused by fragments from the bombs and their casings and contents.
  - The tertiary injuries are caused by blast winds leading to total body disintegration nearby the explosion and evisceration further away. This wind can also make buildings fall and throw people against all kinds of objects. Additionally, the blast wind can also mobilize various objects that can cause penetrating wounds.
  - The quaternary injuries are caused by burns and asphyxia from carbon monoxide or other toxic gases.
- Non-conventional weapons like chemical and biological weapons are banned by international agencies. However, many instances are known where such weapons are used.

3.3 Ballistics

- It is important to know about ballistics which essentially is the science dealing with mechanics that studies the motion and differing behavior of a moving object, specifically with its effects on a target [2]. While internal ballistics, studies the processes that occur inside a gun barrel, and the course of the projectile, it is more important to know about external ballistics which deals with the projectile after it has left the barrel including air resistance, stability, ricochet, and subsequently terminal ballistics, which studies the projectile's effect on the target and human tissues. Terminal ballistics is also known as wound ballistics.
- The basic mechanism of a bullet is a primer encased in a shell. The primer is struck and detonated by a mechanism that produces a flame and rapidly expands large volumes of gas. This force pushes the bullet or shell out of the encasing barrel. Once the bullet leaves the barrel, it spins around its longitudinal axis, and because of this, it 'wobbles' and undergoes different movements called 'yaw'. Air drag may impede the speed and trajectory of the bullet, as may crosswind deflection and raindrops. Finally, the bullet hits an obstacle or target, causing a 'ricochet' and 'pushes' the target. This causes damage to the target or tis-

sue, and if the target is firm enough, the bullet can be deformed or fragmented. The tumbling of the bullet inside a tissue changes its course, angle, and axis till it either exits or stops inside the tissue.

- Hence, large variables determine the characteristics of a projectile or fast-moving object *before* it hits the target. These include velocity at the time of impact, residual velocity (in case of an exit), mass, form, and shape of the projectile, type of weapon, stability of projectile in flight, and any yaw at the moment of impact.
- The energy in the bullet, projectile, or any weapon is determined by kinetic energy, which is KE = ½ mv^2. As the bullet passes through an object, the energy released is as follows: KE (expressed) = ½ $m(v_1^2-v_2^2)$; where v_1 is the velocity of entry and v_2 is the velocity of exit. It is according to the kinetic energy available and the velocity of the bullet that weapons are broadly classified.

3.4 Wound Ballistics

- When a bullet hits a body, it causes a projectile–tissue interaction, resulting in tissue damage and a reciprocal influence of the tissues over the bullet. This depends on the transfer of kinetic energy from the bullet to the tissues. The transferred energy then either compresses, cuts, or shears the tissues, causing crushing, laceration, or stretching. It is the energy transfer that is responsible for the most tissue damage. In tissues, a "permanent wound cavity" is created by the tissue damage after all temporary effects have occurred. This results in a wound channel that the surgeon sees while operating, which is the final result of the crushing and stretching of tissues.
- Several tissue factors are responsible for the damage sustained by a bullet or projectile. The tightness of tissues being bound together and to the fascia or to bones affects the amount of permanent damage. Resistance to crushing, laceration and stretching differs widely among tissues, with tissue elasticity and heterogeneity being important factors in determining the bullet–tissue interaction.
- Elastic tissues, though tolerating stretching well, may still suffer severe crushing. The lung and skin, due to excellent tolerance, leave relatively little residual damage. Skeletal muscle and the empty bowel wall also have good tolerance. The brain, liver, spleen, and kidney, being non-elastic, usually shatter when stretched. Fluid-filled organs react badly owing to the relative incompressibility of the fluid contents; they may even "explode". Nerves and tendons being mobile and blood vessels being elastic, they are usually pushed out of the way by the cavitation. Cortical bones, being dense and rigid, resist stretching.
- Apart from the direct energy transfer, a large projectile like a shell or bomb causes significant damage through sonic waves, compression, and blast effects. These 'shockwaves' may be of short duration but possess a very high amplitude and cause extensive damage to the microvasculature and cellular damage, including the lung, eyes, especially retinal detachment, the hollow viscus of the abdomen, blood vessels, and nervous tissue [3].

3.5 Priority of Trauma Patients and Scorings [4, 5]

- Trauma patients are assessed after a triage, as they usually arrive at the surgical setup in large numbers. Triage is for the purpose of treatment and transport according to the severity. Primary triage is done at the scene of injury or war by the first medical officer, and subsequently, secondary triage is done at the casualty clearing station. Triage is usually repeated prior to transportation away from the scene of injury and repeated again at the hospital.
- The aim of Triage is to identify and treat life-threatening injuries while keeping in mind to do the "best for the most". It's a dynamic process based on the vital signs, mechanism, and

extent of injury. Triage is a dynamic equilibrium process between available needs and resources, where needs are the number of wounded and types of wounds, and resources are the facilities at hand and competent personnel available.

- Triage is at best a multiple-step process: "sift and sort", which is continuous. "Sift" involves placing the patient in a generalized category of wounded patients; "sort" then decides the priority of the injured within that category.
- After checking the pre-hospital clinical course and medical conditions, the patients are given the necessary priority after the triage.

- **Priority 1 (P1) or Triage 1 (T1)**: Where immediate care is needed in the form of life-saving intervention, the allotted color code is red. These are the patients who require care in the 'golden hour' and more so in the 'Platinum Half Hour.'

- **Priority 2 (P2) or Triage 2 (T2)**: Where urgent or intermediate care is needed, requiring significant intervention within a period of 2 or 4 h. the allotted color code is yellow.

- **Priority 3 (P3) or Triage 3 (T3)** : Where delayed medical care is needed. The patient can wait for some hours the allotted color code is green.
- **Priority 4 (P4)** is for the near-moribund patients in whom the surgical results are usually unsalvageable. It also includes patients who are dead. Such patients are not routinely dealt with in an aggressive manner to prevent the expenditure of useful and limited resources and to not waste precious time. Color code black.
- The types of patients who are in P1 cases include injuries of the chest causing tension pneumothorax or major hemorrhage; burns to the face and neck, and injuries requiring urgent tracheostomy; visible massive internal haemorrhage, wounds to major peripheral blood vessels; traumatic amputation; complicated chest injuries and burns >15%.
- P2 includes patients with penetrating head injuries with GCS > 8; visceral injuries with no P1 features, chest injuries without asphyxia; major fractures, and burns 15% involving the head, face, hands, or genitalia.
- P3 includes patients who require delayed surgery, which may affect the outcome. They are often called the 'walking wounded' and usually comprise a large majority of patients. They include minor injuries, spinal injuries, burns under 15%, and closed skeletal injuries. Patients with the pure ocular injuries are included in this. If there is an associated systemic injury, then they are prioritized according to the more serious injury.
- P4 patients are those who are unlikely to survive. These also include those patients who would have a very poor quality of survival, such as penetrating head wounds with GCS 8, quadriplegia, burns >50% of body surface area, major blood loss, and no blood available.
- Immediately after triage, and sometimes accompanying it, is the '**ABCDE**' of the resuscitation system:

  Airway control with stabilization of the cervical spine, usually by the paramedics at the trauma scene
  Breathing
  Circulation and also urgent control of external hemorrhage as a first aid
  Disability or neurological status
  Exposure or undressing of the injured along with protection of the patient from hypothermia
- The 'ABCDE' is now modified to the sequence of 'C-ABCDE' to prevent immediate circulatory collapse and death of patients.

3.6 AVPU Scale

The AVPU scale is used frequently to prioritize patients.

Alert	Awake casualties are lucid, speak normally, and are responsive to their environment (e.g., eyes open spontaneously as one approaches)

Voice responsive	Casualty is able to respond meaningfully when spoken to
Pain responsive	The casualty does not respond to any questions but moves or cries out in response to a painful stimulus
Unresponsive	Casualty shows no response to any stimuli

3.7 Important Scoring Systems and Injury Scales

3.7.1 Red Cross Wound Score (Coupland Et al. [6])

3.7.1.1 Parameters of Wound Score

E	**Entry wound in cm**	
X	**Exit wound in cm**	X = 0 if no exit wound
C	**Cavity**	**Can the cavity take 2 fingers before excision**
		C0 = no
		C1 = yes
F	**Fracture**	**Are any bones fractured?**
		F 0 = no fracture
		F 1 = simple fracture, hole, or insignificant comminution
		F 2 = clinically significant comminution
V	**Vital structure**	**Are the dura, pleura, peritoneum, or major peripheral vessels injured?**
		V 0 = no vital structure injured
		V N = (neurological) penetration of the dura of the brain or spinal cord
		V T = (thorax or trachea) penetration of the pleura or of the larynx or trachea in the neck
		V A = (abdomen) penetration of the peritoneum
		V H = hemorrhage from injury to a major peripheral blood vessel down to the brachial or the popliteal arteries, or carotid artery in the neck.
M	**Metallic body**	**Are bullets or fragments visible on X-ray?**
		M 0 = no
		M 1 = yes, one metallic body.
		M 2 = yes, multiple metallic bodies.

3.7.1.2 Total Scheme of Wound Score

E (entry)	Centimeters
X (exit)	Centimeters
C (cavity)	C 0, C 1
F (fracture)	F 0, F 1, F 2
V (vital structure)	V 0, VN, VT, VA, VH
M (metallic bodies)	M 0, M 1, M 2

After the scoring, the wounds are '**graded**' according to severity (E, X, C, and F) and then '**typed**' according to the tissue type (F and V).

The wounds are **graded** according to the severity of tissue damage.

Grade 1: E +X is less than 10 cm with scores of C 0, F 0 or F 1. (Low energy transfer.)
Grade 2: E +X is less than 10 cm with scores C 1 or F 2. (High energy transfer.)
Grade 3: E +X is 10 cm or more, with C 1 or F 2. (Massive energy transfer.)

The wound are then typed as per the tissue structures of the injuries.

Type ST: Soft-tissue wounds: F 0 and V 0.
Type F: Wounds with fractures: F1 or F2, and V 0.
Type V: Vital wounds putting the patient's life at risk: F 0 and V = N, T, A, or H
Type VF: Wounds with fractures and involving vital structures that put life or limb at risk: F 1 or F 2, and V = N, T, A, or H.

Combining the two results in a classification system divided into 12 categories.

	Grade 1	Grade 2	Grade 3
Type ST	1 ST small, simple wound	2 ST medium soft-tissue wound	3 ST large soft-tissue wound
Type F	1F simple fracture	2F important fracture	3F massive comminution
Type V	1 V small wound threatening life	2 V medium wound threatening life	3 V large wound threatening life
Type VF	1VF: small wound threatening limb and/or life	2VF: important wound threatening life and/or limb	3VF: large wound threatening life and/or limb

3.7.2 Glasgow Coma Scale

The Glasgow Coma Scale (GCS) is used objectively to describe the extent of impaired consciousness in all types of acute medical and traumatic brain injury patients. It was first published by Teasdale and Jennett in 1974 at the University of Glasgow [7].

The GCS is divided into three parameters: best eye response (E), best motor response (M), and best verbal response (V). The total value is 15, and 3 is the worst response. It can be used for all patients older than 5 years of age. The scale is a follows:

Parameters	Response	Scale
Best eye response	eyes opening spontaneously	4
	Eyes opening to command	3
	eyes opening to pain	2
	No eye opening	1
Best motor response	Obeys commands	6
	Localizes pain	5
	Withdraws from pain	4
	Abnormal flexion to pain	3
	Abnormal extension of pain	2
	No motor response	1
Best verbal response	Oriented	5
	Confused	4
	Inappropriate words	3
	Incomprehensible sounds	2
	No verbal response	1

The additive total of the score is calculated, and the severity of traumatic brain injury is assessed.

Severe head injury—GCS 3–8
Moderate head injury—9–12
Mild head injury—13–15

Certain issues of concern for the GCS are preexisting factors like language barriers, intellectual or neurological deficits, hearing loss, or speech impediments. The effects of current treatment include intubated patients and patient under sedation. The effects of other injuries like orbital or cranial fractures, spinal cord damage, or hypoxic-ischemic encephalopathy can also compound the results of GCS.

A GCS–Pupil score (Brenan, Murray, and Teasdale, 2018) was devised to combine the key indicators of traumatic brain injury into a single index [8]

GCS-P = GCS minus PRS

Where PRS = pupil reactivity score, pupils are unreactive to light

Both pupils are 2; one pupil is 1; neither pupil is 0.

3.7.3 Revised Trauma Score (RTS)

The RTS is used as a triage tool based on three parameters: the GCS, systolic blood pressure (SBP), and respiratory rate (RR).

A total score of 1–10 indicates priority T1; 11 indicates T2; and 12 indicates T3. A score of 0 indicates death.

Physiological variable	Value	Score
Respiratory rate (RR)	10–29	4
	>29	3
	6–9	2
	1–5	1
	0	0
Systolic blood pressure (SBP)	>90	4
	76–89	3
	50–75	2
	1–49	1
	0	0
GCS	13–15	4
	9–12	3
	6–8	2
	4–5	1
	3	0

3.7.3.1 Other Scales

The Abbreviated Injury Scale (AIS) is an anatomical scoring system that classifies patients from minor injuries to unrevivable patients. It is not useful when used alone, but it forms the basis of the Injury Severity Score (ISS) and Trauma and Injury Severity Score (TRISS).

The TRISS score determines the probability of patient survival by the combining the ISS and RT score. A logarithmic regression equation is used while calculating.

3.8 Eye Injuries

- The head and neck region comprise 12% of the total body surface area. However, head and neck injuries are seen in over 20% of battlefield casualties in recent warfare [9]. This is most likely due to a decrease in thoraco-abdominal injuries due to the effectiveness of body protective equipment along with an increased incidence of improvised explosive devices. In comparison, there are very limited studies about eye and face protection. Soldiers wearing eye protection should potentially reduce the mean incidence of eye injuries in combat to 0.5% [3, 10].
- The **Birmingham Eye Trauma Terminology System (BETTS)** [11] is the preferred classification for severe bulbar trauma. It is broadly divided into closed-globe injuries and open-globe injuries, with contusions, lacerations, and ruptures.
- The **Ocular Trauma Score** [12, 13] is a more universal evaluation of all eye injuries. It includes the initial raw score (as NPL, PL, or HM), globe rupture, endophthalmitis, perforating injury, retinal detachment, and a relative afferent pupillary defect. It is easy to use, as the six predictive factors (**A** to **F**) are readily assessed, and it can give realistic expectations of the visual potential of an open-globe injury.
- The investigation of choice for facial and eye injuries is a 3D CT scan, after initial hemodynamic and airway stabilization of the patient. The injury is then classified and managed at a tertiary center. However, as peripheral hospitals at a war location would not be equipped with such facilities, it is suggested that basic first aid take the form of irrigation with normal saline solution, topical and systemic antibiotics, tetanus prophylaxis, and analgesics, followed by evacuation to higher centers.
- Ocular war injuries in the Indian scenario have been documented for the Indo-Pak conflict of 1965 and 1971 [14]. Ocular injuries are more common considering that they occupy only 0.1% of the erect frontal silhouette. They are included in head and neck injuries. The main patterns of injuries that were noted were:
  - Incidence of Ocular Injuries

Conflict	% of casualties
World War I	2.1
World War II	2.2
Korean war	4.1
Vietnam war	6.5
Arab-Israel conflict	6.0
Indo-Pak War, 1965	2.9
Indo-Pak War, 1971	3.1

  - Causes of Ocular Injuries: Indo Pak Wars

Cause	1965	1971
Fragments: shells, grenades, and bombs	71%	76%
Gun shot wounds	22%	13%
Mine blasts and explosions	3%	7%
Burns	2%	1.5%
Unspecified forms	2%	2.5%

  - Types of Ocular Injuries

Types of injuries	1965	1971
Perforating injuries	48%	51%
Contusion injuries	40%	38%
Burns and chemical injuries	12%	11%
Intraocular FBS	45%	47%

- The Management protocols included
  - Resuscitation and Management of vital organ injuries.
  - Removal of a completely shattered globe.
  - Subconjunctival and systemic antibiotics, mydriatics, and steroids to reduce iritis and infections.
  - Meticulous repair of eyelid injuries.
  - Detection of foreign bodies by appropriate radiological studies.
  - All other operative procedures, like vitreous surgery, Intraocular Hemorrhage, late reconstruction of the orbit, etc., are undertaken at tertiary centers.
- Combat ocular injuries from January 1992 through December 2004, in which a total of 559 cases were included, were studied [15]. The majority had splinter and shrapnel injuries. 60.36% had open globe injuries, 31.19% had closed globe injuries, and 8.45% had

adnexal injuries. The open globe injuries included perforating and penetrating injuries and ruptures. The closed globe injuries included foreign bodies of the conjunctiva and cornea, traumatic cataract, lacerations, retrobulbar hemorrhage, etc. 15.75% of patients had to undergo evisceration.

3.9 Evacuation Chain and First Aid

- The levels through which a war wounded goes through
- **On the spot: first aid.** It is usually given by a buddy or a paramedic accompanying the soldiers.
- **Collection point: first aid with or without resuscitation** It is usually manned by the regimental doctor, also called the regimental medical officer (RMO); the post is named the Regimental Aid Post (RAP). Others who may be at the site are the Red Cross volunteers, Crescent volunteers or village health and community workers. Resuscitation is done here with the first triage.
- **Intermediate stage: resuscitation with or without emergency surgery** A health center or a makeshift rural hospital may be used for this. In the military, it is termed as Advanced Dressing station (ADS).
- **Surgical hospital: primary surgical treatment** This is also called the forward surgical centre (FSC). The level of facilities and size of the hospital depend on the available resources, funds, and protected area. Most surgical hospitals have a well-equipped OT, basic investigation facilities, an ICU, and a high dependency unit (HDU).
- **Transport system for the transfer of patients from one echelon to another.** Transport is done in the most comfortable, safe, and fastest manner possible. It is either by road ambulance or air ambulances with basic resuscitative measures and an accompanying paramedic.
- **Specialized Center: where definitive surgical treatment of all kinds, including reconstructive procedures; physiotherapy and rehabilitation, both physical and psychological, are available**. These are tertiary centers away from the war zone where specialized surgeries are carried out and the patient undergoes rehabilitation.

3.10 Management of War Wounds [2, 5]

- The factors determining the final outcome of war-wounded patients are the actual injury, which implies the severity of tissue damage and the anatomic structures involved; the general condition of the patient; pre-hospital care; protection, shelter, first aid, triage, and evacuation time; immediate resuscitation; in-hospital triage; initial surgery (being of utmost importance); post-operative nursing, physiotherapy, and rehabilitation. In all of these, the single most important factor is proper wound excision or debridement.
- All patients should receive prophylaxis against tetanus. Penicillin, 5 mega-units 6-hourly intravenous after antibiotic sensitivity, should also be given from the time of admission. This should be followed by oral penicillin, 500 mg six hours a day for a total of 5 days.
- The basic investigations that need to be carried out in all war wounded casualties are as follow
  - Haemoglobin and haematocrit
  - Total and differential white blood cell count
  - Platelet count;
  - Coagulation time, bleeding time, prothombin time, and INR
  - Random blood sugar;
  - Blood smear for malaria (in infested areas only)
  - Urine analysis
  - Blood grouping and cross-matching
  - Plain X-ray of the affected area: chest, skull
  - Pulse oxymetry
- All war wounds usually involve soft tissues, complicated by damage to other structures.

War wounds are often with multiple pathologies: a bomb explosion causing a primary blast injury, penetrating metal, blunt trauma, and burns. It is mandatory for the surgeon to "think anatomy" and identify the path of any projectile. The surgeon must then imagine the possible "pathology". Fractures and peripheral vascular and nerve damage should be identified.

- A golden rule is that war wounds are always dirty and contaminated from the moment of injury because battlefields are dirty places as well. The wounded almost always have no access to basic sanitary facilities, and all precaution should be taken about fundamental hygiene.
- At the operation theater, under anesthesia, dressings and splints are carefully removed. The wound is thoroughly irrigated to remove contamination, usually with normal saline; however, in areas with limited resources, potable tap water can also be used. Full assessment of the wounds may require careful finger exploration by an experienced surgeon. The aim is neither to offer less treatment, causing subsequent sepsis or even death, nor to offer exuberant overtreatment—resulting in loss of normal tissue and subsequent increased disability.
- A two-staged procedure is followed, with the first step being wound debridement. The resulting wound is then left open and undergoes delayed primary closure (DPC) after 5 days, once the exudative phase of trauma-induced inflammation has subsided.
- The principles followed in surgery are
  - Control of haemorrhage
  - Adequate skin incisions and fasciotomies
  - Remove dead and contaminated tissues
  - Respect all tissues and handle them gently
  - Leave the wound unsutured and open
  - Restore physiological function
- Control of haemorrhage is the first priority. Blind clamping in the depths of a blood-filled cavity is never to be done. In such cases, direct local pressure should be exerted while proximal and distal control of the vessels is maintained.
- The next great danger is sepsis. There is an existing rich culture medium comprised of a mixture of dead muscle, hemostasis, bone fragments, dirty skin, and foreign material. In wound debridement, the surgeon removes the dead and damaged, grossly contaminated tissue. This leaves an area of healthy tissue with a good blood supply, capable of combating residual surface contamination, provided the wound is not closed. Skin that is grossly pulped should be removed. Usually 2–3 mm of the skin edge need to be removed at both the wound entry and exit sites. Extension of the skin wound should be made to permit better visualization and also for the proper decompression of deeper tissues. Subcutaneous fat should be excised generously. Shredded fascia should also be trimmed. The fascial incision is left open to prevent congested muscle from swelling and thereby preventing compartment syndrome.
- Bone fragments with no attachment to the periosteum should be discarded. Dirty bone ends are trimmed; periosteum debridement should be conservative and restricted to dirty and unhealthy edges.
- Bleeding should be controlled immediately, followed by repair, and where possible, replacement with a saphenous vein graft.
- All nerves must be preserved. A non-absorbable suture may be placed in the proximal and distal ends of transected nerves and pulled together to facilitate their identification at a future operation. Severed tendons requiring later repair should be marked with a non-absorbable suture.
- A projectile found during wound debridement should be removed; however, healthy tissue should never be dissected in an attempt to find one.
- A perforating bullet wound with a small entry and exit wound and no swelling of intervening tissues can be treated conservatively. Minor surgery is done for multiple superficial wounds caused by "peppering" with tiny fragments of low velocity and low kinetic energy.
- Confusion should not prevail between serial debridement and an incomplete or failed

wound excision. In an incomplete surgical excision, the patient returns to the operating room after 5 days for delayed primary closure. If the wound is found to be infected, it undergoes re-debridement and later suturing.

- In certain cases, the wound needs to be closed, such as injuries to the scalp, head, and neck, and genitals. Soft tissues of chest wounds, and all attempts should be made to close the peritoneum. The synovial membrane should be closed, and the excision of hand wounds should be very conservative. Repaired blood vessels should be covered by viable, healthy muscle.
- After the wound has been adequately excised and cleaned, it must be covered with a bulky absorbent dressing made of dry fluffed-up gauze. The gauze compresses should *not* be packed tightly in the wound.
- Ocular injury is usually associated with other multiple injuries. Triage is based on the associated injury. Open globe injuries have to be differentiated from closed globe injuries. Superficial conjunctival and corneal foreign bodies may be removed by irrigation with saline under topical anaesthesia.
- After irrigation with saline, frequent instillation of antibiotic drops may be instituted to prevent infection in ocular injuries. Eyes may be patched in case of bleeding from lid lacerations or large facial injuries. Eye shields are preferred over patching in open globe injuries to prevent further damage. However, it can be used only in patients with an intact periorbital area. Systemic antibiotics and analgesics are administered. Patient is transferred for further definitive management.
- To sum up, good management of war wounds requires
  - Tetanus prophylaxis, antibiotics, and analgesia
  - Proper wound excision with removal of dead tissue, foreign bodies, debris, and clots with proper hemostasis.
  - Adequate wound drainage and facial decompression; open, healthy wounds; and large absorbent dressings
  - Care of nerves, tendons, and periosteum of bone with limb immobilization
  - Nutrition, nursing, physiotherapy and mobilization of patients with no unnecessary dressing changes
  - Delayed primary suturing wherever required

3.11 Battlefield Surgical Experiences

- KM Rai et al. [16] published a 9 year experience in a single-center, 600-bed military hospital at Srinagar, India, from January 1990 to December 1998. In the Indian state of Jammu and Kashmir, counter-insurgency and militant activities have been witnessed from 1988 on. The study is conducted on casualties sustained by the armed forces personnel and other security forces in India. Casualties were evacuated to the hospital by air or road after receiving treatment from a medical officer, a paramedic, or a buddy at the battlefield prior to evacuation. In some case casualties were received after definitive surgery at a peripherally located hospital by a surgeon. In many cases, however, resuscitation at the site of injury was not rendered due to the element of surprise, the non-availability of medical staff, and the panicked rush of casualties. On arrival, evaluation by the surgical team, triage, and stabilisation at the ICU or surgical ward were done. The mass casualties were received in a large area specifically earmarked. Evaluation was done on RTS and on other factors suggestive of the severity of trauma. Intubation was done, and airway was secured wherever necessary. IV fluids were administered by two 16-gauge cannulae inserted into arm veins (subclavian veins or internal jugular veins). Blood was administered wherever necessary. Reduction in the time interval for initial evaluation, resuscitation, basic radiological investigation, and preparation for the operating room was mandatory. In exceptional cases, exsanguinated patients were wheeled directly into the OT on arrival.

- More than one surgical team operated on the patient quite often--simultaneous craniotomies and laparotomies in a patient with a severe head injury and gunshot wound to the abdomen and shock. Quick and speedy operations were followed. In contradiction to the Red Cross trauma policy of delayed primary closure, a policy of selective primary closure following debridement of the wound was adopted. Contraindications to selective primary closure were grossly contaminated wounds, wounds older than 12 hours, and wounds in the perineal region or the skin edges that could not be approximated.
- The minimum number of annual casualties received and managed were 380 in 1998, and the maximum number was 946 in 1994. A total of 5737 casualties were managed in a 9-year period, of which 44.37% were bullet wounds and 55.63% were fragment and splinter wounds. There was a relatively high number of abdominal injuries, which also included injuries to the back, spine, flanks, perineum, groin, and abdominal wall.
- The overall mortality in the series was 3.62%, steadily decreasing from 4.2% to 2.4% in the last year. The lessons learned were evacuation to a proper trauma center by the fastest means, aggressive resuscitation, and prompt surgery. War wounds can be closed primarily after debridement in a few selected patients. Craniotomies for severe head injuries are justifiable, with a CT scan being mandatory for the management of such patients. A policy of laparotomy in all cases of penetrating injury to the abdomen gives good results. Colonic injuries can be treated primarily with the surgery in most instances. The presence of super-specialists in a forward-looking hospital in a developing country is not mandatory for proper utilization of human resources. Finally, a dedicated and motivated team, adequately trained and experienced, can deliver good results even under trying circumstances.

3.12 Author's Personal Experience at a High Altitude Peripheral Surgical Setup in War

In the year 1999, India detected militants and infiltration along the high mountainous ridges of 14,000 to 17,000 feet in the northern region of the country. The infiltration was noticed by the Indian Army in the first week of May 1999, and subsequently, an armed conflict occurred on the high-altitude, barren mountains along the Line of Control from 03 May to 26 July, 1999. My experience of managing battle casualties at a remote peripheral field hospital in a high-altitude area from 22 May to 26 July,1999, is now elucidated. Certain peculiarities specific to the management of these casualties in a high-altitude, remotely located peripheral hospital are specified.

- The field hospital was a peripheral hospital situated amongst a nearly barren mountainous terrain in the northern part of India. Communication facilities to base hospitals were limited and time-consuming. The entire setup was within range of the enemy's medium artillery gun fire. Evacuation facilities for post-care were by road to Base hospital, dependent on the availability of transport ambulances, helicopters and on the weather & enemy artillery shelling.
- The Battle Casualties usually arrived in the evening hours. In the battlefield regimental aid post, the injured were stabilized. Injection Tetanus Toxoid, basic first aid—wound dressing, analgesics, splintage of fractures and a single dose of antibiotics were given. Subsequently they were evacuated to the hospital by ambulances by road or air ambulances. The arrival of casualties, usually would be in the evening, and the management would commence thereafter and continue through the night.
- On arrival of the casualties, they were checked for active bleed along with monitoring of the vital parameters. Triage was carried out as per

the international guidelines, with monitoring by the ABC.

- The patients were then worked up for surgery after getting the basic laboratory parameters. The following investigations were done:
  - Hemoglobin, total count, differential count, bleeding time, clotting time
  - Blood sugar (random), blood urea, and serum creatinine
  - Blood grouping, cross-matching of donors
  - X-ray of the affected region
- The standard intravenous fluid started was Ringer lactate.
  - Hemaccel (a colloidal solution) was administered for patients with systolic BP > 90 mmHg and for patients in hypovolemic shock awaiting blood.
  - Normal Saline was administered to patients with head injuries.
- Blood was demanded for all cases of shock, penetrating chest injuries, hemoperitoneum, and all cases of continuous blood loss.
- Antibiotics started were: Inj Ampicillin 500 mg IV 6 hrly after a sensitivity test; Inj Gentamicin 80 mg IV 8 hrly; Inj Metronidazole 500 mg IV 8 hrly; Inj Cloxacillin 500 mg IV 6 hrly after a sensitivity test (for all cases of bone injuries).
- Analgesics administered were Inj Pethidine 50 mg IM, or Inj Pentazocine 30 mg IM; and Inj Diclofenac Na 75 mg IM was administered for cases of head injury.
- Intraoperative and postoperative blood requirements were arranged with the military soldiers of the local regiments; these men underwent immediate grouping and cross-matching as and when blood administration was felt necessary. Blood so collected was immediately administered.
- In the post-op period, only very minor cases were discharged from the field hospital. All other cases were evacuated to the base hospital in Leh by road or helicopter and the major cases were evacuated by helicopter to the base hospital in Srinagar. A helicopter facility was being provided as per the weather and availability of aircrafts.

3.13 Results and Discussion

- A total of 300 casualties were managed in 60 days, of which the majority underwent surgery. All patients were young male soldiers in the age range of 19 to 39 years.
- Surgery was done under GA with passage of ETT (oral), NTT (nasal), or DA. Some cases with minor wounds were done under LA.

The various types of cases seen and managed at the set-up were gunshot wounds, splinter injuries, mine blasts, falls, road traffic accidents, and war psychosis.

3.14 Few Cases

Case I

A 32-years-old soldier with a splinter injury in the (L) Axilla was explored and found to have a laceration in one of the branches of the axillary artery, which was ligated. There was no injury to the brachial plexus, and the patient did not develop features of gangrene of the left upper limb 48 hours after the surgery.

Case II

A 34-years-old man sustained a splinter injury to the back. Exploration revealed a fracture to the 10th and 11th ribs (L), a pleural tear and extensive damage to the L paravertebral muscles, a splenic laceration, and a contusion of the stomach wall. Splenectomy, pleural repair, layered muscle repair, and (L) ICD were done.

Case III

A 26-years-old soldier sustained GSW (L) flank. Laparotomy revealed a lacerated descending colon, an extensive retroperitoneal hematoma, and a fracture of the iliac crest. A single-layer interrupted colon repair was done.

Case IV

A 22-years-old soldier had sustained a splinter injury to the abdomen. Laparotomy revealed a hemoperitoneum of 4 L. The splinter tract had torn the stomach, shattered the pancreas, and caused laceration of the superior mesenteric vessels and laceration of the liver. Surgery included pancreatic bed hemostasis, repair of the superior mesenteric vessels, liver laceration repair. Patient developed DIC and subsequently died 6 h after the surgery.

Case V

A 39-years-old soldier sustained a splinter injury back®. The splinter had traveled to the left side, fractured his eighth rib and caused a laceration of the lung. Exploration of the splinter tract and a limited thoracotomy were done with bilateral (ICD).

Case VI

A 23-years-old soldier has a splinter injury to his arm and a cold, clammy, and pulse-less® hand. Exploration revealed a shattered brachial artery in spasm. Artery mobilization and end-to-end anastomosis were done with 5–0 polypropylene. Fig. 3.4, below

Case VIII

THE ***POW Case***: A 27-years-old soldier of the Pakistan army (5 NLI), the only POW, had sustained multiple GSW of the (R) leg and GSW® mandible. Wound debridement and thorough bone and wound cleaning were done. The leg was salvaged, and the patient was later handed over to Pakistan on Independence Day.

3.15 Ocular Injuries

One percent of cases had ocular injuries, which were associated with head injuries. One case had penetrating globe injury, which was managed by normal saline wash, injectable analgesia, and antibiotics. One case had conjunctival hemorrhage with a mild decrease in visual perception. He was managed with topical antibiotics (Ciprofloxacin drops). The third case had chemosis and a lacerated eyelid; the eyelid was sutured. All cases were evacuated to a tertiary center. All the ocular injury cases had multiple associated injuries, as seen in Figs. 3.1, 3.2, 3.3, 3.4, 3.5, 3.6, 3.7, and 3.8 below.

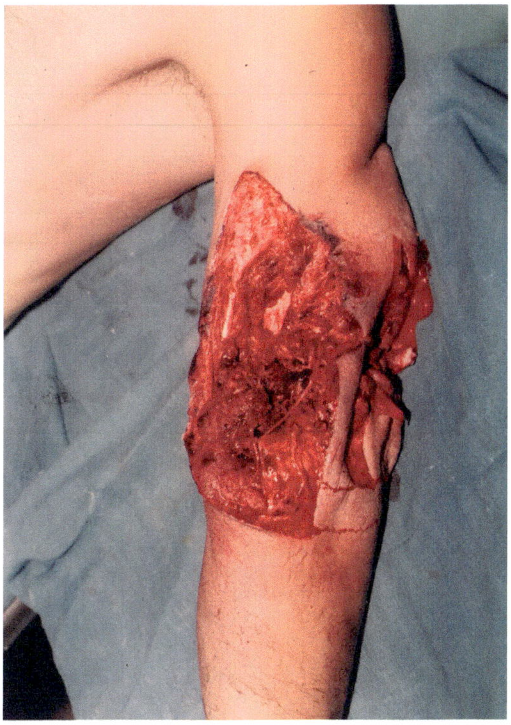

Fig. 3.1 Splinter injury left arm with fracture humerus

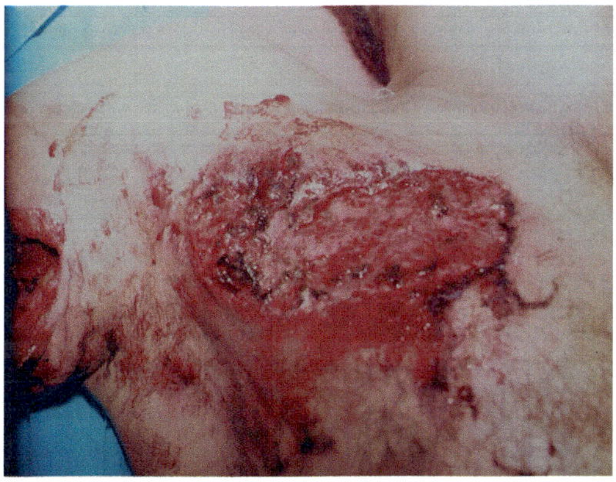

Fig. 3.2 Degloving injury right chest wall

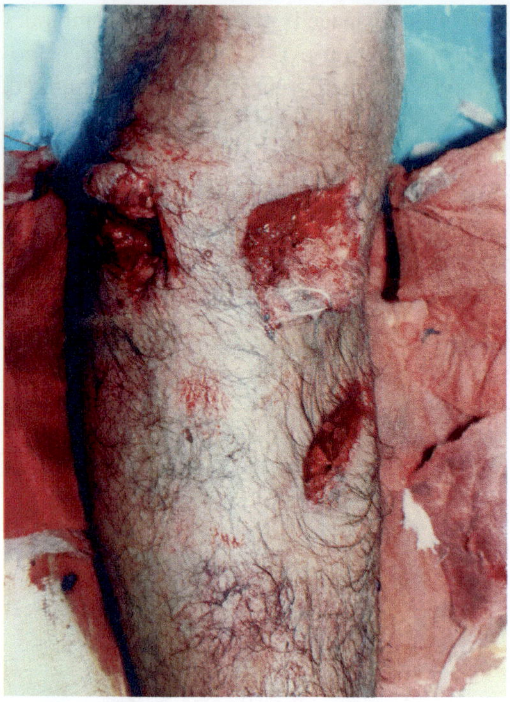

Fig. 3.3 Multiple splinter injury right leg

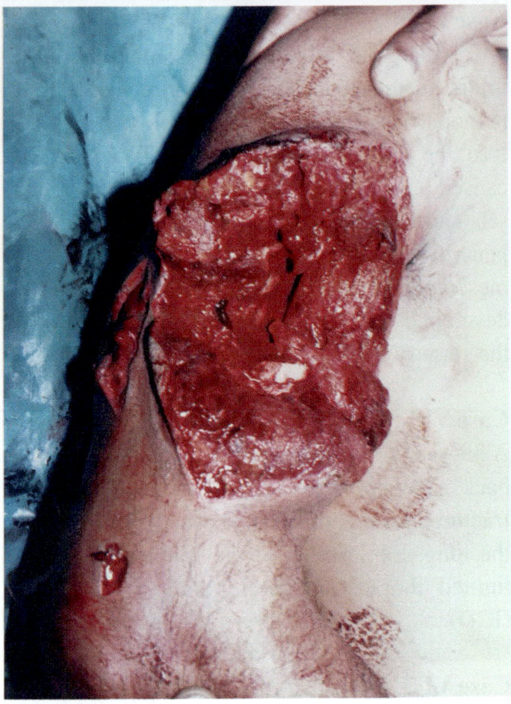

Fig. 3.5 Degloving splinter injury right arm. No fracture or neurovascular damage

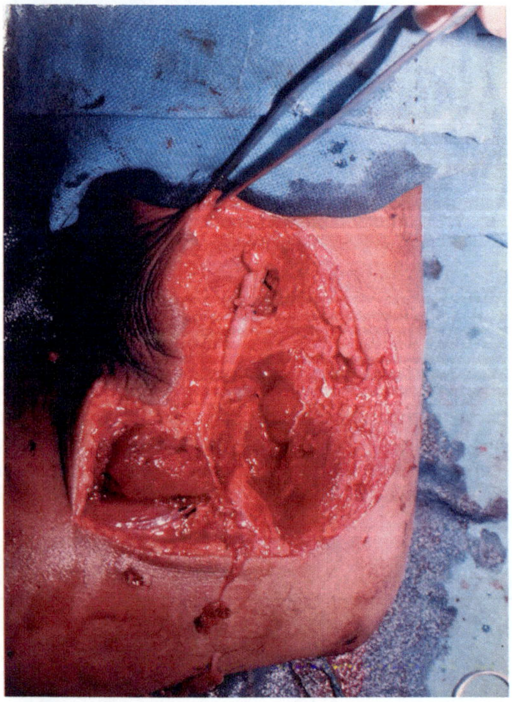

Fig. 3.4 Splinter injury right Brachial artery. Anastomosis with 5–0 polypropylene

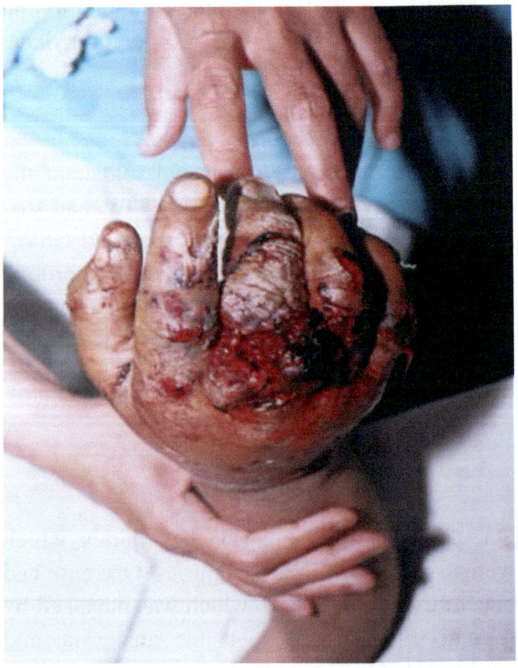

Fig. 3.6 Mine blast right hand

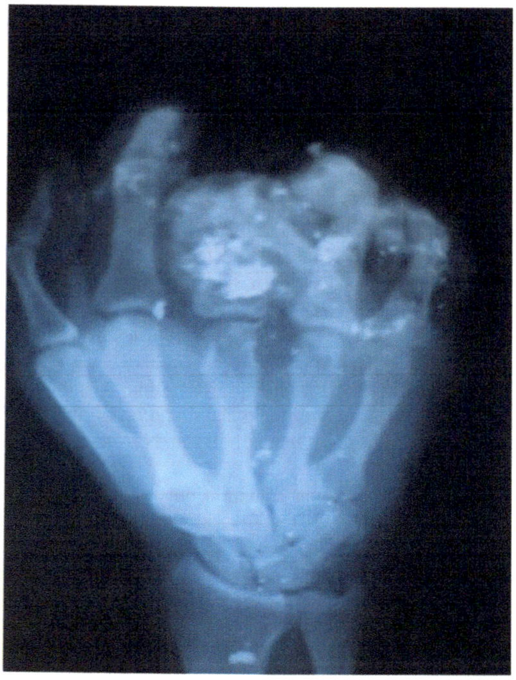

Fig 3.7 X ray of the right hand with destroyed proximal phalanx of third digit.

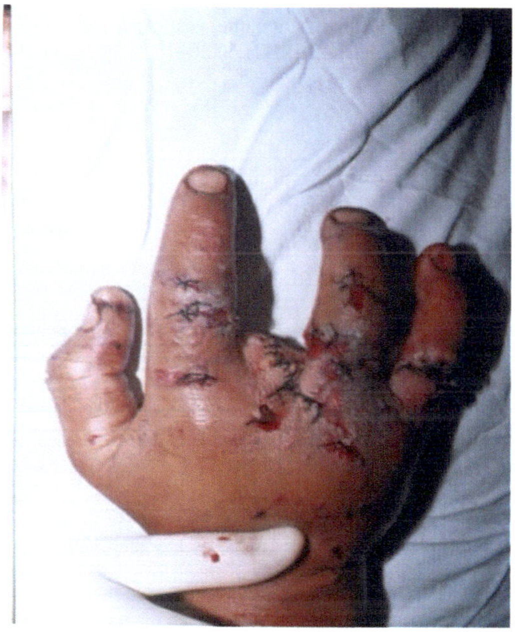

Fig. 3.8 The completed surgery

Comparable results with other areas of conflicts are as under

War	Gunshot wounds	Splinters	Others
World war I	40	60	–
World war II	10	85	5
Korea	31	69	–
Vietnam war	46	54	4
Arab Israel	18	66	16
Irish conflict	58	24	18
Yugoslavia	41	64	5
Croatia	24	76	–
OP desert storm	5	95	–

Distribution of war wounds (%)

War	Head and neck	Thorax	Abdomen	Extremities
World war II	25	13	9	53
Korea	19	8	7	53
Vietnam	15	8	5	55
Desert storm	13	6	9	90
Croatia	16	12	4	76
Yugoslavia	21	9	8	62

Ocular trauma in a conflict situation or on the battlefield is often associated with polytrauma and head injuries. Few of the battlefield injuries encountered have been shown in the figures. In such situations, life-saving measures take precedence. However, the moment the patient is stabilized, an ocular evaluation is a must. And an endeavor for early transfer to a hospital with ophthalmology facilities should be made.

3.16 Conclusion

War scenarios and casualties are highly unpredictable and do not follow the routine dictums of life. The situation is a high-tension one that requires an organized, motivated, and stress-free handling. Casualties are more often than not received in large numbers at once and require efficient triage according to their seriousness. Scoring systems are awarded to assess their morbidity and scale of injury. The management requires doing the most for the patient in the minimum amount of time and resources. Strict adherence to the basic principles of surgery is maintained, keeping in mind sepsis, thorough wound irrigation, and wound debridement, often 'imagining' the anatomy and pathology of the travelling projectile and the weapon. Evacuation and Tertiary Center Management are reserved for complicated cases, ocular injuries, neurovascular surgery, and reconstructive surgeries.

References

1. Williams NS, O'Connell PR, McCaskie AW. Trauma. In: Bailey and love's—short practice of surgery. 27th ed. Boca Raton, FL: CRC; 2018.
2. ICRC. War surgery. Working with limited resources in armed conflict and other situations of violence, vol. 1. Geneva: ICRC; 2010.
3. Breeze J, et al. Face, neck, and eye protection: adapting body Armour to counter the changing patterns of injuries on the battlefield. Br J Oral Maxillofac Surg. 2011;49(8):602–6.
4. Lecky F, et al. Trauma scoring systems and databases. British Journal of Anaesthesia. 2014;113(2):286–94
5. Ryan JM, et al. Field surgery on a future conventional battlefield: strategy and wound management. Ann R Coll Surg Engl. 1991;73:13–20.
6. Coupland RM. The red cross classification of war wounds: the E.X.C.F.V.M. scoring system. World J Surg. 1992;16(5):910–7.
7. Teasdale G, Jennett B. Assessment of coma and impaired consciousness. A practical scale. Lancet. 1974;297872:81–4.
8. Jain S, Iverson LM. Glasgow coma scale. [updated 2020 Jun 23]. In: StatPearls [internet]. Treasure Island, FL: StatPears Publishing; 2020.
9. Gibbons AJ, Breeze A. The face of war: the initial management of modern battlefield ballistic facial injuries. J Mil Veterans Health. 2011;19(2):15–8.
10. Biehl JW, et al. Penetrating eye injuries in war. Mil Med. 1999;164(11):780.
11. Kuhn F, et al. Birmingham eye trauma terminology (BETT); terminology and classification of mechanical eye injuries. Ophthamol Cin N Am. 2002;15:139.
12. Scott R. The ocular trauma score. Community Eye Health J. 2015;28(91):44.
13. Kuhn F, Maisik R, et al. The ocular trauma score (OTS). Ophthalmol Clin N Am. 2002;15(2):163–5.
14. Boparai MS, Sharma RC. Ocular war injuries. Indian J Ophthalmol. 1984;32:277–9.
15. Verma S, Waikar S, Sharma V, et al. Ocular trauma in counter insurgency and proxy war environment: epidemiological study, 1992–2004. Med J Armed Forces India. 2021;77(4):390–6. https://doi.org/10.1016/mjafi.2020.02.001.
16. Kumud R, et al. Treatment of casualties in a forward Hospital of Indian Army: nine-year experience. Med J Armed Forces India. 2004;60:20–4.

Open Globe Injuries: Initial Evaluation and Primary Repair

4

Parthasarathi Moulick

Open-globe injuries are a common occurrence in armed conflicts, with young people being most affected, and they are an important cause of visual loss worldwide [1]. Males sustain open globe injuries more often than females [2]. All ophthalmologists should be well versed in primary repair, as these initial actions and interventions determine the need for future reconstruction and visual rehabilitation. A good, meticulous repair of an open-globe injury is important, and all ophthalmologists must have the knowledge and skills in dealing with such types of injuries.

The patient should be assessed initially for any life-threatening injury, and thereafter ocular injuries should be assessed. Severe pain or nausea should be addressed to decrease lid squeezing and Valsalva manoeuvre effects.

Initial assessment of visual function is important and should be documented since it is directly related to visual prognosis [3] and is also important from a medicolegal perspective.

Poor visual acuity and a relative afferent pupillary defect as assessed during the initial examination carry a poor prognosis [4].

Taking a proper history of injury will elicit about the type of injury and the material which has caused the injury. Kuhn et al. described an Ocular Trauma Score **(OTS)** system that can prognosticate the visual outcome of the injured person [5].

P. Moulick (✉)
Ophthalmology, Apollo Multispeciality Hospitals Ltd, Kolkata, India

4.1 The Ocular Trauma Classification System for Open-Globe Injuries

Type	Grade (Visual Acuity)[a]
A. Rupture	A. >= 20/40
B. Penetrating	B. 20/50 to 20/100
C. Intraocular foreign body	C. 19/100 to 5/200
D. Perforating	D. 4/200 to light perception
E. Mixed	E. No light perception[b]
Pupil	*Zone*
Positive: Relative afferent pupillary defect in affected eye	1. Isolated to cornea(including the corneo-scleral limbus)
Negative: Relative afferent pupillary defect absent in affected eye	2. Corneoscleral limbus to 5 mm posterior to sclera
	3. Posterior to the anterior 5 mm of sclera

[a]Measured at distance (20 ft., 6 m) using the Snellen chart with correction and pinhole when appropriate.
[b]Confirmed with a bright light source and fellow eye well occluded

The presence or absence of an afferent defect should be documented by the examiner after checking the pupillary reflex [6]. Slit-lamp examination using different illumination techniques should be done to appreciate the extent of the cor-

S. Waikar (ed.), *Ocular Trauma in Armed Conflicts*, https://doi.org/10.1007/978-981-19-4021-7_4

neal injury and lens status. Opacification of the lens is indicative of a ruptured lens capsule. Initial assessment of a corneoscleral injury entails a detailed history, medications, and interventions done after the injury. Also, visualization of the posterior segment should be tried if it is possible to do so and documented.

The examiner should inquire about the mode, duration, time, and object of the injury. Also the, possibility of intraocular foreign bodies, concomitant microbial contamination, etc. should be assessed. Evaluation for occult globe injury is a must in every case of ocular injury. After a thorough evaluation of the anterior segment and the extent of injury, certain investigations are mandatory.

X-rays are taken from both the AP and lateral views to rule out any foreign bodies and fractures of the bone.

If there is suspicion of an open globe injury, then a CT scan is the imaging modality of choice. Magnetic resonance imaging should not be done when we are suspecting a metallic foreign body.

If the injured eye requires assessment of the posterior segment, then ultrasonography could be done gently with care to avoid further damage to the injured eye.

If the wound is infected, the cultures taken from the margins of the wound and devitalized excised tissue.

4.2 Surgical Indications

Surgery is best performed as early as possible unless there is a delay due to the medical condition of the patient. Surgery is indicated when there is a loss of normal anatomic structure or functioning of the eye, as well as if there are partial and/or full thickness lacerations with aqueous leakage and intraocular tissue prolapse.

Small lacerations (<2 mm) with minimal gape, self-sealing wounds, no evidence of intraocular penetration, and no sign of necrosis or infection can be managed with bandages contact lenses or tissue adhesives (Table 4.1).

Cases with good tissue approximation can be given topical broad-spectrum antibiotics, cycloplegics, and antiglaucoma medications. Patients should be advised to refrain from any strenuous activity, and their eyes should be protected by an eye shield.

Meticulous planning for surgery should be done so that maximum tissue is conserved and iatrogenic damage is minimized. Other special equipment, like phacoemulsification and vitrectomy machines, should be kept standby on hand with complex procedures.

Retrobulbar or peribulbar anaesthesia may increase the intraocular pressure (IOP) with the extrusion of intraocular contents. Therefore, general anaesthesia is preferred in open globe injuries.

The following items are mandatory for performing ocular surgery:

- Microsurgical tooth forceps
- Microsurgical tying forceps
- Non locking needle holder
- Vannas scissors
- Iris repositor
- 9-0/10-0 Monofilament nylon suture
- Muscle retractors
- Viscoelastic
- Cellulose sponges
- Tissue glue
- Irrigation aspiration cannula
- Phacoemulsification, automated vitrectomy units

Table 4.1 Management of full thickness corneal laceration

Size of wound	Nature of wound	Management
<2 mm	Nondisplaced self sealing wound	Bandage contact lens (BCL)
	Nonselfsealing/stellate/tissue loss	BCL + glue
<2 mm in noncooperative/mentally challenged individuals		Primary surgical repair
>2 mm		Primary surgical repair

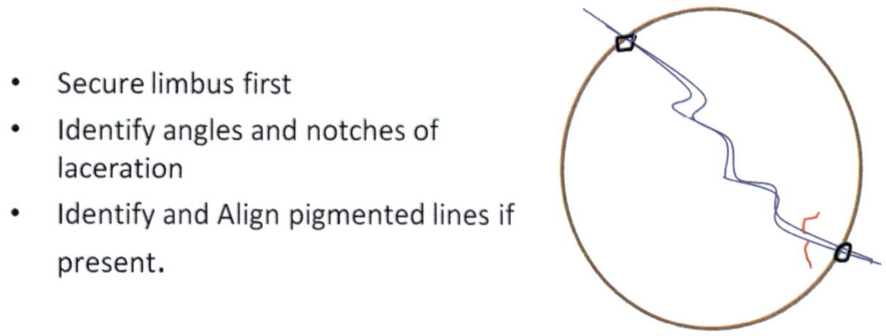

Fig. 4.1 Limbus, angles of the wound and epithelial pigmentation lines identified to facilitate anatomic realignment

4.3 Principles of Surgical Repair of Corneal Laceration

A surgeon should aim for certain surgical goals, which include watertight wound closure, avoidance of misalignment, restoration of normal anatomical relationships, and restoration of optimal visual function.

During the initial slit lamp examination, the ophthalmologist should identify the landmarks like the limbus, stellate edges, pigmentation lines in the epithelium, and sharp angles of laceration (Fig. 4.1), as these features will aid in locating the edges of the wound correctly and restoring the displaced tissue to the correct anatomical location.

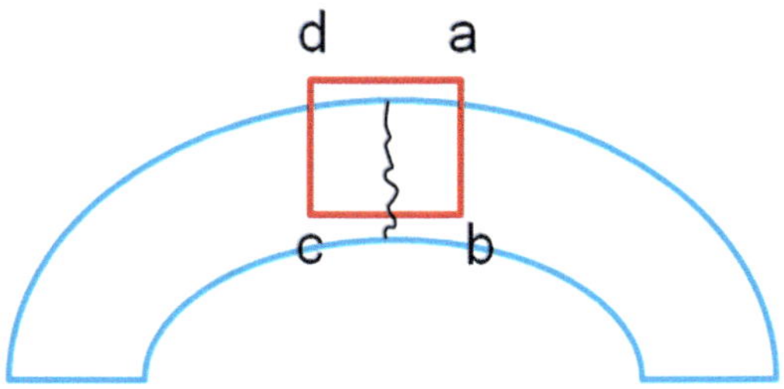

Fig. 4.2 Suturing of a perpendicular laceration. Distance from the entry (**a**) to the exit site (**d**) of the wound margin is equal to the posterior placement of the suture (**b**, **c**)

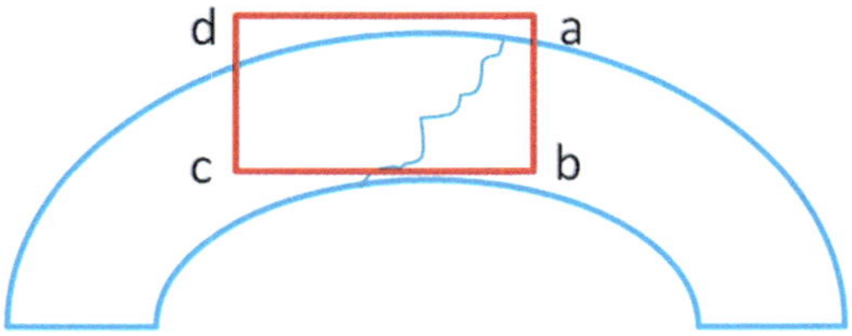

Fig. 4.3 Suturing of a shelved laceration. The distance from the anterior margin of the wound to the suture entry site (**a**) is not equal to the exit site (**d**). The distance from the entry (**b**) and exit site (**c**) should be equal from the posterior margin of the wound

4.4 Surgical Technique

The surgeon should ensure that there is good apposition of the wound. Since perpendicular wounds are likely to gape under normal IOP, they should ideally be sutured. Shelved areas of the wound are usually self-sealing and may not require suturing. However, as far as possible, the visual axis should be spared from suturing.

The management of prolapsed intraocular contents is a very important step. If the prolapsed uveal or retinal tissue is viable, it should be reposited back gently with viscoelastic and fine instruments. Infected or necrosed tissue, if extruded, should be excised. However, the surgeon should try to preserve as much tissue as possible for post-trauma reconstruction [7]. Since the cornea is not elastic, any unnecessary removal of tissue will result in the need for tight sutures that can have a significant torque effect, resulting in high astigmatism.

To avoid wound gape and leakage, corneal sutures should be placed perpendicular to the lacerations because oblique sutures produce tissue torque and wound slippage. The suture entry and exit sites should be equidistant from the wound margins in vertical lacerations for good apposition (Fig. 4.2). In beveled or shelved lacerations, to prevent wound overriding and tissue distortions, the sutures should be centered on the posterior aspect of the wound margins instead of taking the bites equidistant from the anterior aspect of wound margins (Fig. 4.3).

4.4.1 Suturing of the Cornea

For suturing the cornea, a spatulated needle is used, and monofilament suture (nylon or polypropylene) is preferred because of its low tissue reactivity. To avoid tissue injury, especially near the central part of the cornea, a no-touch technique is employed after placing the tip of the needle perpendicular to the anterior surface.

Since full-thickness sutures can lead to intraocular infection, it will be ideal to place the corneal sutures at 90% depth in the stroma and of equal depth and length on both sides of the wound. Suture passes should be approximately 1.5 mm to 2 mm in total length [8]. This may not be possible in macerated or oedematous tissue, where one has to incorporate healthy tissue in each suture pass to avoid pull-through of the suture when tied. Interrupted sutures create a zone of compression extending away from the suture and a plane of compression in the tissue enclosed within the suture loop. Wound closure is achieved when the compression zones adjoin. Long suture bites allow a greater distance between sutures, while smaller bites require more closely placed sutures and overlap the zones of compression.

The smallest possible knot (granny-style knot) should be made while tying the suture. In order to facilitate burying of the knot, it should be trimmed short and superficially buried in the tissue, on the side away from the visual axis. If the sutures are not buried, then the patients will have intense irritation and watering, leading to difficulty opening their eyes. It may lead to papilla formation in the upper tarsal conjunctiva [9].

- Longer sutures, especially near the visual axis, lead to greater tissue distortion and therefore more astigmatism. Therefore, corneal lacerations should be closed with long, tight sutures in the corneal periphery and shorter, minimally compressive sutures in the corneal center thus causing peripheral flattening and central steepening (Rowsey-Hays technique) (Fig. 4.4).
- To avoid wound override, the suture placements in a perpendicular laceration must be of equal length from the anterior and posterior perspectives, whereas in a shelved laceration, passage of suture should be of equal length as seen from the posterior aspect and not from the anterior view.
- In traumatic corneal wounds, running sutures are avoided since they straighten the curvilinear wounds because of the continuous nature of compression and also because they tend to flatten the overlying corneal surface through the length of the suture. Moreover, placing the integrity of the entire wound on a single suture is a risky proposition in the case of running sutures.

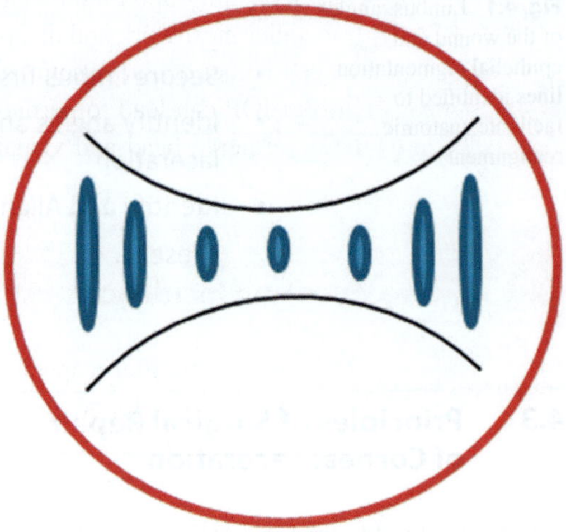

Fig. 4.4 Long tight compression suture placed in the periphery leads to flattening of the periphery and steepening of the centre of the cornea. Short spaced, minimally compressive suture bites are then placed in centre to preserve the central steepening as much as possible leading to a flattened periphery with a spherical center. (The Rowsey – Hays technique of wound closure)

4.5 Simple Full Thickness Corneal Laceration

These types of wounds usually do not involve the limbus, and there is no iris or vitreous incarceration or traumatic damage to the lens. These types of lacerations can be either perpendicular or shelved, and the two types require slightly different approaches to suturing for appropriate wound apposition [10].

A laceration of less than 2 mm can be managed with the help of BCL and/or glue provided the following criteria are fulfilled:

- There is no intraocular tissue in the wound.
- No other ocular structures are involved.
- No foreign bodies in wound.
- Self-sealing wound.

BCL should be left in place until the wound stabilizes. Glue can be natural or synthetic. It is extremely important to dry the corneal surface prior to the application of adhesive [11]. Fibrin glue requires a longer time for adhesive plug formation, but it provides faster healing and significantly less corneal vascularization as compared to cyanoacrylate glue, which sets immediately on exposure to air as a result of anionic polymerization. A thin film of glue should be applied after debriding any loose or necrotic tissue. A bandage contact lens should be applied immediately after gluing. The glue remains in place for several days to weeks if properly applied on a firm bed that has been debrided of necrotic tissue. Further surgical intervention will be required if the anterior chamber does not reform in 24 hours or if iris or lens incarceration supervenes. The managenent of various types of full-thickness corneal wounds is given in Table 4.1.

4.6 Suturing of Zigzag Incision

Closure of a zagged wound requires initial suturing of the linear aspect of the wound individually (Fig. 4.5). If properly done, the apices will self-heal, thereby avoiding additional trauma to the tissue from instrumentation. If there is a requirement for closure of the apical portions of the wound, then a mattress suture technique can be used.

4.6.1 Stellate Laceration Closure

During closure of stellate laceration, after initial closure of straight arms of laceration with interrupted sutures, the stellate portion is closed last by two different techniques. The Eisner method of purse strings or the Akkin method can be applied. In the former, a partial-thickness incision is made between the arms of the laceration, and a purse-string suture is passed through these grooves and tightened optimally to approximate the apices of the wound [12]. Overtightening should be avoided since it may lead to forward displacement of the apices and wound leakage. The knot should be buried after tying. In the Atkin technique, the suture is passed through the tissue and over the apices of the wound to attach the tissue. If there is a tissue loss, then a partial-thickness lamellar patch can be applied, either from a donor or from autologous tissue if donor tissue is not available.

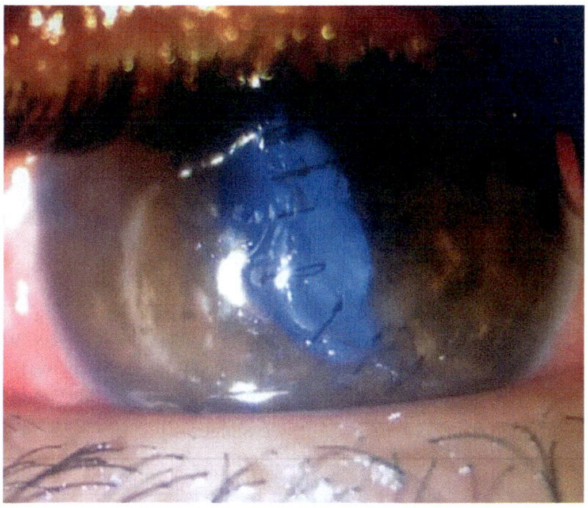

Fig. 4.5 A zigzag corneal laceration with shelved edges sutured at each linear aspect. Associated traumatic cataract managed at secondary stage (Courtesy Dr Amit Sethi)

4.7 Corneoscleral Lacerations

When there is a corneoscleral wound, identifying the limbus is the most important step since apposition should be done here first. Thereafter, repair of the corneal aspect followed by the scleral portion should be done. Large wounds with iris prolapse should be managed under general anaesthesia. Thorough irrigation should be done to remove foreign bodies, if any. Prolapsed iris tissue should be handled with extra care, and every effort should be made to

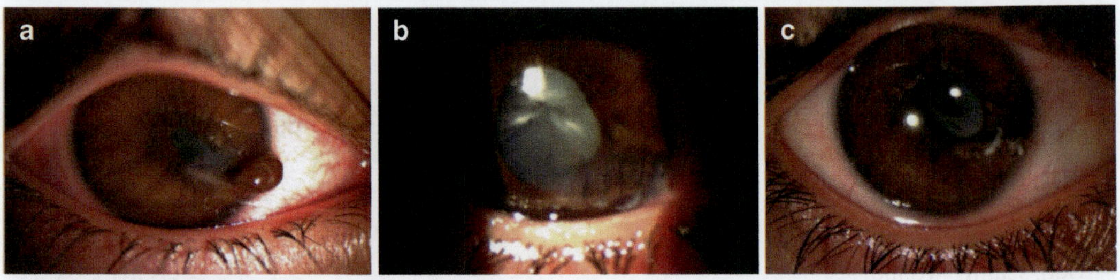

Fig. 4.6 (**a**) Corneoscleral wound with prolapse of uveal tissue. (**b**) Postoperative picture of same patient showing sutured linear full thickness corneal laceration and traumatic cataract. (**c**) Postcataract surgery picture of same patient with PCIOL and dense Posterior capsular opacification with central capsulotomy opening. Patient regained visual acuity of 6/9. (Courtesy Dr.(Col) Shrikant Waikar & Dr Sriharsha Lanka)

preserve it (Fig. 4.6a, b). If the uveal tissue is devitalized or macerated, then it should be removed to prevent infection or epithelial ingrowth (Fig. 4.7a, c). A cleanly incised wound with adherence of iris tissue to the posterior margins of the wound can be easily managed by putting suture and sweeping the iris with the help of a fine iris repositor or Sinskey hook through a side port entry under the cover of a viscoelastic. The repositioning of the iris should be done gently so as to prevent iatrogenic dialysis. Also, care should be taken to prevent corneal endothelial and lens injury during the procedure. Suturing of the cornea should ideally be done with 10-0 monofilament nylon suture in a spatulated needle passing through 90% depth. The anterior chamber should be kept formed with air or viscoelastic. However, viscoelastic should be thoroughly removed after the completion of the surgery. Associated lenticular injury is best left to be managed by secondary repair (Fig. 4.6c) unless there is an associated anterior capsular tear with cortical matter in the anterior chamber, which needs to be managed at the time of primary repair (Fig. 4.6).

4.8 Scleral Lacerations

Scleral lacerations can extend posteriorly (Figs. 4.7b, 4.8), and sometimes the complete extension of the laceration is not always visible, so careful exploration of the wound is required (Fig. 4.8). Before suturing the sclera, one should clear the tenons and conjunctiva completely off the wound edges to prevent their involvement (Fig. 4.7d).

To prevent prolapse of intraocular contents, the sclera should be closed in a step-wise fashion (hand-on-hand technique). If the limbus is involved, then it should be approximated first with 8-0 or 9-0 nylon interrupted sutures. When dealing with separate edges, any extruded intraocular contents may be repositioned by the assistant with a spatula. After passing the needle through the proximal wound edge, the surgeon regrasps the needle and passes it through the distal wound edge. If the wound intersects a muscle insertion, the muscle may be disinserted (preferably by a double-armed 6-0 vicryl suture) to continue closure of the defect and reattached it once the wound is closed. Prolapsed vitreous should be excised to minimize traction on the vitreous base and retina. In these cases, a detailed fundus examination is essential to rule out tractional detachments. If there is loss of tissue, then a scleral patch graft may be used.

For larger defects of the sclera, non-absorbable sutures (8-0 Mersilk) should be used, and for smaller wounds, 7-0 or 8-0 Vicryl absorbable sutures will be appropriate. The sclera can be closed in a step-wise fashion, the so-called "close as you go" technique. This technique involves a limited anterior dissection, exposing of a small portion of the sclera defect prior to further posterior dissection. Scleral lacerations that extend far posteriorly (near the optic nerve) are best managed by observation, as the surgical approach may increase tissue prolapse and cause additional damage. The orbital soft tissue serves to tampon-

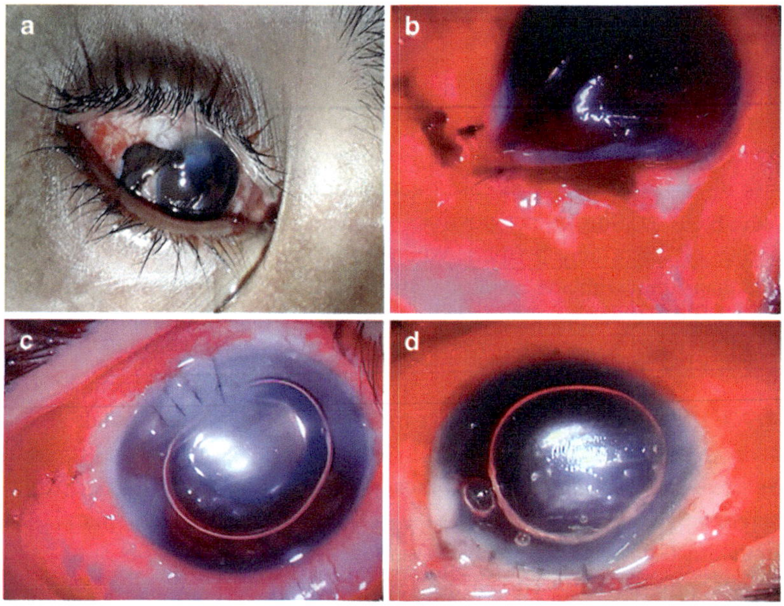

Fig. 4.7 (**a**) Showing open globe injury (OGI) right eye in zone 1 and (**c**) showing repaired OGI, (**b**) showing OGI right eye in zone 3 and (**d**) showing repaired OGI. (Courtesy Dr. Vipin Rana)

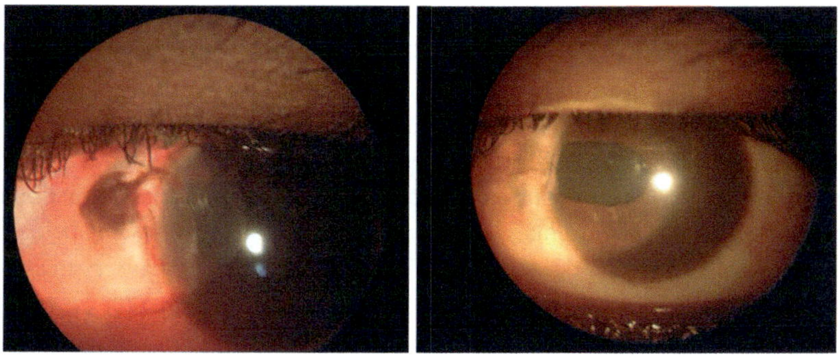

Fig. 4.8 Open globe injury zone 2 with uveal prolapse and postoperative picture with good visual outcome. (Courtesy Dr. (Col) Shrikant Waikar)

ade the wound as it heals. The prognosis in these cases is guarded.

4.8.1 Non Perforating Corneal Injuries

Checking the wound leak is essential by putting 2% fluorescein in it and performing Seidel's test. If found to be negative, then it should be rechecked by applying pressure. The following actions should be taken:

- If the wound is non-gaping and non-overriding, the pressure patching after putting on antibiotic eye ointment can be done.
- If there is a deeper laceration and for the stability of the wound, a bandage contact lens (BCL) may be used for supporting the wound and enhancing epithelialization.
- Partial thickness avulsion of the cornea with a flap remaining attached at its base can be managed by passing a few sutures for proper approximation.

If multiple small fragments or edges are present, a bandage soft contact lens placed immediately at the end of surgery can be helpful to keep the tissue in place as well as for substantial postoperative patient comfort [13]. The aim is to ensure a smooth surface after the healing of the wound with minimal astigmatism.

4.9 Management of Tissue Loss

If tissue loss cannot be managed with glue, then an autologous graft can be used since an autograft precludes the need for donor tissue and avoids the risk of graft rejection or disease transmission. If autologous grafting is not possible, then donor cornea or sclera may be used. Wounds that are less than 5 mm with non-necrotic stroma can benefit from the above-mentioned procedure.

4.9.1 Effects of Suture Placement

Sutured incisions flatten the cornea under the suture but steepen it at closure to the visual axis. In contrast, unsutured incisions flatten the entire cornea with a loss of corneal power. A simple appositional suture would be adequate if no wound gaping is present. However, to overcome the elastic tendency of the globe and prevent wound leaking, tissue compression is required. Longer sutures have greater lateral zones of tissue compression, as the zone of tissue compression along the incision is roughly equal to the length of the suture. Longer and deeper sutures penetrate the deeper stroma, closing any posterior wound gaping and decreasing the possibility of iris or adhering to the raw posterior surface. Shorter corneal sutures tend to allow wound leakage between the sutures since the zones of tissue compression are similarly narrow.

4.9.2 Suture Tightening

Control of astigmatism may be optimized by the use of slipknots. However, the square knot provides good closure. A double half-hitch slipknot is used to adjust wound tension optimally, followed by a square knot to secure closure.

4.10 Suture Removal

Sutures should be removed from the corneal laceration when adequate interface fibrosis has been attained. Sutures that loosen spontaneously because of wound contractions and are providing no further tensile strength to the cornea should be removed before epithelial breakdown, corneal melting, or infection occur.

4.11 Prognostic Factors

The following factors are usually found to have a poor prognosis: poor acuity at the first visit, presence of RAPD, vitreous loss, lens involvement, retinal detachment, and posterior extension of the wound. Wounds that were smaller than 5 mm have a good prognosis for the visual outcome compared to patients with wounds that were larger than 5 mm [14, 15].

4.12 Conclusion

Corneoscleral injury management has greatly improved over the years with advances in diagnostic and therapeutic techniques and improvements in knowledge of the pathophysiology of eye trauma and its prognostic factors. OTS calculated at the initial evaluation may have predictive value in patients with open globe injuries. However, corneoscleral injury management will always remain a challenge for every ophthalmologist.

References

1. Parver LM. Eye Trauma. The neglected disorder. Arch Ophthalmol. 1986;104:1452.
2. McCormack. Penetrating injury of the eye (editorial). Br J Ophthalmol. 1999;83:1101–2.
3. Esmali B, Elner SG, Schork A, Elner VM. Visual outcome and ocular survival after penetrating trauma. Ophthalmology. 1995;102:393–400.
4. Isaac DL, Ghanem VC, Nascimento MA. Prognostic factors in open globe injuries. Ophthalmologica. 2003;217:431–5.
5. Kuhn F, Pieramici DJ. Ocular Trauma Principles and Practice 2002; Chapter 2: Page 7.
6. Mittra RA, Mieler WF. Controversies in the management of open-globe injuries involving the posterior segment. Surv Ophthalmol. 1999;44:215–25.
7. Hersh PS, Kenyon KR. Anterior segment reconstruction following ocular trauma. Int Ophthalmol Clin. 1988;28:57.

8. Brightbill FS, Mcdonnell PJ, McGhee CNJ. Corneal surgery: theory, technique and tissue. Amsterdam: Elsevier; 2009.
9. John B, Raghavan C. Open Globe injuries—primary repair of Corneoscleral Injuries. Kerala J Ophthalmol. 2010;22(3):225–34.
10. Melki S, Azar DT. 101 pearls in refractive, cataract and surgery. 2nd ed. Thorofare: SLACK Incorporated; 2006.
11. Mohan S, Aggarwal A, Panda A, Bhartiya S. DOS times. Repair of corneoscleral perforations. 2008;14(2):21–6.
12. Vote BJ, Elder MJ. Cyanoacrylate glue for corneal perforations: a description of a surgical technique and a review of literature. Clin Exp Ophthalmol. 2000;28(6):437–42.
13. Eisner G. Eye surgery. New York, NY: Springer; 1990. p. 97–103.
14. Rofail M, Lee GA, O'Rourke P. Prognostic indicators for open globe injury. Clin Exp Ophthalmol. 2006;34(8):783–6.
15. Sternbey P Jr, de Juan E Jr, Michels RG, Aver L. Multivariate analysis of prognostic factor in penetrating ocular injuries. Am J Ophthalmol. 1984;98(4):467–72.

Corneal Rehabilitation and Anterior Segment Reconstruction

5

Bhaskar Srinivasan, Geetha Iyer, Shweta Agarwal, Chetan Rao, and Sripriya Krishnamurthy

5.1 Introduction

Ocular war injuries are of significance not only on humanitarian grounds but also for being a potential cause of loss of vocation. Most of these unfortunate patients become unfit for further military operations and even for most civilian assignments. The incidence of eye injuries in combat operations has steadily increased from 0.65% in Crimea to 2% in World War 2, to 9% in Vietnam to almost 14% in Operation Desert Storm. 22.5% of the evacuated patients by the US army from Iraq and Afghanistan were due to eye disease; [1]. Though the eye contributes only 0.27% of the erect frontal silhouette, the incidence of ocular injuries is approximately 10%, almost 50 times higher than that expected based on surface area alone [2]. Due to the increased use and efficacy of fragmented ammunition (land mines) and the use of armored protective fighting vehicle warfare suits that limit the exposed area to the head and neck region, almost 30% of facial and cranial gunshot wounds result in ocular injury, with nearly 50% of them resulting in permanent visual dysfunction [2]. Adequate combat eye protection helps reduce these numbers, but the issues of misting, restricted field of view, and frequent scratches have demotivated its users [3]. Blast injuries are amplified in a closed or secure place and cause more injuries [4]. In the Oklahoma City bombing, 8% of survivors had ocular injuries. In the World Trade Center blast, eye injuries were the second most common cause of injury in survivors after inhalational lung injury [4]. Triage is essential in the management of trauma in combat injuries. Life-threatening injuries are the first to be addressed. Medical management is sufficient for mild ocular injuries, whereas an open globe injury requires prompt closure of the wound to achieve globe integrity. The presence of a posterior segment complication requires a referral to a higher center after the primary wound repair. The management strategy in the chronic phase involves assessment of the corneal condition, lens status, and posterior segment status to plan for visual rehabilitation. This chapter deals with decreased vision secondary to corneal injuries and measures to correct them and improve the vision and quality of life of patients.

B. Srinivasan (✉) · G. Iyer · S. Agarwal
C J Shah Cornea Services, Sankara Nethralaya, Chennai, India

C. Rao
Bhagwan Mahaveer Vitreoretinal Services, Sankara Nethralaya, Chennai, India

S. Krishnamurthy
SMT Jadhavbai Nathmal Singhvee, Glaucoma Services, Sankara Nethralaya, Chennai, India

S. Waikar (ed.), *Ocular Trauma in Armed Conflicts*, https://doi.org/10.1007/978-981-19-4021-7_5

Reduced vision due to corneal causes in the medium/late phase after ocular trauma is due to

1. Corneal scar.
2. Irregular astigmatism.
3. Corneal decompensation.
4. Corneal scar/oedema along with posterior segment complications
5. Limbal stem cell deficiency.

5.1.1 Corneal Scar

A corneal scar in the visual axis causes a decrease in vision. Slit-lamp evaluation should include the extent of the scar, the depth of the scar, and the density of the scar. An anterior segment OCT is useful to identify the depth of the scar and to measure corneal thickness. Potential acuity meter testing and a rigid gas-permeable contact lens help ascertain vision potential. If vision improves with contact lenses, this could be an alternative before proceeding with any surgery.

Based on the depth of the scar treatment options include

1. Phototherapeutic Keratectomy
2. Superficial lamellar keratoplasty
   (a) Manual superficial lamellar keratoplasty
   (b) Microkeratome assisted anterior lamellar keratoplasty
   (c) Femtosecond laser-assisted anterior lamellar keratoplasty
   (d) Hemi automated anterior lamellar keratoplasty
3. Deep anterior lamellar keratoplasty
4. Penetrating keratoplasty

5.1.1.1 Phototherapeutic Keratectomy

Superficial corneal scars are amenable to an excimer laser ablation (phototherapeutic keratectomy, PTK). PTK is best performed when the stromal involvement of the scar is limited to 10-20% depth. PTK results in a refractive change that is corrected with glasses. The use of intraoperative topical mitomycin (0.02%) on the bed reduces the possibility of haze formation. A postoperative bandage lens is placed until the epithelial defect heals. Topical low potency steroids (Loteprednol/Fluorometholone) and antibiotics are continued during the postoperative period. The use of ultraviolet protective glasses in the early postoperative period could reduce the possibility of haze formation.

The advantages of PTK include the precise control of ablation depth, ease of the procedure, fast postoperative recovery, and the option of a repeat treatment if required [5, 6].

5.1.1.2 Superficial Lamellar Keratoplasty

Deeper corneal scars need anterior lamellar keratoplasty.

Manual Superficial Lamellar Keratoplasty

Create an initial groove using a guarded trephine of predetermined depth or a suction trephine. Using crescent or lamellar dissectors, peel the recipient's cornea off to achieve a smooth interface. The presence of a residual scar necessitates further dissection to reach a transparent recipient bed. The donor cornea is mounted on an artificial anterior chamber to facilitate the dissection using DSEK dissectors. The donor cornea is trephined, and the anterior lamellar cap is sutured on the recipient bed. Problems with manual lamellar keratoplasty stem from the manual dissection of both the donor and recipient corneas. The residual interface haze can result in suboptimal visual recovery.

Microkeratome Assisted Lamellar Keratoplasty

Once the depth of the scar is ascertained, a microkeratome with a predetermined depth blade is used to create a free anterior corneal cap of the donor and recipient's corneas. The donor cornea is then placed on the recipient's bed and secured with sutures. The advantage of a microkeratome procedure is the smooth interface and ease of the surgery. The problem with microkeratome-based surgery is the possible mismatch between donor and recipient tissue. A-2 step microkeratome-assisted ALK, as proposed by Tan et al., might be useful to achieve better tissue approximation [7].

Femtosecond Assisted Lamellar Keratoplasty: (FALK)

With the femtosecond laser, the corneal tissue can be precisely cut within a few microns. Based on the predetermined depth of the scar on optical coherence tomography (OCT), we can plan the depth of the femtosecond laser ablation. A similar tissue is cut from the donor cornea and placed on the recipient's bed. The lamellar cap is placed on the recipient's bed along with a bandage lens if the thickness is 200 microns or less. Tissues thicker than 200 microns are sutured with 10.0 nylon sutures [7, 8].

Hemi Automated Lamellar Keratoplasty (HALK)

This combines the manual dissection of the recipient bed based on a predetermined depth with a microkeratome-assisted dissection of the donor tissue of the appropriate size. The advantage is a smoother interface as compared to manual dissection.

Deep Anterior Lamellar Keratoplasty: DALK is performed in eyes with a deep corneal scar without endothelial involvement or in the presence of multiple foreign bodies at various depths, causing photophobia. Only attempt a Big Bubble DALK if there is no apparent damage to the Descemet's membrane and endothelium. Other techniques of DALK, such as manual layer-by-layer dissection, the Malbran peeling technique and fluid-assisted technique advocated by Sugita, and Melles technique, can be performed to bare the Descemet's membrane or reach close to the Descemet's membrane [7, 9].

Figure 5.1 shows a case of corneal scarring and symblepheron that was managed by symblepheron release and amniotic membrane transplantation along with DALK.

The patient had corneal astigmatism that was addressed by topography-guided photorefractive keratectomy.

Penetrating keratoplasty (PK): Eyes with a full-thickness corneal scar affecting the visual axis or eyes with corneal decompensation undergo a full-thickness corneal transplant. Keratoplasty is combined with additional surgeries such as cataract extraction, intraocular lens implantation, antiglaucoma surgery, and vitreoretinal surgery in select cases.

PK with cataract surgery: The presence of corneal decompensation or scars with cataractous changes warrant a combined surgery. Operative consideration includes the amount of corneal haze or edema and lens status. The power of the IOL to be placed is calculated using the axial length and the standard keratometry value. If visualization permits phacoemulsification, intraocular lens implantation is performed, followed by keratoplasty. In cases with a disorganized anterior segment or very poor visibility, the recipient cornea is trephined, and open-sky extracapsular cataract extraction with IOL implantation is performed followed by keratoplasty. In the case of aphakia, the option of scleral fixation or a glued IOL exists.

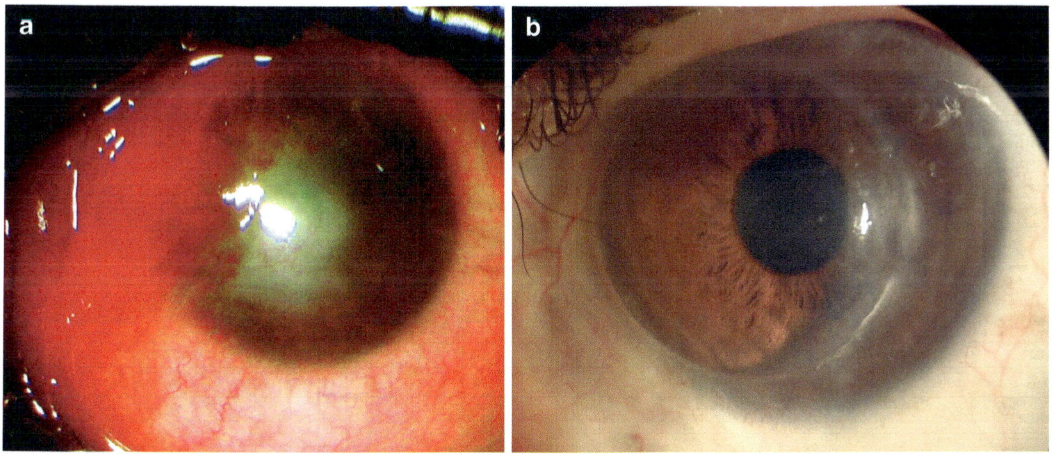

Fig. 5.1 (**a**) Corneal scar with symblepheron (**b**) The patient underwent deep anterior lamellar keratoplasty with amniotic membrane grafting. For astigmatism, he later underwent photorefractive keratectomy

To precisely place the scleral-fixation or a glued IOL, the scleral grooves or flaps or the area for the intrascleral haptic fixation needs to be marked before trephination of the cornea. Another option is to perform a corneal transplant first and subsequently plan cataract surgery after suture removal. The benefit of a staged procedure is a better refractive outcome; however, the drawback is the delayed visual recovery and the risk of endothelial damage due to the cataract surgery [10].

Figs. 5.2 and 5.3 depict the images of both eyes of 2 patients, one eye of both patients was rehabilitated with Penetrating keratoplasty and the other required Catarct surgery (a) eye that underwent penetrating keratoplasty along with cataract surgery.

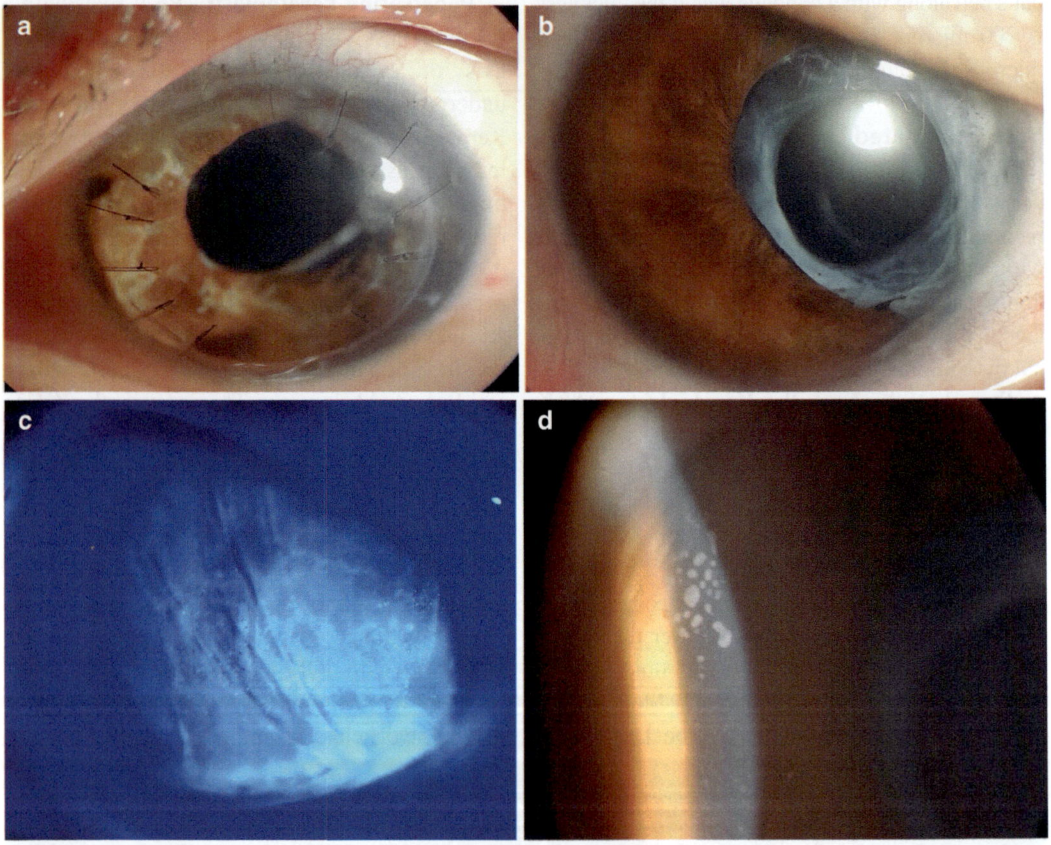

Fig. 5.2 Blast injury to both eyes (**a**) eye underwent penetrating keratoplasty with cataract surgery and a 2-year follow-up with a BSCVA 20/30. (**b**) Had cataract surgery with Capsular tension ring. This eye also had flap striae (**c**) subsequent to the trauma, primary wound repair, and epithelial ingrowth (**d**) that was stable

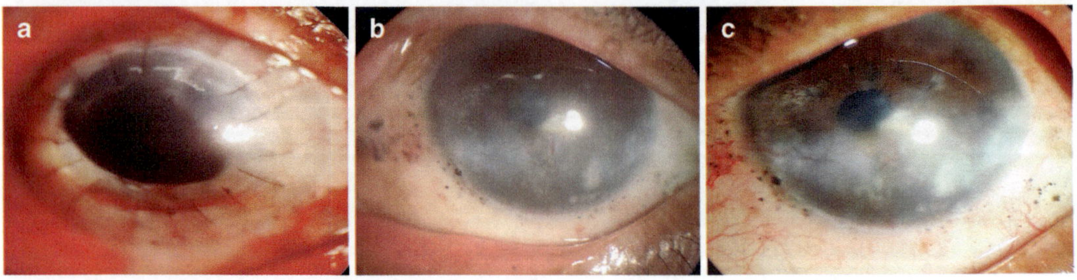

Fig. 5.3 Blast injury (**a**) underwent Penetrating keratoplasty with lensectomy and vitrectomy (**b**) Other eye of the same patient with scar and cataract (**c**) Postoperative picture after phacoemulsification with intraocular lens implantation

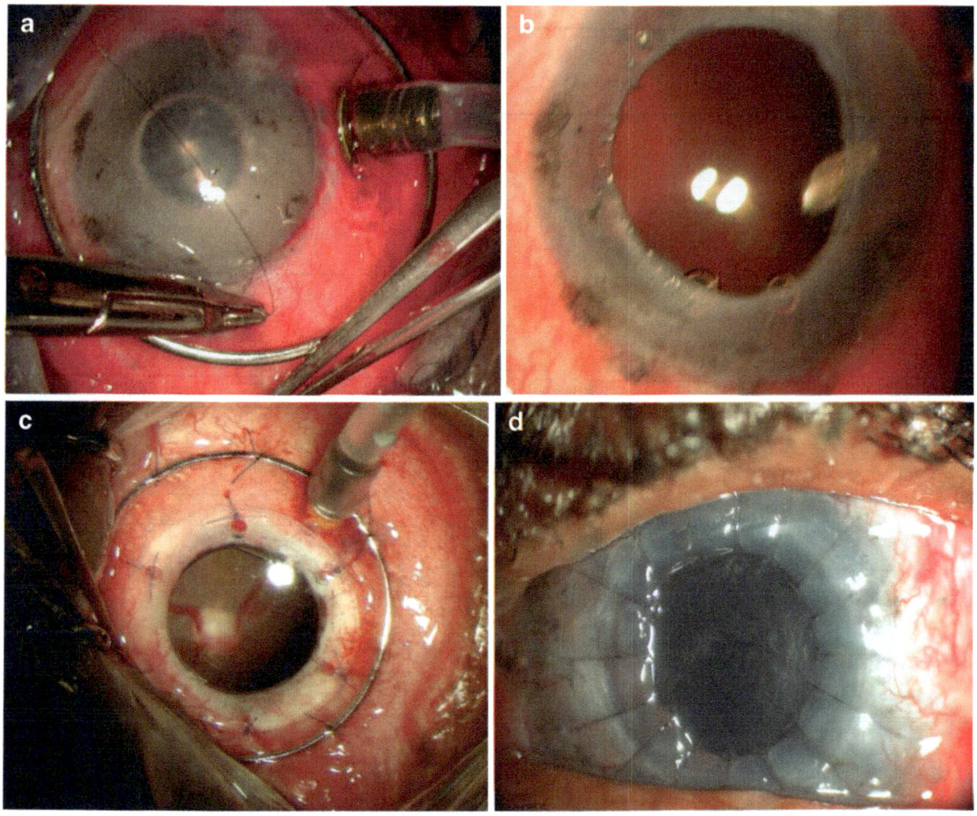

Fig. 5.4 Steps in Combined PK with Vitreoretinal Surgery. (**a**) Sclerotomy ports are made and infusion cannulas are secured. (**b**) Cornea trephined and position of infusion canula confirmed. (**c**) A temporary Landers keratoprosthesis is secured, and retinal surgery is performed. (**d**) Keratoprosthesis replaced by donor cornea

5.1.1.3 PK with Antiglaucoma Surgery

Patients with raised intraocular pressure and corneal opacity or edema need better control of intraocular pressure before corneal transplant. Graft survival is better if surgery is performed after adequate intraocular pressure control. Surgical options for IOP control include trabeculectomy, glaucoma drainage devices (valved or non-valvular), and diode laser cyclophotocoagulation. If an anterior segment is formed, then a trabeculectomy or Ahmed glaucoma device can be placed before the transplant. If the anterior segment is significantly disorganized or the pressure is high despite a trabeculectomy or a glaucoma valvular device, diode laser cyclophotocoagulation can be tried. When combining transplant with surgery for IOP control, it is preferable to create scleral flaps or secure the glaucoma valvular device to the sclera before the corneal trephining. The glaucoma valvular device is placed in the anterior chamber, significantly away from the corneal graft. If possible, a pars plana positioning of the tube is preferred [11].

5.1.1.4 PK with Vitreoretinal Surgery

Surgical steps in the case of a combined PK with vitreoretinal surgery include sclerotomies, corneal trephination, and suturing a temporary keratoprosthesis (a Lander's or an Eckardt's) to achieve a closed globe status and allow good visualization using a wide-angle viewing computer for the retinal procedure. The keratoprosthesis is then exchanged with a donor cornea [12, 13]. Another option is to perform keratoplasty and then perform vitreoretinal surgery through the grafted cornea. However, there is increased surgical trauma to the transplanted endothelial cells. Figures 5.4 and 5.5 enumerate the steps in performing a combined keratoplasty and vitreoretinal surgery.

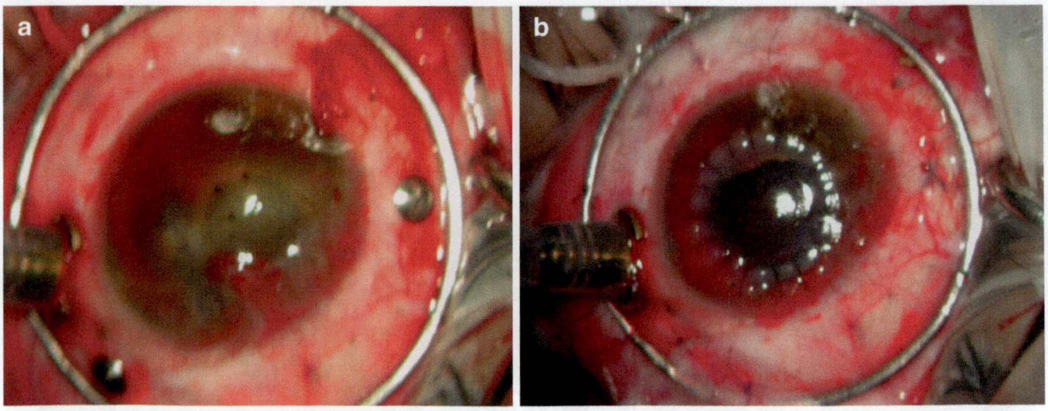

Fig. 5.5 (**a**) The patient had a corneal scar with an intraocular foreign body (IOFB). (**b**) Underwent penetrating keratoplasty with lensectomy with IOFB removal

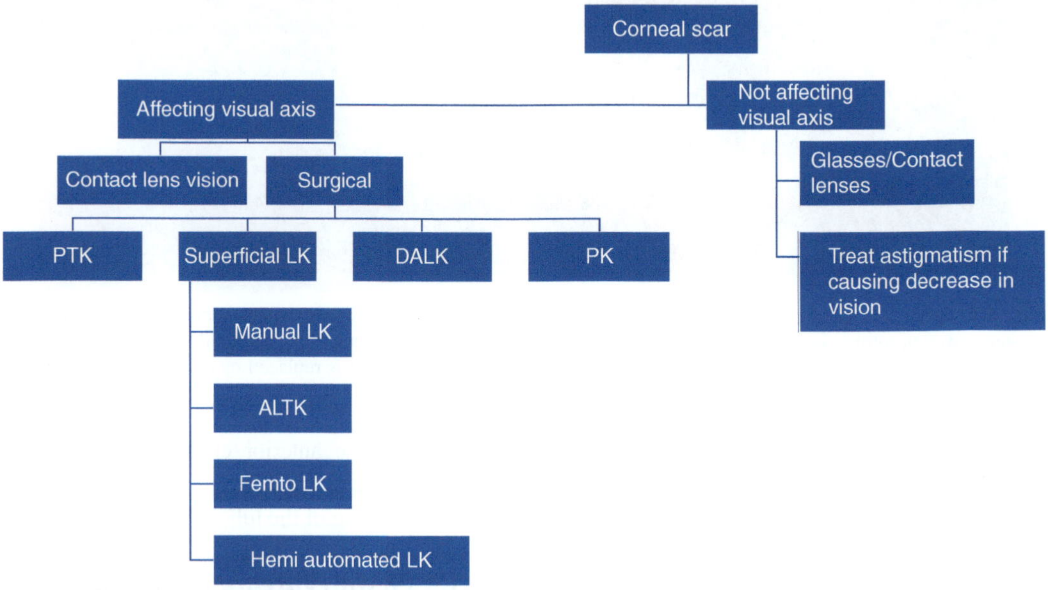

Fig. 5.6 Algorithmic approach to corneal scars

The algorithmic approach to corneal scars is enumerated in Fig. 5.6.

5.2 Corneal Irregular Astigmatism

Corneal scars and foreign bodies cause irregular astigmatism that compromises visual acuity. The simplest option would be to consider dispensing a rigid gas-permeable contact lens to improve vision. If the patient desires the best spectacle-corrected or uncorrected vision, then the choice would be corneal topography-guided or corneal aberrometry-guided laser ablation to improve the corneal curvature—correction of corneal irregularity results in a refractive change. Refractive correction is performed in two steps: the first step improves the corneal curvature, and the second step aims to correct the refractive error. A very high degree of irregular astigmatism is not amenable to laser correction and needs DALK/PK [14, 15].

Figure 5.7 depicts the irregular corneal topography in the eye with a corneal scar and sym-

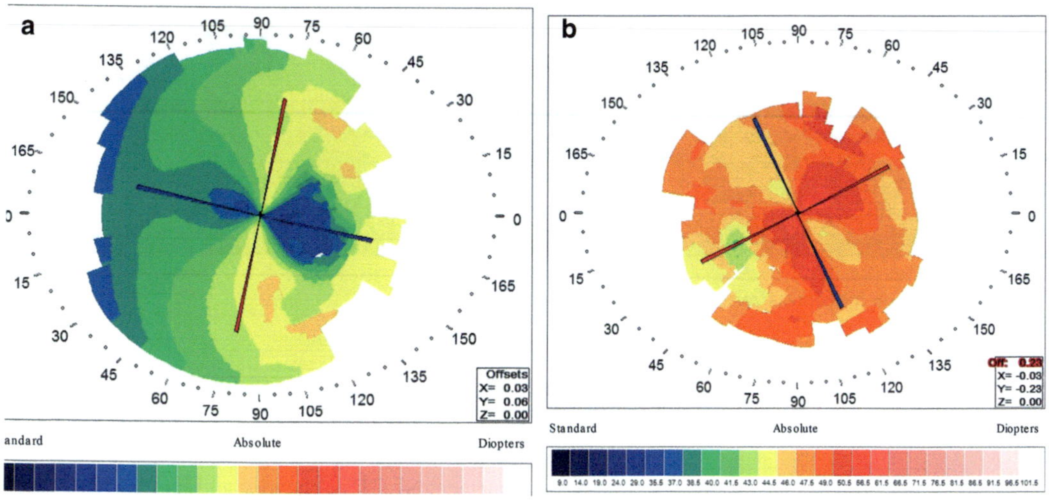

Fig. 5.7 (**a**) Corneal topography showing the nasal area flattening at the site of the corneal scar with symblepharon. (**b**) Corneal topography shows Post-keratoplasty astigmatism, the patient underwent topography guided Photorefractive keratectomy

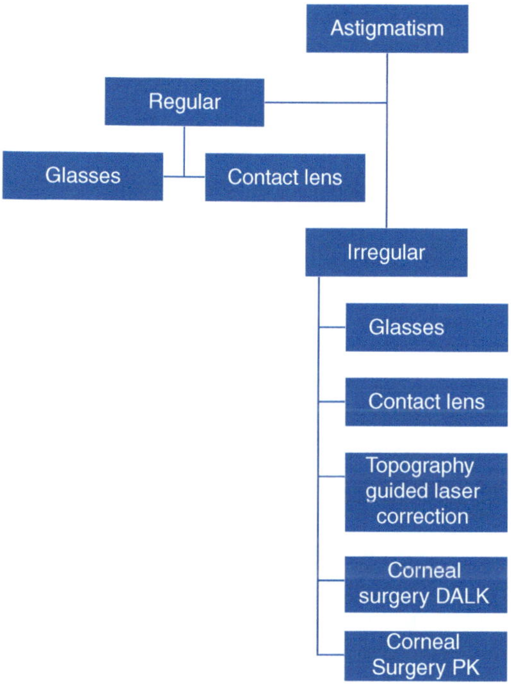

Fig. 5.8 Algorithmic approach to astigmatism management

blepharon secondary to a blast injury in Fig. 5.7a, and irregular astigmatism post-keratoplasty is depicted in Fig. 5.7b.

The algorithmic approach to managing astigmatism in these eyes is enumerated in Fig. 5.8.

5.3 Corneal Decompensation/ Perforation

Corneal decompensation with significant corneal scarring or irregularity would need penetrating keratoplasty. Corneal decompensation without a substantial scar and with normal curvature, such as decompensation post-surgery, can undergo endothelial transplants such as Descemet's stripping automated endothelial keratoplasty.

Corneal decompensation with retained silicone oil is a special consideration. Retained silicone oil can cause endothelial dysfunction. Penetrating keratoplasty (DSAEK) can be combined with silicone oil removal in select cases. A penetrating keratoplasty with an exchange or top-up of silicone oil is performed in cases with a high risk of hypotony, recurrent detachment, or phthisis. However, these grafts will fail in due course.

One-eyed patients with multiple failed grafts and retained silicone oil are suitable candidates for Boston type 1, type2, or modified osteo-odonto-keratoprosthesis. Good anatomical and functional success has been reported with keratoprosthesis in eyes with retained silicone oil. A primary PK in these eyes gives a reasonable estimation of visual potential before proceeding with keratoprosthesis [16].

Indication for Corneal transplant
- Corneal scar with irregular astigmatism not corrected with rigid gas permeable contact lens
- Corneal decompensation
- Corneal perforation
- Corneal scar with posterior segment complication
- Multiple intrastromal Foreign bodies in cornea causing glare

Fig. 5.9 Indication for corneal transplant

The indications of a corneal transplant are enumerated in Fig. 5.9.

5.4 Limbal Stem Cell Deficiency

In combat injuries, limbal deficiency occurs after ocular burns due to blast or secondary to chemical warfare (mustard gas)-induced ocular surface damage. The treatment of limbal deficiency depends on whether it is unilateral or bilateral and on the state of vision in the other eye. In the case of unilateral limbal deficiency, autologous limbal tissue from the other eye is used. The technique of conjunctival limbal autograft is well described and accepted. However, the concerns about damage to healthy eyes and improvements in the method of stem cell-based cultures led to the concept of ex vivo cultivation of limbal stem cells on fibrin or amniotic membrane and its use as a cultivated sheet for ocular surface restoration.

The success of ex vivo LSCT almost mirrored that of CLAU without the risk to the donor site.

The drawbacks, however, included cultivating cells in the laboratories, which required certification and expertise to grow cells, and the added cost of the treatment. In 2012, Sangwan et al. published their outcome of cultivating the limbal cell directly on the amniotic membrane integrated on the patient's ocular surface, and they called the technique Simple limbal epithelial transplantation (SLET) [17]. It utilized the benefit of taking a tiny bit of tissue from the donor site, cutting it into small bits, and placing them strategically in the amniotic membrane placed on the cornea to achieve epithelization of the ocular surface. SLET is cheaper and can be performed by any ophthalmologist trained in the concept of this surgery. After stabilization of the ocular surface, the residual corneal scar is addressed with a lamellar or penetrating keratoplasty. In some instances, lamellar or penetrating keratoplasty is combined with a stem cell transplant (CLAU, ex vivo LSCT, or SLET). In the case of a bilateral limbal deficiency, the option is to use autologous mucosa as a source of epithelial cells, and the midterm results of cultivated mucosal epithelial transplantation (COMET) are favorable [18]. Mucosal epithelium, however, doesn't have the same properties as the corneal epithelium, concerning transparency and vascularization [18]. The other option is to use a donor limbal source such as a keratolimbal allograft or conjunctival limbal allograft from cadaveric tissue or a live, related donor. Live-related donors have their tissues matched more closely to reduce the risk of rejection [19]. Recently, the use of allo limbal cells has been used as a source of epithelial healing like that described in SLET (allo SLET) in acute chemical injuries with faster epithelial recovery [20]. Few cases report of a similar procedure in the chronic phase, i.e., Allo SLET for visual rehabilitations, are encouraging. Allografts need systemic immunosuppression, at least for the first few years, for the tissue to survive [21–23].

5.4.1 Keratoprosthesis

Patients with multiple failed grafts or bilateral limbal deficiency can be visually rehabilitated with keratoprosthesis. The Boston type 1 keratoprosthesis is the most common keratoprosthesis used worldwide. The basic design is a nut and bolt type of keratoprosthesis wherein the PMMA optic and the titanium/PMMA backplate sandwich a corneal graft. The assembled cornea with the keratoprosthesis is sutured to the recipient cornea. The refractive power of the lens is based on the axial length of the eye and the lens status (aphakic or pseudophakic). A bandage contact lens is placed on the eye after the surgery. The bandage contact lens helps protect the ocular surface from desiccation and reduces the risk that the donor carrier melts in the keratoprosthesis. Patients are continued indefinitely on topical fluoroquinolone and topical vancomycin to minimise the risk of infective keratitis. A moist eye with a good blink is one of the essential prerequisites for a type 1 Boston keratoprosthesis. Eyes with significant lid scarring, exposure of the surface, or keratinisation are not candidates for the type 1 Boston keratoprosthesis. These eyes are better suited to the Boston type 2 keratoprosthesis or the MOOKP (modified Oseto Odonto Keratoprosthesis). The Boston type 2 keratoprosthesis is similar to the type 1 except that, by design, there is a protrusion of the front plate to accommodate the lids. The lids are sutured to each other to cover the keratoprosthesis completely as a through the lid keratoprosthesis. A type 2 keratoprosthesis is usually combined with a pars plana vitrectomy and an Ahmed glaucoma valve placement routinely as prophylaxis since it is more difficult to open the lids again for subsequent surgery.

MOOKP remains the gold standard for long-term visual retention in eyes with severe damage to the ocular surface. It involves the use of a canine tooth as a haptic for the PMMA optic cylinder. This is done in three stages. The first stage consists of complete iris and lens removal (ICCE) with or without a corneal graft based on corneal thickness. The second stage involves draping the ocular surface with a buccal mucous membrane graft and preparing the osteo-dental lamina by removing and shaping the canine teeth and fixing the PMMA to the teeth. This complex is allowed to develop a vascular covering by being placed in the subcutaneous pouch for a few months. Later, the osteodentoalveolar lamina is removed from the cheek and placed under the mucosal flap as an epicorneal keratoprosthesis, wherein only the posterior part of the optic nerve enters the eye. Osteo keratoprosthesis is similar to MOOKP except that it uses the tibial bone as the haptic to carry the PMMA optic cylinder instead of the canine tooth. Of the three commonly used keratoprosthesis for end-stage ocular surface disease or severe burns with lid deformity, the MOOKP has the best long term anatomical and functional success [24–28].

The algorithmic approach to severe ocular surface damage, unilateral or bilateral is presented in Figs. 5.10 and 5.11.

Figure 5.12 depicts a chemical injury with an impending perforation that was managed by a large diameter corneoscleral lamellar graft with amniotic membrane transplantation and fornix formation to achieve tectonic stability.

Figure 5.13 depicts the management of a post-blast corneal perforation with PK with vitreoretinal surgery and subsequently a Boston type 1 keratoprosthesis.

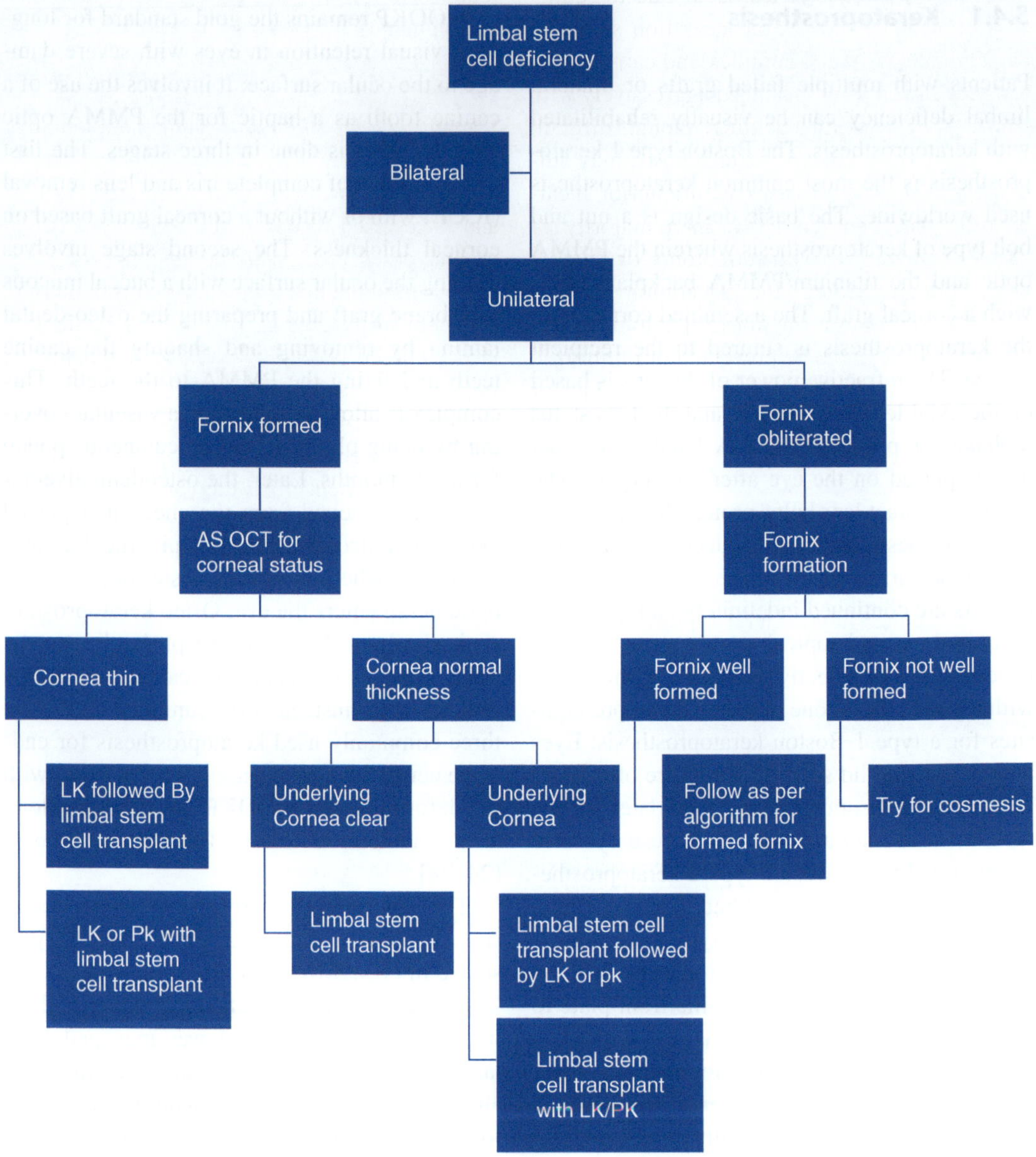

Fig. 5.10 Management of severe unilateral ocular surface injuries with unilateral limbal deficiency

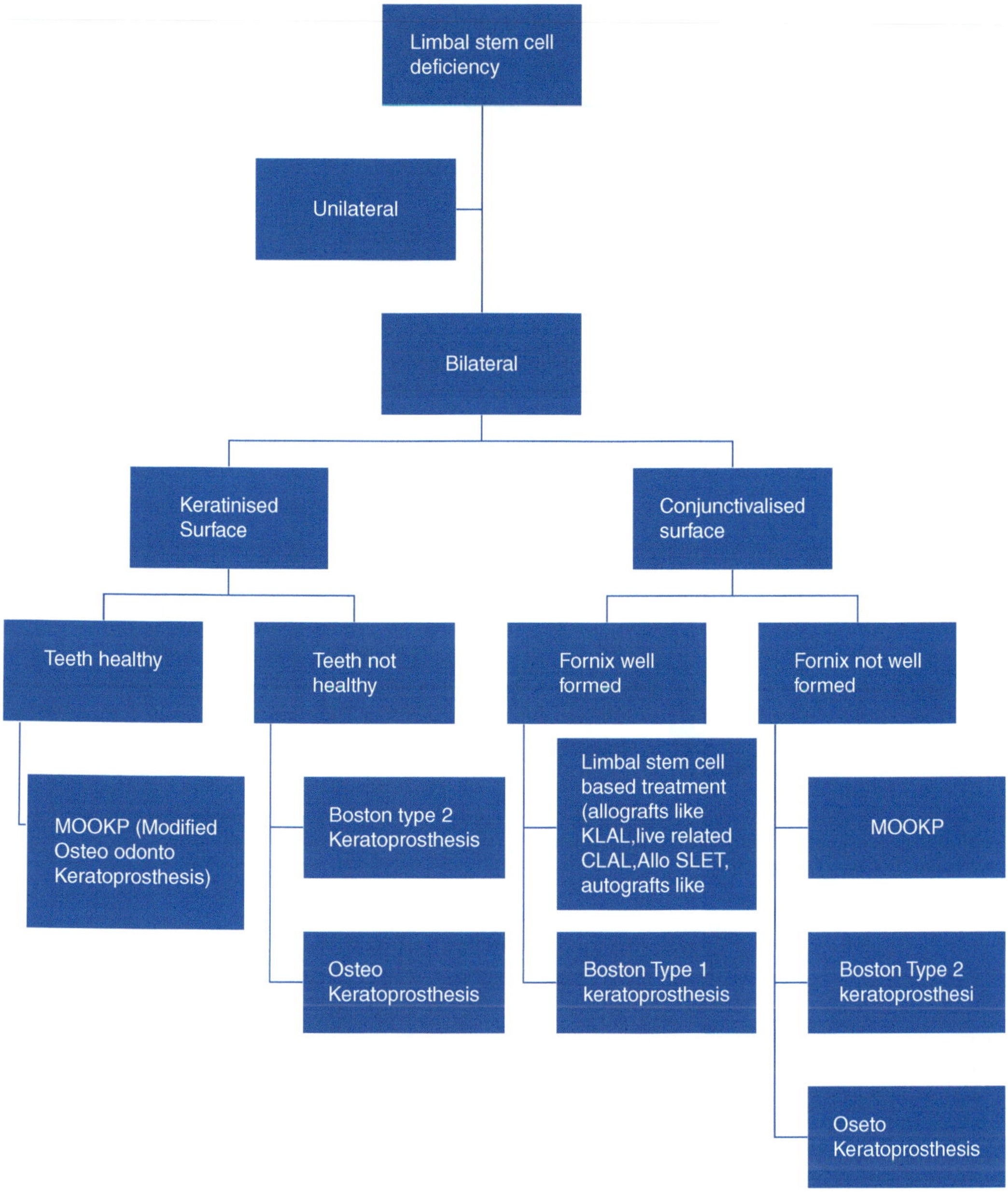

Fig. 5.11 Management of severe ocular injury and bilateral limbal stem cell deficiency

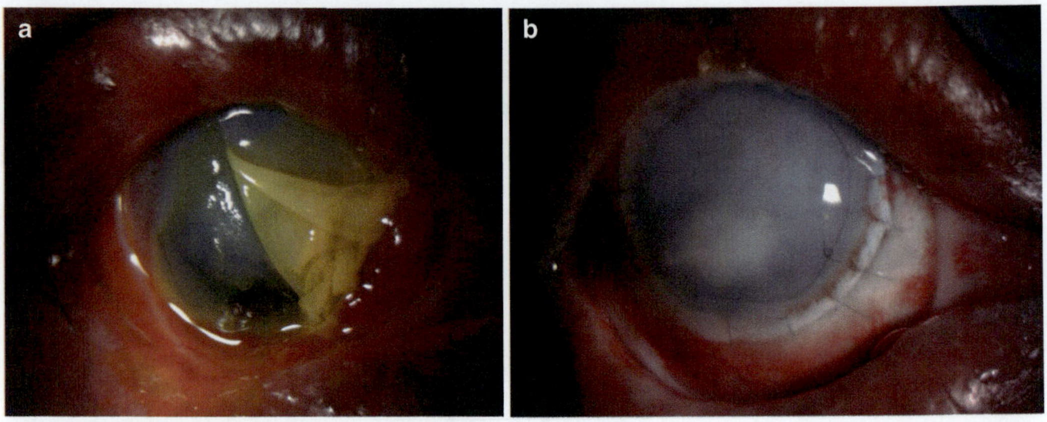

Fig. 5.12 (**a**) Patient with thermal injury with impending perforation and a loose or disintegrating amniotic membrane with a persistent corneal defect. (**b**) Symblepheron release with amniotic membrane transplantation and large corneoscleral Lamellar keratoplasty for tectonic glove integrity

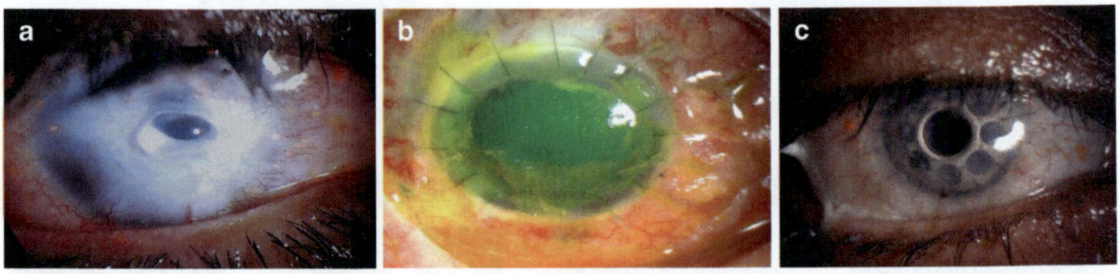

Fig. 5.13 (**a**) Blast injury with corneal scarring and perforation (**b**) underwent PK with vitrectomy and lensectomy with silicone oil injection. to assess it visual potential. (**c**) Subsequently underwent Boston type 1 keratoprosthesis with silicone oil exchange

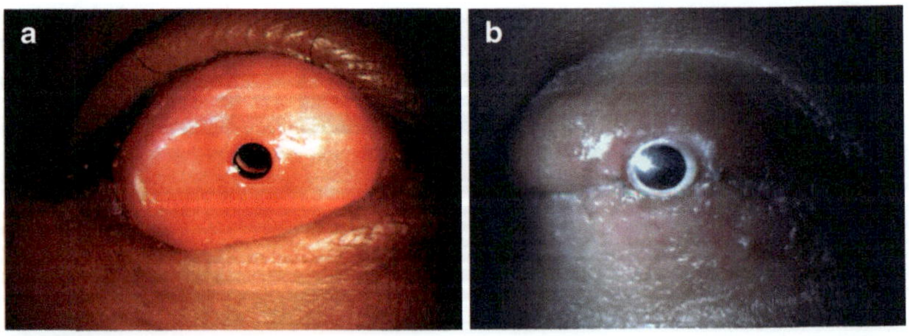

Fig. 5.14 (**a**) Final appearance of an eye with MOOKP (**b**) Final appearance of an eye with a Boston type 2 keratoprosthesis

Figure 5.14 depicts the final appearance of different types of keratoprosthesis in eyes with severe ocular trauma.

Take Home Points

Examine the cornea in detail to identify the cause of decreased vision.

Use investigative modalities like topography, tomography, and ASOCT to help establish the surgical plan.

In cases of ocular surface failure with limbal stem cell deficiency, assess the other eye's limbal stem cells and vision to determine between limbal stem cell-based treatment and keratoprosthesis.

Keratoprosthesis is generally limited to patients with bilateral visual loss.

References

1. Abbotts R, Harrison SE, Cooper GL. Primary blast injuries to the eye: a review of the evidence. J R Army Med Corps. 2007;153(2):119–23. https://doi.org/10.1136/jramc-153-02-10.
2. Erickson BP, Feng PW, Ko MJ, Modi YS, Johnson TE. Gun-related eye injuries: a primer. Surv Ophthalmol. 2020;65(1):67–78. https://doi.org/10.1016/j.survophthal.2019.06.003.
3. Weichel ED, Colyer MH. Combat ocular trauma and systemic injury. Curr Opin Ophthalmol. 2008;19(6):519–25. https://doi.org/10.1097/ICU.0b013e3283140e98.
4. Morley MG, Nguyen JK, Heier JS, Shingleton BJ, Pasternak JF, Bower KS. Blast eye injuries: a review for first responders. Disaster Med Public Health Prep. 2010;4(2):154–60. https://doi.org/10.1001/dmp.v4n2.hra10003.
5. Al AK, Jain V, Hantera M, et al. Phototherapeutic keratectomy outcomes in superficial corneal opacities. Ophthalmol Eye Dis. 2011;3:1–6. https://doi.org/10.4137/oed.s5985.
6. Rathi VM, Vyas SP, Sangwan VS. Phototherapeutic keratectomy. Indian J Ophthalmol. 2012;60(1):5–14. https://doi.org/10.4103/0301-4738.91335.
7. Singh NP, Said DG, Dua HS. Lamellar keratoplasty techniques. Indian J Ophthalmol. 2018;66(9):1239–50. https://doi.org/10.4103/ijo.IJO_95_18.
8. Tan DTH, Ang LPK. Modified automated lamellar therapeutic keratoplasty for keratoconus: a new technique. Cornea. 2006;25(10):1217–9. https://doi.org/10.1097/01.ico.0000248388.39767.42.
9. Maharana PK, Sahay P, Singhal D, Garg I, Titiyal JS, Sharma N. Component corneal surgery: an update. Indian J Ophthalmol. 2017;65(8):658–72. https://doi.org/10.4103/ijo.IJO_582_17.
10. Seitz B, Langenbucher A, Viestenz A, Dietrich T, Küchle M, Naumann GOH. Cataract and keratoplasty—simultaneous or sequential surgery? Klin Monatsbl Augenheilkd. 2003;220(5):326–9. https://doi.org/10.1055/s-2003-39429.
11. Lee JY, Sung KR, Tchah HW, et al. Clinical outcomes after combined Ahmed glaucoma valve implantation and penetrating keratoplasty or pars plana vitrectomy. Korean J Ophthalmol. 2012;26(6):432–7. https://doi.org/10.3341/kjo.2012.26.6.432.
12. Mayalı H, Kayıkçıoğlu Ö, Altınışık M, Bıçak F, Kurt E. Clinical results in patients with combined penetrating keratoplasty and vitreoretinal surgery using Landers wide-field temporary keratoprosthesis. Turk J Ophthalmol. 2019;49(5):270–6. https://doi.org/10.4274/tjo.galenos.2019.87059.
13. Lee DS, Heo JW, Choi HJ, Kim MK, Wee WR, Oh JY. Combined corneal allotransplantation and vitreoretinal surgery using an Eckardt temporary keratoprosthesis: analysis for factors determining corneal allograft survival. Clin Ophthalmol. 2014;8:449–54. https://doi.org/10.2147/OPTH.S60008.
14. Alió JL, Belda JI, Osman AA, Shalaby AMM. Topography-guided laser in situ keratomileusis (TOPOLINK) to correct irregular astigmatism after previous refractive surgery. J Refract Surg. 2003;19(5):516–27.
15. Lin DTC, Holland SR, Rocha KM, Krueger RR. Method for optimizing topography-guided ablation of highly aberrated eyes with the ALLEGRETTO WAVE excimer laser. J Refract Surg. 2008;24(4):S439–45. https://doi.org/10.3928/1081597X-20080401-22.
16. Iyer G, Srinivasan B, Gupta J, et al. Boston keratoprosthesis for keratopathy in eyes with retained silicone oil: a new indication. Cornea. 2011;30(10):1083. https://doi.org/10.1097/ICO.0b013e318213a8b5.
17. Sangwan VS, Basu S, MacNeil S, Balasubramanian D. Simple limbal epithelial transplantation (SLET): a novel surgical technique for the treatment of unilateral limbal stem cell deficiency. Br J Ophthalmol. 2012;96(7):931–4. https://doi.org/10.1136/bjophthalmol-2011-301164.
18. Cabral JV, Jackson CJ, Utheim TP, Jirsova K. Ex vivo cultivated oral mucosal epithelial cell transplantation for limbal stem cell deficiency: a review. Stem Cell Res Ther. 2020;11(1):301. https://doi.org/10.1186/s13287-020-01783-8.
19. Movahedan A, Cheung AY, Eslani M, Mogilishetty G, Govil A, Holland EJ. Long-term outcomes of ocular surface stem cell allograft transplantation. Am J Ophthalmol. 2017;184:97–107. https://doi.org/10.1016/j.ajo.2017.10.002.
20. Agarwal S, Srinivasan B, Gupta R, Iyer G. Allogenic simple limbal epithelial transplantation versus amniotic membrane grafting in the early management of severe-grade ocular chemical injuries-a retrospective comparative study. Am J Ophthalmol. 2020;217:297–304. https://doi.org/10.1016/j.ajo.2020.05.001.
21. Deng SX, Borderie V, Chan CC, et al. Global consensus on definition, classification, diagnosis, and staging of limbal stem cell deficiency. Cornea. 2019;38(3):364–75. https://doi.org/10.1097/ICO.0000000000001820.
22. Sacchetti M, Rama P, Bruscolini A, Lambiase A. Limbal stem cell transplantation: clinical results, limits, and perspectives. Stem Cells Int. 2018;2018:8086269. https://doi.org/10.1155/2018/8086269.
23. Iyer G, Srinivasan B, Agarwal S. Algorithmic approach to management of acute ocular chemical injuries-I's and E's of management. Ocul Surf. 2019;17(2):179–85. https://doi.org/10.1016/j.jtos.2019.02.002.
24. Iyer G, Srinivasan B, Agarwal S, et al. Keratoprosthesis: current global scenario and a broad Indian perspective. Indian J Ophthalmol.

2018;66(5):620–9. https://doi.org/10.4103/ijo.IJO_22_18.
25. Iyer G, Srinivasan B, Agarwal S, Barbhaya R. Visual rehabilitation with keratoprosthesis after tenonplasty as the primary globe-saving procedure for severe ocular chemical injuries. Graefes Arch Clin Exp Ophthalmol. 2012;250(12):1787–93.
26. Salvador-Culla B, Kolovou PE, Arzeno L, Martínez S, López MA. Boston keratoprosthesis type 1 in chemical burns. Cornea. 2016;35(6):911–6. https://doi.org/10.1097/ICO.0000000000000837.
27. de la Paz MF, Salvador-Culla B, Charoenrook V, et al. Osteo-odonto-, tibial bone and boston keratoprosthesis in clinically comparable cases of chemical injury and autoimmune disease. Ocul Surf. 2019;17(3):476–83. https://doi.org/10.1016/j.jtos.2019.04.006.
28. Iyer G, Srinivasan B, Agarwal S, et al. Boston type 2 keratoprosthesis-mid term outcomes from a tertiary eye care Centre in India. Ocul Surf. 2019;17(1):50–4. https://doi.org/10.1016/j.jtos.2018.08.003.

6 Management of Lenticular Injury

Keiki Mehta

Ocular trauma is unfortunately a fairly commonplace more frequently in men and those who take part in active activities. A study from the World Health Organization has estimated that up to 55 million eye injuries occur annually. And unfortunately, over 1.6 million people may lose their sight. The final visual outcome depends on the quantum of damage which has taken place, and which layers of the eye have been affected by the trauma, which is especially important in battlefield situations where the incidence of both blunt and penetrating injuries are high. For the purposes of this chapter the author will restrict himself to the lens as it is affected in trauma, and its subsequent management. Trauma can affect the lens in various ways. It could be displaced from its normal position, partially or it may be completely displaced. Injury to the lens can also lead to other problems like phacomorphic glaucoma wherein the anterior–posterior diameter of the lens swells to such a degree that it can block the iridocorneal angle. Occasionally the injury can be so severe that the lens capsule itself may rupture leading to cortical remnants in the anterior chamber which can impair or even block aqueous outflow and may even result in an inflammatory response termed as phaco antigenic glaucoma.

Detection of the subluxation lens.

K. Mehta (✉)
Mehta International Eye Institute, Mumbai, India
e-mail: drkeiki@mehtaeyeinstitute.com

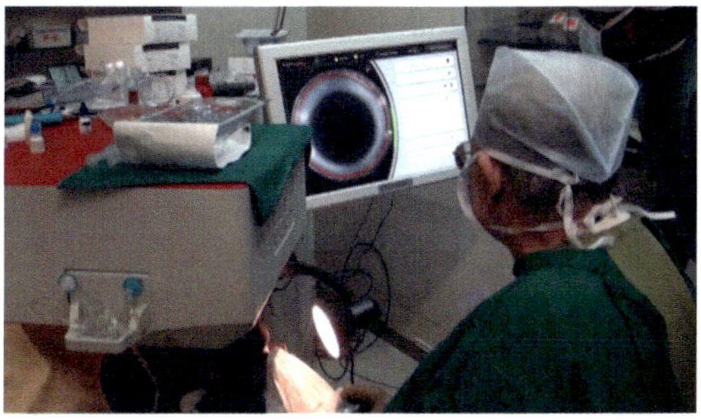

Fig. 6.1 Patient on the CATALYS FLACS system

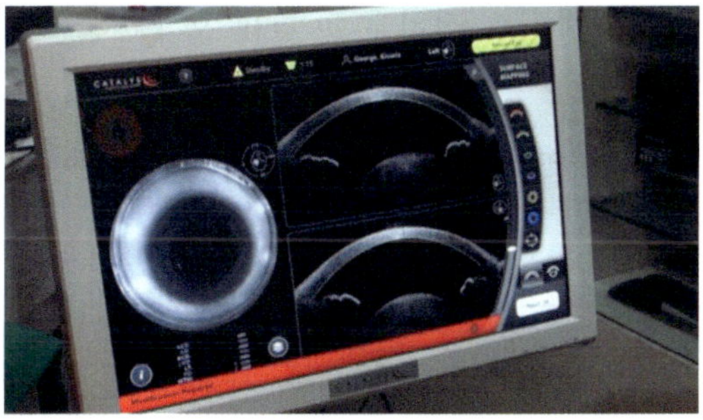

Fig. 6.2 The subluxated lens is clearly seen. Note the large gap between the iris and the capsule

Perhaps the earliest signs of subluxation are a decentralized nucleus, with the lens edge being visible. Irregular depth of the anterior chamber is always considered as suspicious sign as is an irido-lenticular gap made more obvious by lateral illumination (Figs. 6.1 and 6.2).

S. Waikar (ed.), *Ocular Trauma in Armed Conflicts*, https://doi.org/10.1007/978-981-19-4021-7_6

The presence of phakodonesis is an important confirmatory sign.

Other signs which may lead to a diagnosis are marked astigmatism, decreased vision, and monocular diplopia.

Subluxation in children is usually accompanied with a sudden change in power and inability to get adequate vision even with spectacle lenses. It is important to recognize it early, as early surgery with visual rehabilitation will prevent the formation of amblyopia The surgeon should carefully preoperatively assess the eye if he feels there are any signs of zonular weaknesses, as it indicates point of penetration of a FB, or the location of a focal capsular defect. One should be particularly careful if the lens subluxation is at the 6 o'clock position as this may simply indicate a 360° zonular damage.

If gonioscopy is possible preoperatively or if a surgical gonioscope is available, it will give valuable information.

6.1 Presurgical Considerations

The first step is to determine whether a traumatic cataract has resulted from blunt or penetrating trauma. Check the intraocular pressure. If no obvious opening or tear is visible and the IOP is low, indicates an open wound which may even be hidden in the sclera under the conjunctiva. Often a penetrating wound, if small, tends to conceal itself and may self-seal and the intraocular pressure may become normal. All eyes following trauma with low IOP to be taken as having a penetrating injury and a precaution has to be taken to look for it in detail. As a regular routine, A and B scans should be done to assess ocular status. A scan is required as it may become necessary to replace the ocular lens with an IOL. B scan is mandatory to look for any intraocular retained foreign body or cortical material if the posterior capsule has given way. Often the capsular break can be diagnosed by the "fish tail" sign on B scan sonography where on movement of the eye the break in the posterior cortex shows movement left and right coinciding with the leakage of cortical material. Recognizing the retained cortical and lenticular material is essential as it will induce a fairly severe reaction, and even rise of IOP, and may mimic endophthalmitis.

The patient's physical status should be ascertained in detail prior to surgery especially if he has hypertension as the presence of a raised blood pressure would precipitate per-operative complications like expulsive haemorrhage, while the presence of any background or uncontrolled diabetes may lead to increased incidence of post op infection.

The choice of anaesthesia is dependent partially on the patient's status and on the facilities available at the surgical facility or hospital. However, as a regular routine in penetrating injuries, general anaesthesia, using the positive pressure insufflation technique is considered the safest as it maintains a soft eye during surgery which may become lengthy if complications ensue. Giving retrobulbar or peribulbar anaesthesia is contraindicated in a penetrating injury as the increased pressure will lead to loss of contents especially if the wound is large.

Pre-surgically, wash using Povidone iodine solution (Betadine) solution is perhaps the safest way to prevent any further risk of infection and to sterilize ocular adnexa prior to entering the eye.

Irrespective of whether you plan on removing the subluxated lens during phacoemulsification or a vitrectomy and follow-up with or without subsequent sutured/loop fixated IOL, of primary importance is closing the corneal or any scleral wounds so the eye can be pressurized to normal levels. This simple step is often forgotten leading to acute difficulties in lens removal, in a soft soggy eye or even vitrectomy with a persistent leaking wound which will precipitate complications like vitreous prolapse and even haemorrhage in the globe.

Corneal wounds should be closed with 10-0 nylon as parallel interrupted stitches rather than continuous. The tension applied to the stitch depends on whether it is a young or an older patient. In younger children, it is always better to use a higher tension in the stitch rather than simply approximating the tissue, since the tissues are soft, they tend to leak subsequently if any pressure is applied to the globe.

Always keep an intraocular lens (IOL) as standby in case the lens has been damaged and you plan on removing the subluxated lens. The implant you keep as a standby should be the one which you would suture or fixate as per your requirement. It is often impossible to use an A scan on a traumatized eye. Simpler to evaluate the power of the other normal eye and apply the A scan reading to the injured eye. An important indicator of significant difference in the two eyes will be the spectacle number of the patient. If the power in both eyes was the same prior to injury the other normal eye's biometry will suffice to decide on the power of the implant in the traumatized eye.

If the anterior capsule is ruptured in the traumatized eye, it is always better to stain it with Trypan Blue as it tells you the extent of the rupture of the anterior capsule. If the tear is only in the central zone one should consider on carefully converting the opening to continuous curvilinear capsulorhexis. Since the anterior zonules are also very likely to be affected extreme care should be taken not to pull or tug on the lens capsule. A second option rather than trying to do a rhexis, more so if the zonules seem to be affected, is to use Vanna's scissor and cut the capsule in a round manner. Availability of a femtosecond laser assisted cataract surgery (FLACS) makes anterior capsulotomy easy to do with a high level of safety and will be discussed later.

Though most surgeons would say that hydrodissection should be avoided, the author is of the view that it has a great deal of advantage as it permits the nucleus edge to be luxated out of the bag, thus sparing the compromised zonules. Subsequently careful rotation of the nucleus partially out of the bag will make phacoemulsification a simple task without applying any stress or pull on the zonules.

An often-asked question is whether one should use peristaltic or venturi system in phacoemulsification. The author's personal preference is peristaltic, as it is far safer since vacuum is only triggered when the tip is occluded. Slow Motion (Slo-Mo) phacoemulisfication can be done using low flow, low aspiration rate, low vacuum vehicle can be utilized.

If the lens is comparatively clear especially in a young adult, a still safer alternative is to use coaxial cannulas, or the Daljit Singh biaxial cannula.

Naturally with the presence of vitreous in the anterior chamber phacoemulsification cannot be utilized. If you find that the posterior capsule is broken a safe method of managing the displaced lens, is to first place an intraocular lens in the bag if intact, or on the surface of the anterior capsule, if not, and then rotate the nucleus on the lens and then do a slow motion phacoemulsification on the surface which is a technique advocated by Dr. Amar Agarwal termed the Scaffold method. Another simpler technique, long advocated by the author is simply inject an 8 mm punched out HEMA soft +5.00 D contact lens on the anterior surface of the iris, rotate the lens or its fragments on its anterior surfacer and then subsequently phacoemulsification the nucleus off. Subsequently, the soft lens can be easily removed (Images 6.1, 6.2, 6.3, 6.4, 6.5, 6.6, 6.7, 6.8, and 6.9).

Vitrectomy is indicated in all cases where the B scan sonography shows a luxated lens in the posterior chamber, or presence of lens or cortical remnant. Carefully doing this procedure eliminates not only the antigenic reaction which tends to occur, and often an associated rise in IOP subsequently but will permit the eye to recover faster with sharper visual acuity.

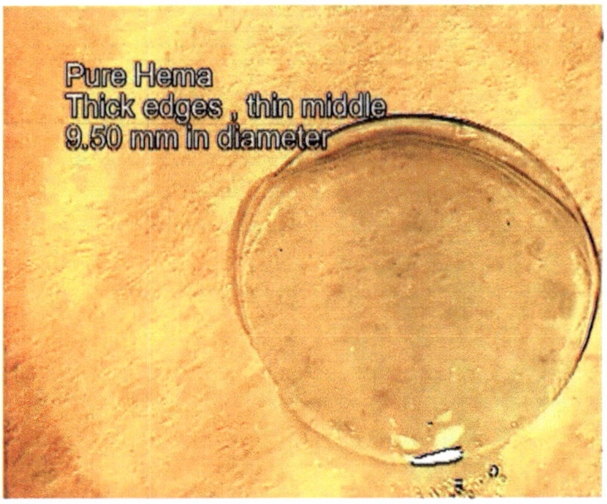

Image 6.1 A +5D contact lens is punched out to 9.5 mm in diameter

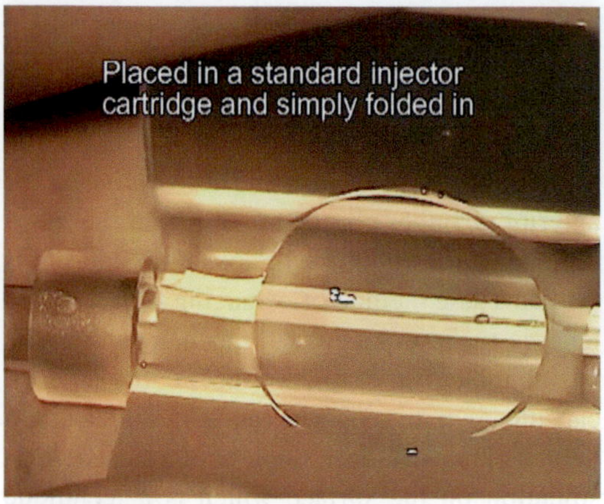

Image 6.2 Placed in standard injector

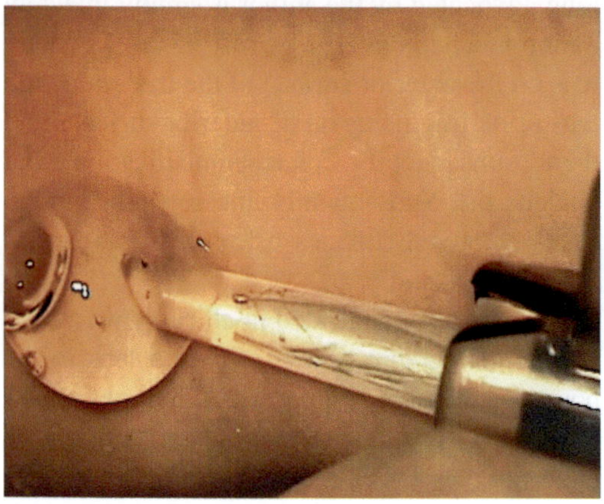

Image 6.3 Prepared for injection

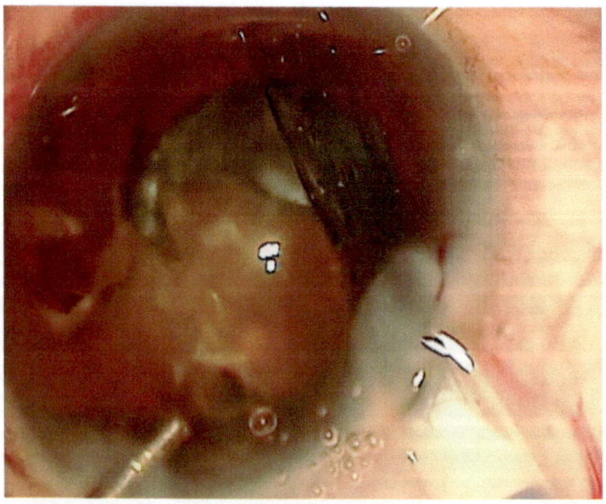

Image 6.4 The lens is injected anterior to the iris

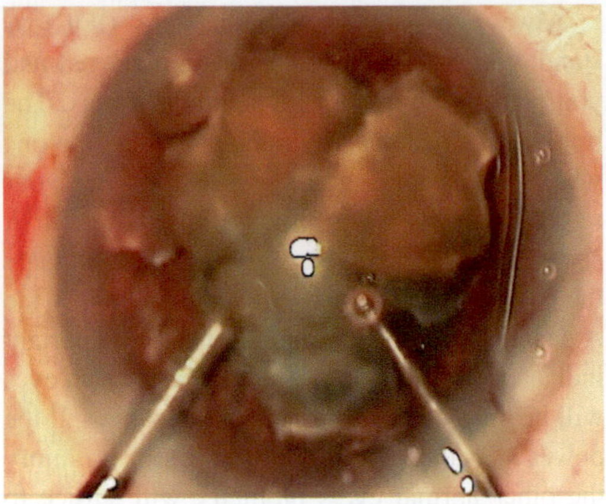

Image 6.5 The lens fragments folded anterior to the lens

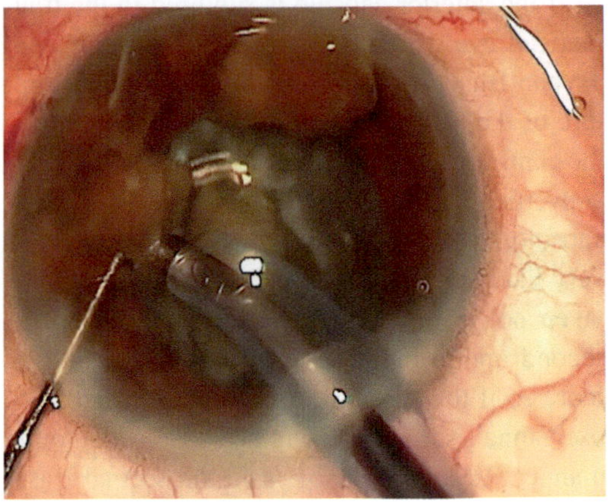

Image 6.6 Phacoemulsification done over the lens with complete safety

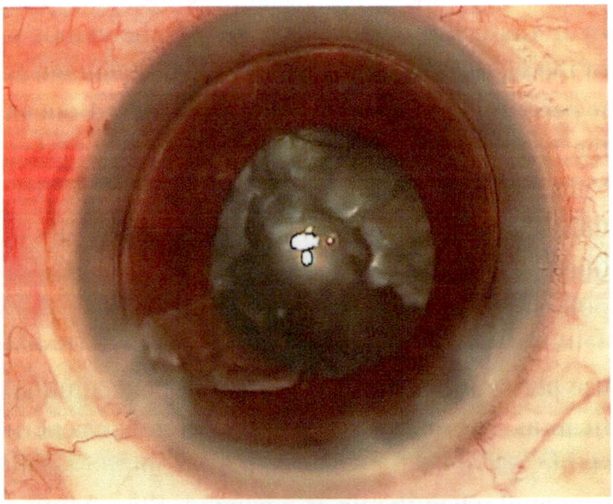

Image 6.7 The final appearance prior to removal of the Hema lens

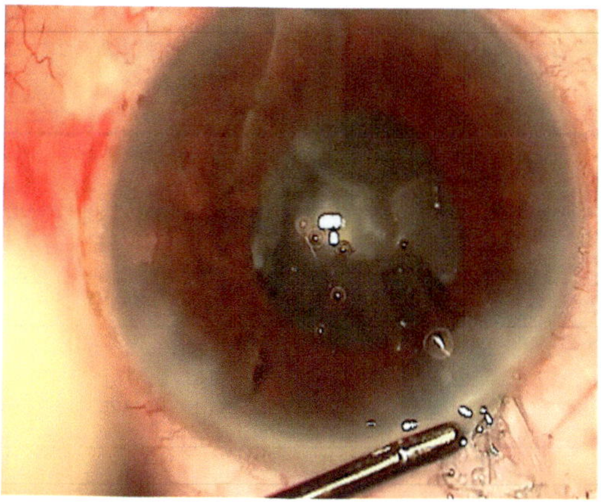

Image 6.8 Lens being removed

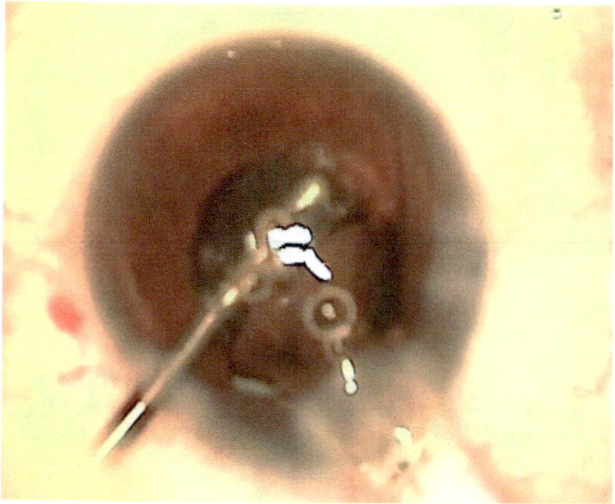

Image 6.9 IOL injected anterior to a repositor and placed on the anterior capsule

If there is vitreous in the anterior chamber due to a broken posterior capsule, remove all the vitreous carefully, always using the pars plana technique, and subsequently injecting Triamcinolone acetonide in the A/C which will show the residual vitreous and which can subsequently, with vitrectomy, be completely removed.

It is essential to vitrectomize all strands especially if they are adhering to the wound edges, as it will significantly reduce the complications such as pupillary distortion, iritis, vitritis, and tractional retinal detachment. In addition, it also prevents infection since vitreous in the sutured wound acts as nidus for further infection.

Hyphema if present in the anterior chamber or in the posterior chamber should be evacuated fully as there is always a risk of the intraocular pressure rising leading to hematocornea (blood staining) of the cornea or secondary glaucoma. A simple tip to prevent later hyphema developing during surgery is to admix two drops of epinephrine in the dispersive viscoelastic.

An intraocular lens should be placed in at the primary stage, unless there has been excessive trauma, or the patient is physically unfit for a lengthy surgery, in which case it could be considered as a second stage placement. Perhaps the best and simplest technique is to sclerally suture the lens into place, or use the Agarwal technique of sclerally buried loop placement or the newer and perhaps even more simpler Yamane technique which requires no sutures and simplifies placement.

If there is only a small rent in the posterior capsule, it is ideally converted into a round posterior rhexis, and placing a hydrophilic lens like (Rayner) either in the bag if undamaged or in the anterior capsule. A hydrophilic lens is preferred as in future if any retinal repair needs to be done, silicone oil can be used safely.

At the completion of surgery should assess for any leakage with air injection and later with fluorescein applied on the conjunctiva and wound edges. At the end of the surgery, the author highly recommends the use of injectable undiluted moxifloxacin injection which severely reduces the risk of infection.

Femtosecond Laser Assisted Cataract Surgery (FLACS) and Subluxation Management

Femtosecond laser assisted cataract surgery certainly has proven to be a great help in regular cataract surgery (Fig. 6.1). When FLACS came into being it was viewed as a technology which would significantly help reflect the outcomes especially with premium lenses. The ability to always make a perfect rhexis (Fig. 6.3) so that the lens fixation would be perfect was considered to be a tremendous advantage. In essence preparing the anterior capsulotomy in a single stroke and at the same time fragmenting the lens significantly reduces the quantum of manipulation (Fig. 6.4). The ability to make precise incisions and to accurately do precise toric correction proved to be a great boon.

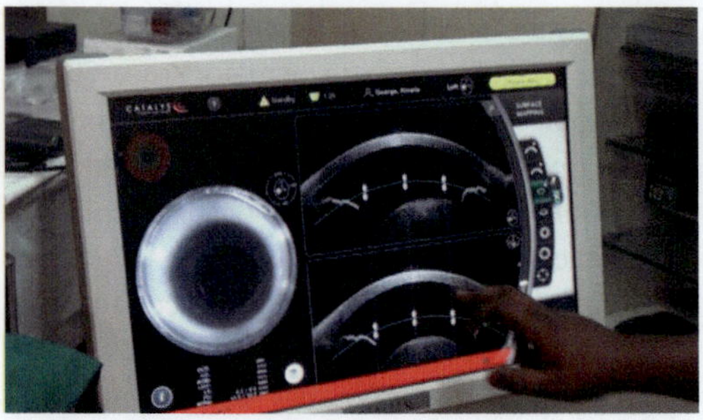

Fig. 6.3 Prior setting the anterior capsulotomy onto the anterior capsule

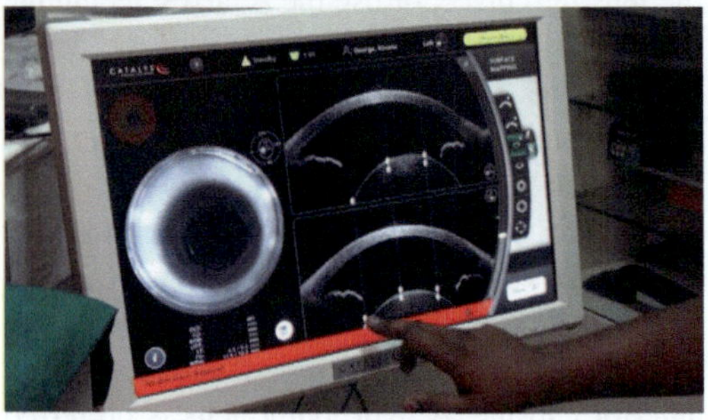

Fig. 6.4 Capsular setting completed so that the laser may fire accurately

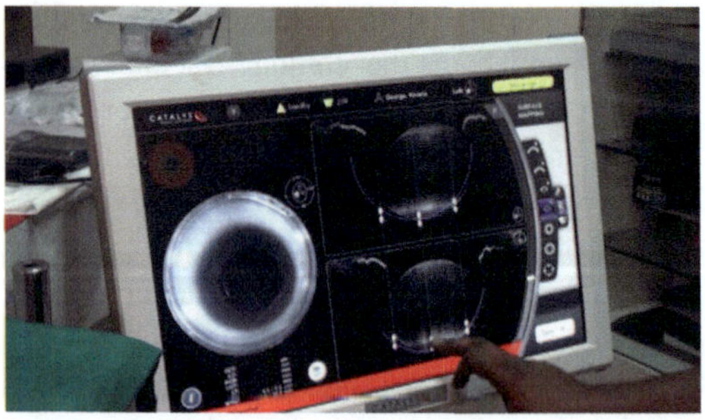

Fig. 6.5 Posterior capsular area set. Note: a subluxated lens is always much thicker than a normal lens

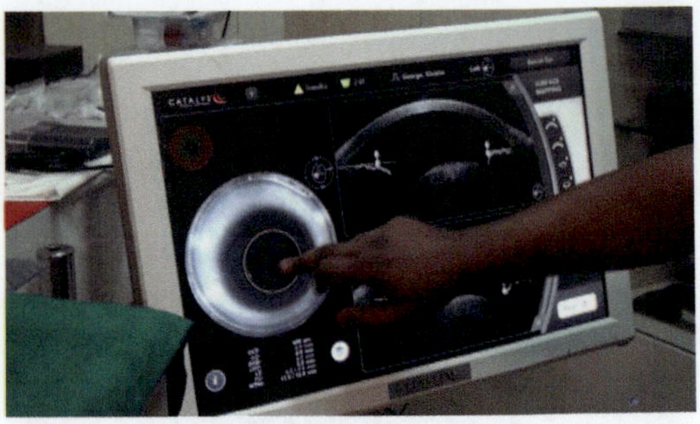

Fig. 6.6 Setting the pupil by simply moving the ring with the hand

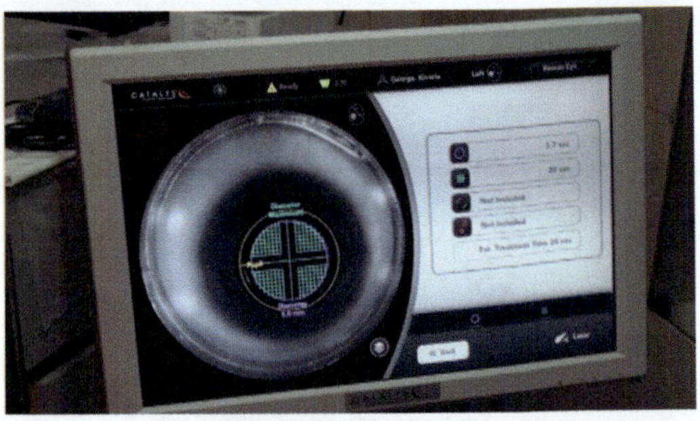

Fig. 6.7 Setting the diameter at 5 mm prior laser firing

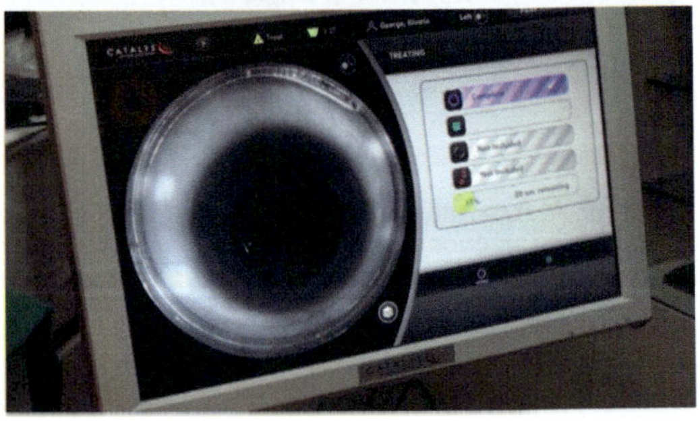

Fig. 6.8 Capsulotomy completed

It would thus stand for reason that subluxation lenses (Fig. 6.2) would be an ideal indication for the use of this advanced technique (Fig. 6.5). As long as the lens remained in the pupillary centre it is possible by simply adjusting the parameters on the FLACS machine and to pre-fragment the lens (Figs. 6.6 and 6.7) preplace incision and all this with no pressure on the eye, and with no stress on the compromised zonules. A number of authors commented on its use on Marfan's syndrome and the significant success achieved using this technique (Figs. 6.8 and 6.9).

It is interesting the presence of vitreous has no effect on femtosecond laser application and hence as long as the instrument setting is perfect an excellent capsulotomy can be done. Simultaneously placing precise corneal incisions can also be done without any pressure on the globe. Thus femtosecond laser offers the unique advantage of a closed chamber technique which

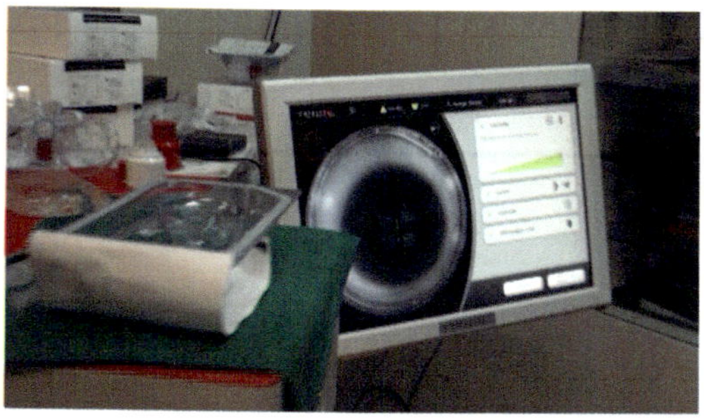

Fig. 6.9 Laser completed

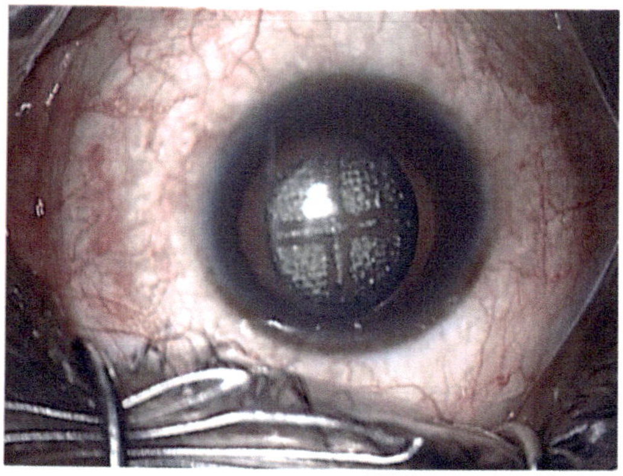

Fig. 6.10 Patient prior phacoemulsification, showing the centring of the capsulotomy

permits the procedure to be done with a modicum of safety.

Subsequent to the application of the laser, the rhexis needs to be completed taking great care as tags are likely to be there (Fig. 6.10). Ideally, following the commencement of rhexis, at a point opposite the subluxated zone, placement of zonular support hook should be placed. Since capsular tags are to be expected, the capsular hooks will support the capsule (Figs. 6.11 and 6.12) not only by holding the lens up but by placing it on a level lain so that the rhexis can be done smoothly.

The lens can be easily aspirated or emulsified using the Slo-Mo phacoemulsification technique (Fig. 6.13) as described earlier. If the subluxation is less than 6 o'clock hours following placement of a capsular tension should be adequate to stabilize the bag. However if the capsule is broken and the subluxation is more extensive an attempt to inject a capsular ring unless the surgeon is very

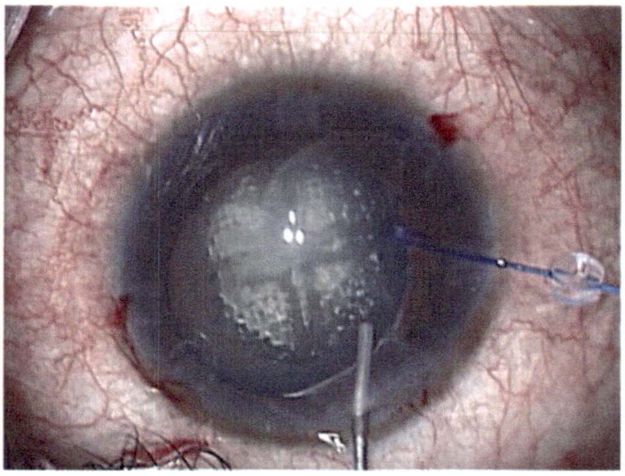

Fig. 6.11 Placement of hooks to stabilize and raise the anterior capsule to iris plane

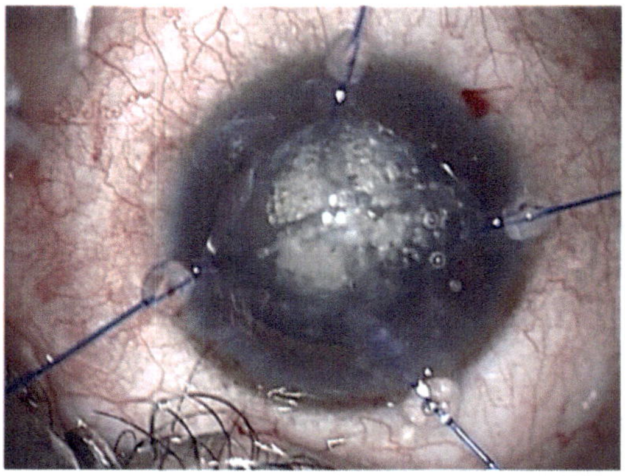

Fig. 6.12 4 hooks placed to stabilize the lens

experienced will lead to a total avulsion of the bag, converting a simple case into a catastrophic endeavor. Whenever there is doubt, a Capsular Tension ring, Cionni (Figs. 6.14 and 6.15), with either a single or a double eyelet should be chosen and the eyelet sutured to the sclera; however, if any doubt arises the ring may be sutured to the sclera (Fig. 6.16).

The author highly recommends the use of a Rayner pattern IOL (Figs. 6.17, 6.18, and 6.19) which can fit comfortably and keep the bag expanded. Subsequently one must assess the vitreous for any tractional bands which may have been left over causing pupillary notches. If the face has been broken vitrectomy is essential to remove vitreous as tractional bands will over time lead to a retinal detachment obviating a successfully conducted case.

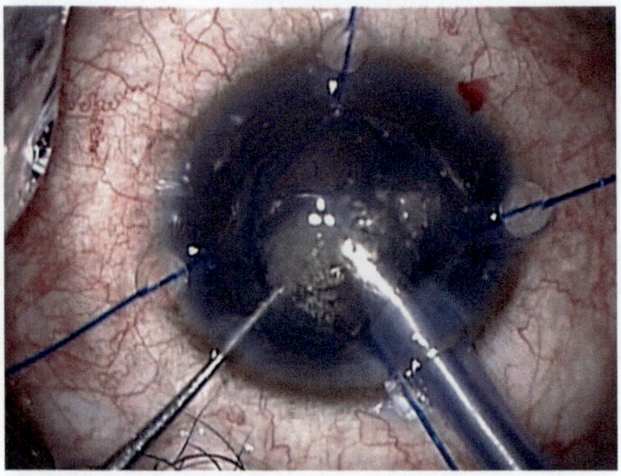

Fig. 6.13 Slow motion phacoemulsification

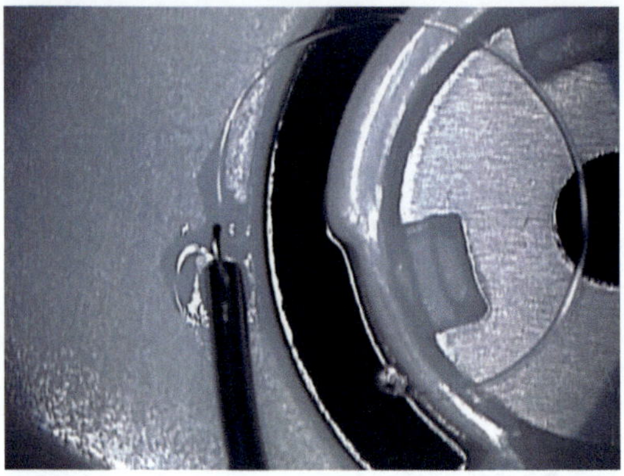

Fig. 6.14 Preparation of capsular ring for injection

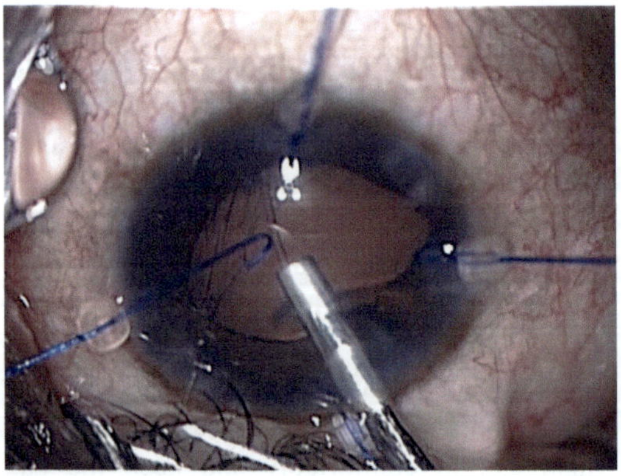

Fig. 6.15 Injection of capsular ring

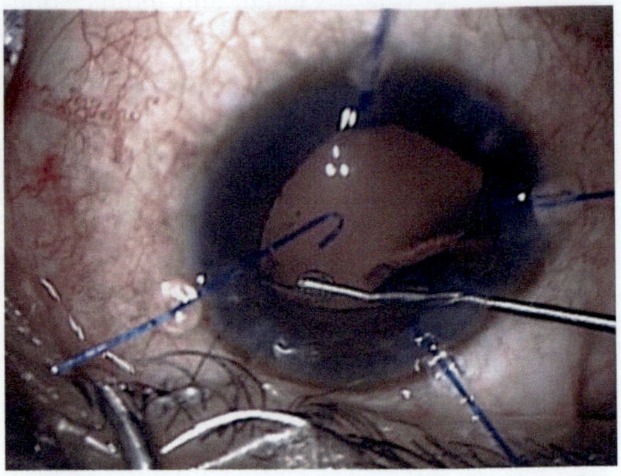

Fig. 6.16 Final placement of the ring being dropped into position

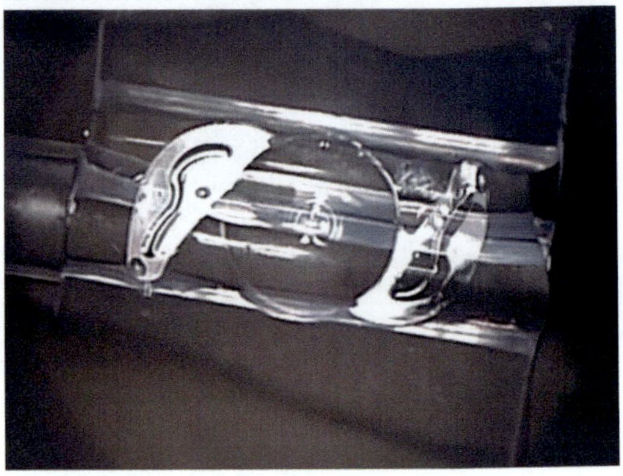

Fig. 6.17 Rayner multifocal IOL being prepared for insertion

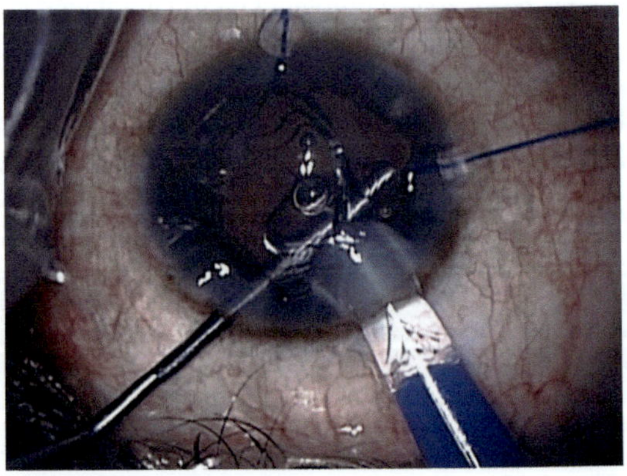

Fig. 6.18 IOL being inserted in the eye

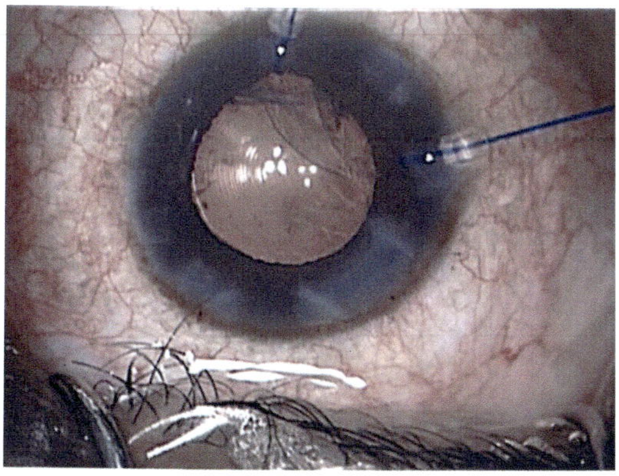

Fig. 6.19 Final placement before closure

Particular care should be taken if the trauma has occurred in the child since children are inveterate rubbers and can subluxate lens again if inadequately sutured.

Thus, application of FLACS immensely simplifies managing this difficult situation and enhances the surgical and visual outcome.

6.2 Summary

The surgical management of a subluxation traumatic lens presents the ophthalmic surgeon with multiple challenges and options. From the detailed clinical evaluation to a properly planned surgical approach with application of the newer techniques and devices will ensure the best possible outcome.

The continuous enhancement of surgical techniques and new prosthetic devices has led to an incremental improvement in the subsequent results and reduction of complications. Post-operative care and long-term follow-up of these patients are mandatory to maintain an excellent surgical outcome and to minimize complications.

Glaucoma in Trauma

7

Madhu Bhadauria and Rahul Bhardwaj

7.1 Background

Glaucoma following trauma is unique as it is caused by a heterogeneous group of challenging and potentially devastating mechanisms like blunt, sharp, or blast injuries. A variety of pathological mechanisms increase the intraocular pressure (IOP) in the early phase or years after the trauma. Ocular trauma can be divided into closed globe injuries (CGI) and open globe injuries (OGI). There are other types of traumatic insults that also lead to an injured globe, causing secondary glaucoma, like chemical injuries, blast injuries, and surgery. Transient or prolonged elevations in IOP occur depending upon the extent of damage to the trabecular meshwork and disorganization and damage to other ocular structures. A long-term increase in IOP can lead to permanent damage to the optic nerve head and visual functions.

7.2 Prevalence and Incidence

The risk of developing glaucoma after a specifically closed globe contusion was found to be 19% in one study [1]. Another study found the corresponding risk of penetrating ocular injury to be about 3% [2]. In the United States trauma registry of 1998, 58% of ocular trauma subjects were less than 30 years of age [3]. Young males are prone to ocular trauma, with male-to-female ratios ranging from 3.4: 1 to 13.2: 1 [3].

The causes and circumstances of ocular injury can vary widely according to geographic, socioeconomic, occupational, and cultural factors. For instance, in Los Angeles County, California, violent assault accounts for 41% [4] of ocular injuries. In the past, a majority of ocular trauma originated in the workplace or in settings of violent conflict, but in recent years, there has been an increase in ocular injuries secondary to leisure activities and motor vehicle accidents [3]. Among 32 patients hospitalized for sport-related ocular injury, ball games were the most common cause, smaller the ball more, the more damage it causes as it fits in the socket [5]. A golf ball or shuttlecock is far more dangerous than football. An increasingly common source of severe blunt ocular trauma is airbag injuries related to motor vehicle accidents [6].

When armed forces are used against civilians in political unrest, actions can result in a dramatic increase in the incidence of eye injuries. Injuries can be specifically brutal from tear-gas canisters and rubber-coated bullets [7]. In armed forces conflicts like insurgency and war, the types of injuries are splinters from mine blast and bomb blasts. These mechanisms may lead to closed or open globe injury and may be further associated

M. Bhadauria (✉) · R. Bhardwaj
Regional Institute of Ophthalmology, Eye Hospital Sitapur, Sitapur, UP, India

S. Waikar (ed.), *Ocular Trauma in Armed Conflicts*, https://doi.org/10.1007/978-981-19-4021-7_7

with the effect of blast making damage more than if one mechanism were responsible. An Andhra Pradesh Eye Study in rural southern India showed a high incidence of injury among workers at the workplace (55.9%), followed by injuries at home (21.7%). Laborers or industrial workers are performing hazardous duties in factories and construction sites without adequate safety standards.

A study by Kamalkar et al. found post-traumatic IOP elevation occurred in 15% of pediatric eyes, more common with closed globe injuries compared to open globe injuries. In a closed-globe injury group, nearly 25% of patients required glaucoma surgery and 63% required medical management. High-risk populations like the military, police, and athletes playing contact games and ball games are more susceptible than the general population [8].

7.3 Mechanisms of Glaucoma Secondary to Closed Globe Injury

7.3.1 Early Onset

Common mechanisms of raised IOP after CGI are angle recession, hyphema, inflammation, and lens-related factors. Another possible mechanism could be uveal effusion leading to shallowing of the anterior chamber and liberation of retinal photoreceptors in **Schwartz–Matsuo syndrome**, typically accompanied by important IOP fluctuations [9].

7.3.2 Hyphema

Hyphema is defined as the presence of blood in the anterior chamber. The annual incidence of traumatic hyphema has been estimated at 12 injuries per 100,000 people, with males being affected three-to-five times more frequently than females [10]. Sports-related injuries account for 60% of ocular trauma resulting in hyphema [11].

CGI causes high-impact compression followed by expansion, leading to rupture of iris stromal or anterior ciliary body blood vessels and bleeding into the anterior chamber. Based on the extent of blood in the anterior chamber and the type of treatment required, hyphema is graded as under (Figs. 7.1 and 7.2).

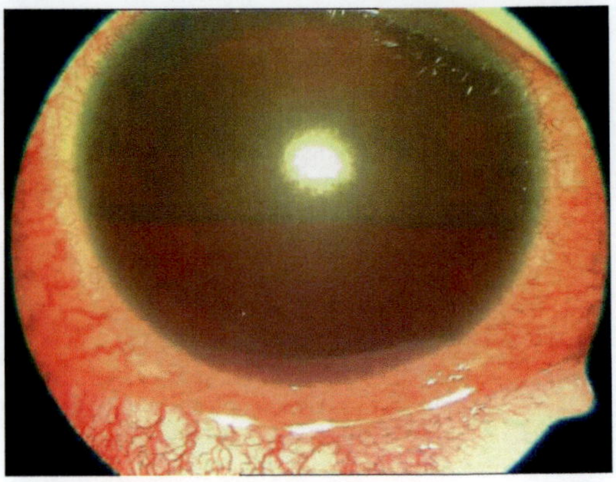

Fig. 7.1 Hyphema half chamber

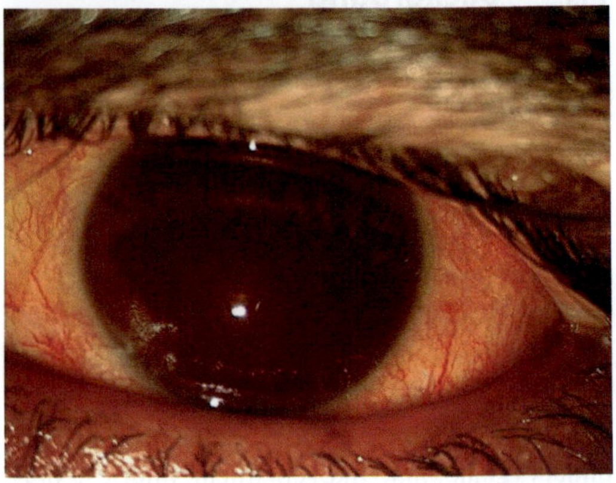

Fig. 7.2 Full chamber hyphema

Hyphema grading	
Grade I	Less than one-third filling of the anterior chamber
Grade II	One-third to one-half of the anterior chamber
Grade III	One-half to near total filling of the anterior chamber
Grade IV	Hyphema corresponds to complete filling of the anterior chamber

The degree of IOP elevation has been shown to be related to the extent of hyphema [11]. In healthy children and adolescents, pressures up to 50 mmHg can be tolerated well for 5 days without permanent optic nerve damage [12].

However, patients with sickle hemoglobinopathy can only withstand an IOP of 24 mmHg for

24 h (**Goldberg's rule**) before permanent damage to the optic nerve occurs [13].

Secondary hemorrhage typically occurs two to five days after the initial injury, as the initial clot begins to retract and lyse [14]. Potential predisposing factors for rebleeding include: those with high IOP at first examination (>22 mmHg) [14], sickle cell disease or trait [15], African-American race without hemoglobinopathy [16], use of antiplatelet and anticoagulant medications, and systemic bleeding dyscrasias [17]. The real threat to glaucoma damage depends on the degree and duration of elevated IOP and rebleeding. In one study of 235 cases, the prevalence of glaucoma was 13.5% in eyes with grade II hyphema, 27% in eyes with grade III hyphema, and 52% of eyes developed glaucoma with total hyphema [18]. About 60–94% of eyes with traumatic hyphema are found to have associated angle recession [19] (Figs. 7.3 and 7.4).

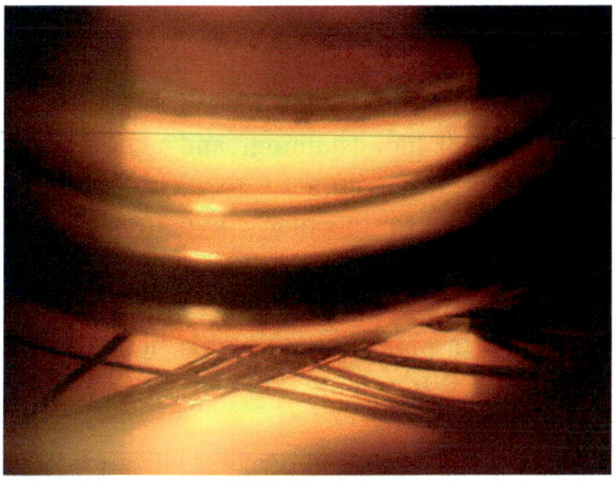

Fig. 7.3 Angle recession

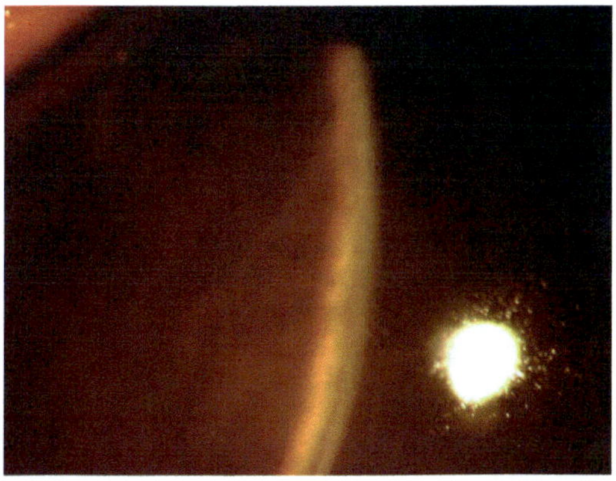

Fig. 7.4 Blood staining of cornea

7.3.3 Management

Immediate patching of the eye with an eye shield, restriction of activity (even reading), and elevation of the head of the bed by 30° are the best ways to start treatment. Before patching, it is important to ascertain that there is no abrasion on the cornea. If no abrasion is seen, the eye is patched with prednisolone and atropine eye drops and lubricant. In the presence of an abrasion, prednisolone eye drops are withheld until the abrasion heals. The Patient is supported by adequate medicine for pain and vomiting. Acetazolamide is a standard drug that is given for IOP control in all the hyphema in cases of AC > 1/3 filled with blood. However, it is extremely important to ascertain the history of sickle cell disease and sulpha allergy due to a cross-drug reaction with acetazolamide. H/O drug intake like aspirin or antiplatelets should also be asked in elderly patients. Hospitalization is suggested for high intraocular pressure on initial examination, delayed presentation, hyperactive children, or large hyphema (filling >50% or more of the anterior chamber). Systemic diseases like hemophilia and associated body trauma [17].

Medical management focuses on the prevention of secondary hemorrhage and raising IOP. Cycloplegia with cyclopentolate or homatropine provides pain relief and prevents the development of posterior synechiae [17]. The prednisolone acetate may lower the risk of rebleeding and reduce inflammation. Oral antifibrinolytics, including aminocaproic acid and tranexamic acid, stabilize anterior chamber blood clots and delay clot retraction so that rebleeding is reduced [20]. Once patching is removed, topical antiglaucoma medications like beta blockers or Alpha 2 agonists can be used. In sickle cell patients, IOP has to be aggressively controlled in the first 24 hours. A carbonic anhydrase inhibitor or mannitol is typically avoided in patients with sickle cell disease because of the risk of sickling caused by metabolic acidosis or volume depletion.

Surgical interventions are aimed at anterior chamber clot evacuation in patients with large persistent hyphema (≥Grade III for >10 days), early corneal bloodstaining, and uncontrolled IOP despite maximal medical therapy. Uncontrolled intraocular hypertension is defined as >60 mmHg for 2 days, >50 mmHg for 5 days, >35 mmHg for 7 days, or >25 mmHg for >24 h in patients with sickle hemoglobinopathy [17, 20].

7.4 Delayed Onset Glaucoma

7.4.1 Angle Recession

Angle recession occurs due to separation between the longitudinal and circular muscle fibers of the ciliary body. Intractable secondary open-angle glaucoma may develop even many years later, up to 15 years following trauma, and raised IOP may be seen even in the contralateral eye (Figs. 7.5 and 7.6). In the presence of a hyphema, an angle recession should be suspected in the majority of eyes [19]. The angle recession itself does not cause outflow obstruction, but represents a visible marker of invisible degenerative damage. However, the total number of patients who develop glaucoma following an angle recession is only 7–9% [21, 22]. The risk of glaucoma appears to be greater if more than 180° or 240° of angle recession is present. Raised IOP in the contralateral eye of the patient's angle recession may be up to 50% [23, 24]. However even 360 degree angle recession in the absence of raised IOP does not require treatment.

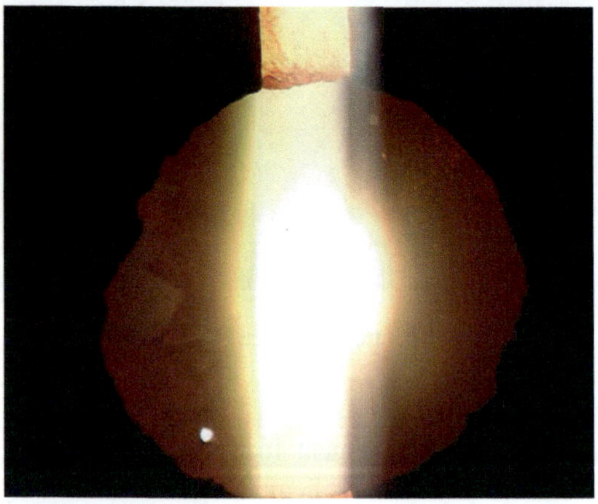

Fig. 7.5 Traumatic sphincter rupture

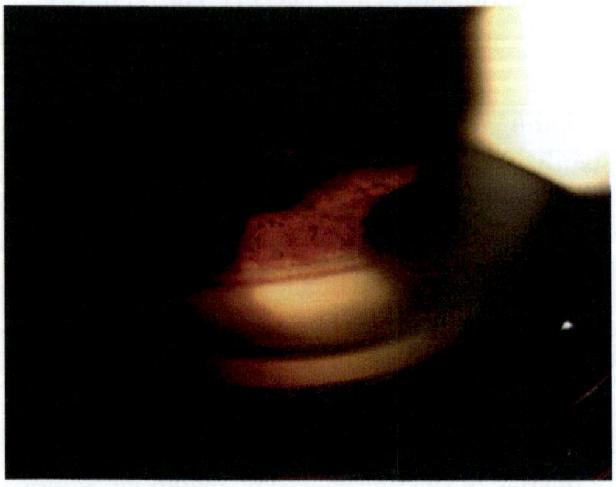

Fig. 7.6 Angle recession

7.4.2 Management

Antiglaucoma medicines that increase outflow and/or laser trabeculoplasty usually have a poor response due to damaged trabecular meshwork [25, 26]. Aqueous suppressants are generally used to lower elevated IOP. Trabeculectomy augmented with antimetabolites is the first-line surgical therapy and is associated with the greatest reduction of IOP and the fewest postoperative glaucoma medications [27, 28] (Figs. 7.7 and 7.8).

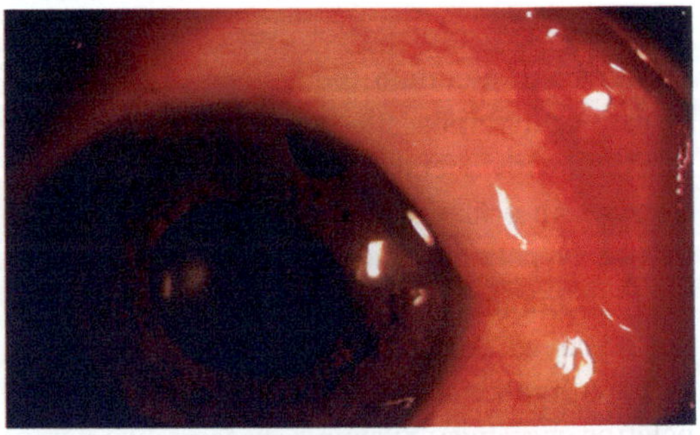

Fig. 7.7 Diffuse bleb with shallow AC

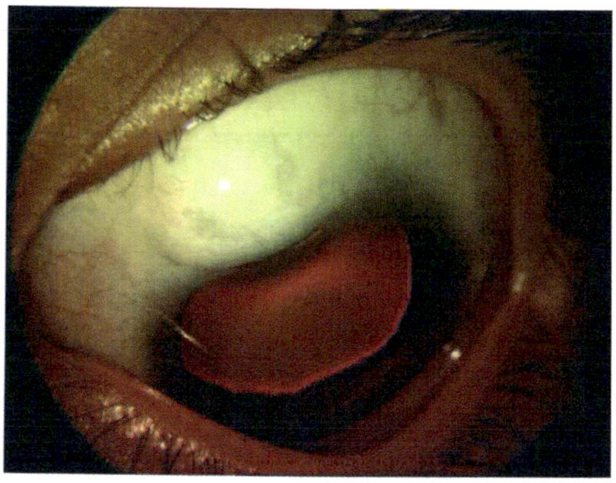

Fig. 7.8 Small localized bleb with subluxation of lens

7.5 Ghost Cell Glaucoma

First described by Campbell [29], this type of glaucoma occurs in patients who have had a vitreous hemorrhage. The hemoglobin is absorbed, and the rigid shells of RBCs travel to the anterior chamber and block the trabecular meshwork, leading to a raised IOP. A tan-colored pseudohypopyon forms once these cells precipitate. A **'candy-striped' sign** is present when a mix of fresh red blood cells and ghost cells layers out. The diagnosis is confirmed by demonstrating thin-walled, hollow erythrocytes with a shrunken appearance in an anterior chamber aspirate specimen under phase contrast or light microscopy [30] (Fig. 7.9).

7.5.1 Management

In most cases, raised IOP lasts for several months, and treatment with topical aqueous suppressants is sufficient to control IOP. Cases with dense hemorrhage or pressure not adequately controlled by medical therapy may require an anterior chamber wash or vitrectomy to remove all the remaining ghost cells. In refractory cases, anterior chamber lavage and removal of the blood source (vitrectomy in the presence of vitreous hemorrhage) are indicated. In the event that the lens is ruptured or dislocated, it may need to be removed out simultaneously, as lens proteins or position may also play a part in the IOP rise (Figs. 7.10 and 7.11).

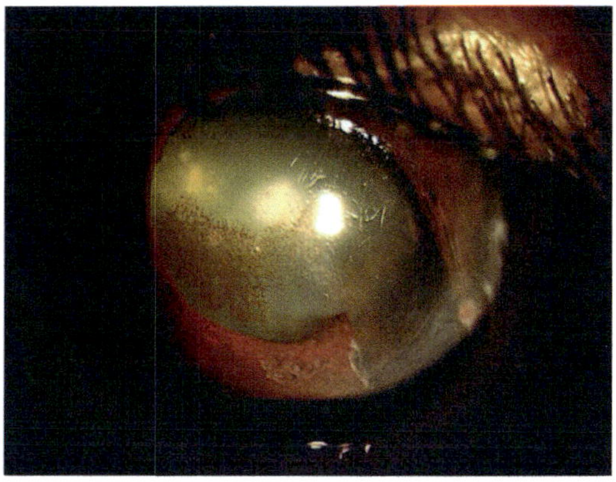

Fig. 7.9 Post penetrating Injury loss of Iris pigment on lens, shallow AC

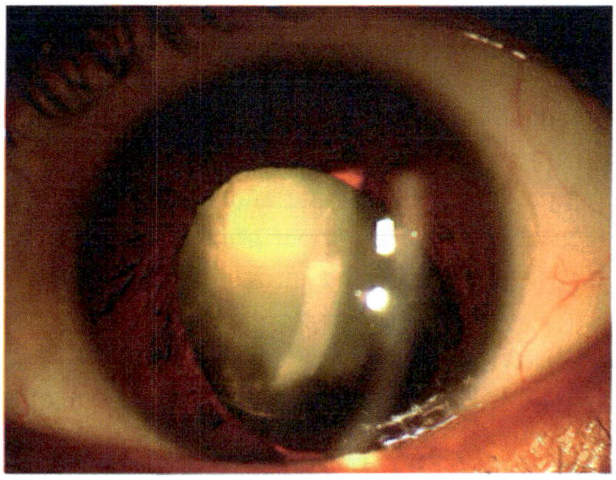

Fig. 7.10 Traumatic subluxation with cataract

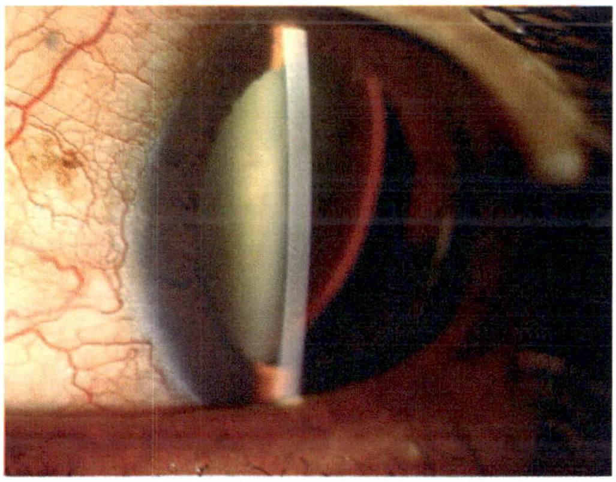

Fig. 7.11 Traumatic posterior subluxation

7.6 Penetrating Trauma

Glaucoma following penetrating injury occurs usually after a few weeks or months. The origin of penetrating injuries can be blunt force, sharp objects, or lacerations of the globe. A gonioscopic evaluation needs to be done to discover an unsuspected foreign body at the angle as and when the eye is safe enough for the procedure.

7.6.1 Mechanisms of Glaucoma Secondary to Penetrating Trauma

Secondary angle closure due to peripheral anterior synechiae is the most common mechanism for the development of glaucoma in penetrating eye injuries.

Epithelialization of the anterior chamber can occur in cases of improper primary surgery and may lead to glaucoma through several mechanisms, including growth over the trabecular meshwork and peripheral anterior synechiae formation [31]. Iron released from intraocularly retained iron objects is toxic to the trabecular meshwork, leading to decreased outflow and elevated IOP (siderosis). Copper may be oxidized within the eye, causing similar trabecular changes as with iron but with less frequency (chalcosis) (Figs. 7.12 and 7.13).

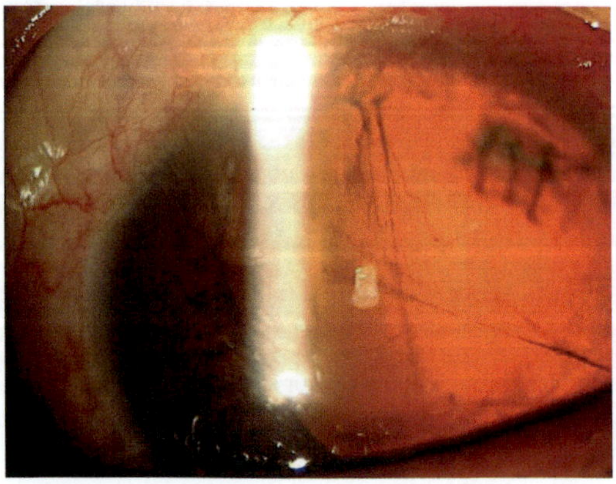

Fig. 7.12 Corneal wound repair with aphakia

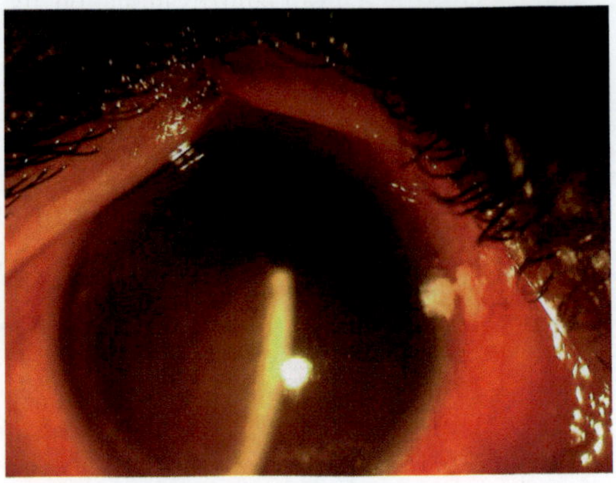

Fig. 7.13 Blood staining cornea

7.6.2 Management

The management consists of globe closure with rapid removal of the foreign objects, if any. Corticosteroids oral as well as topical need be given to avoid severe inflammation, cyclitic membranes and sympathetic ophthalmia. Antibiotics in appropriate dosage are given for endophthalmitis prophylaxis. Raised IOP can be treated with beta-adrenergic antagonists, carbonic anhydrase inhibitors, alpha-2-agonists, and hyperosmotic agents. Filtering surgery is required for uncontrolled IOP. Glaucoma drainage devices are required in eyes that have very badly damaged conjunctiva or a deformed anterior segment.

7.7 Chemical Injuries and Secondary Glaucoma

7.7.1 Alkali Burns

Alkaline substances may penetrate into the eyeball within seconds of contact, causing severe damage to the anterior segment structures. These types of burns may produce characteristic IOP changes with an initial rapid rise, which has been attributed to anterior segment shrinkage and increased uveal blood flow [32, 33]. These effects may be prostaglandin-mediated. Trabecular meshwork may undergo irreversible damage, as a direct consequence of the original alkali burn or due to secondary angle closure as a result of peripheral anterior synechiae. Pupillary block due to inflammation leading to iris bombe and angle closure may be yet another reason for IOP rise in the late phase.

7.7.2 Management

Raised IOP in the early phase can be controlled with beta-adrenergic antagonists, carbonic anhydrase inhibitors, alpha-2-agonists, and hyperosmotic agents. The damage caused by alkali burns is mostly due to a severe inflammatory reaction. Topical corticosteroids must be used for the first two weeks but are contraindicated beyond that period because of the risk of stromal lysis [34]. Surgical intervention should be the last option in these patients, and if required, a glaucoma drainage device is the best possible option as a primary procedure, as trabeculectomy does not work due to associated damage to the ocular surface. Acid burns cause coagulation of surface tissues, so penetration inside the eye is less, but if high concentrations of acid are the cause, it behaves almost like alkali.

7.7.3 War Time Injuries and Glaucoma

During war, most of the injuries are penetrating or blast, and both are lethal to the eye. Blast injury is associated with contusion, and if impact is less, the globe remains intact, but severe tissue trauma occurs as a result, and glaucoma is seen more often than contusion or closed globe injury in civil set-ups. Another association of blast is the chemical and physical burning of the ocular surface, making the conjunctiva unhealthy for glaucoma surgery. Penetrating injuries are more common and have a higher morbidity due to the severity of the damage and the often-delayed treatment. If these eyes survive with a high IOP, initial treatment is done with antiglaucoma medications like betablockers, alpha-2 agonists, and topical CAI inhibitors. Prostaglandins are withheld until inflammation subsides completely. As and when surgery is needed, the main choice remains between glaucoma drainage devices and cyclodestructive procedures.

References

1. De Leon-Ortega JE, Girkin CA. Ocular trauma-related glaucoma. Ophthalmol Clin N Am. 2002;15(2):215–23.
2. Girkin CA, McGwin G Jr, Morris R, et al. Glaucoma following penetrating ocular trauma: a cohort study of the United States Eye Injury Registry. Am J Ophthalmol. 2005;139(1):100–5.
3. May DR, Kuhn FP, Morris RE, et al. The epidemiology of serious eye injuries from the United States Eye Injury Registry. Graefes Arch Clin Exp Ophthalmol. 2000;238(2):153–7.
4. Liggett PE, Pince KJ, Barlow W, et al. Ocular trauma in an urban population. Review of 1132 cases. Ophthalmology. 1990;97(5):581–4.
5. Gracner B, Kurelac Z. Gonioscopic changes caused by blunt eyeball injuries in sports. Klin Monatsbl Augenheilkd. 1985;186(2):128–30.
6. Lesher MP, Durrie DS, Stiles MC. Corneal edema, hyphema, and angle recession after air bag inflation. Arch Ophthalmol. 1993;111(10):1320–2.
7. Eldaly MA, Abdelhakim MA, Zaki RS, et al. Eye trauma during the 2011 Egyptian revolution. Graefes Arch Clin Exp Ophthalmol. 2013;251(3):661–5.
8. Kalamkar C, Mukherjee A. Incidence, clinical profile, and short-term outcomes of post-traumatic glaucoma in pediatric eyes. Indian J Ophthalmol. 2019;67(4):509–14.
9. Matsuo T. Photoreceptor outer segments in aqueous humor: key to understanding a new syndrome. Surv Ophthalmol. 1994;39(3):211–33.
10. Kennedy RH, Brubaker RF. Traumatic hyphema in a defined population. Am J Ophthalmol. 1988;106(2):123–30.
11. Crouch ER Jr, Crouch ER. Management of traumatic hyphema: therapeutic options. J Pediatr Ophthalmol Strabismus. 1999;36(5):238–50; quiz 79–80.
12. Read JE, Goldberg MF. Blunt ocular trauma and hyphema. Int Ophthalmol Clin. 1974;14(4):57–97.
13. Cohen SB, Fletcher ME, Goldberg MF, et al. Diagnosis and management of ocular complications of sickle hemoglobinopathies: part V. Ophthalmic Surg. 1986;17(6):369–74.
14. Rahmani B, Jahadi HR, Rajaeefard A. An analysis of risk for secondary hemorrhage in traumatic hyphema. Ophthalmology. 1999;106(2):380–5.
15. Nasrullah A, Kerr NC. Sickle cell trait as a risk factor for secondary hemorrhage in children with traumatic hyphema. Am J Ophthalmol. 1997;123(6):783–90.
16. Lai JC, Fekrat S, Barron Y, et al. Traumatic hyphema in children: risk factors for complications. Arch Ophthalmol. 2001;119(1):64–70.

17. Brandt MT, Haug RH. Traumatic hyphema: a comprehensive review. J Oral Maxillofac Surg. 2001;59(12):1462–70.
18. Coles WH. Traumatic hyphema: an analysis of 235 cases. South Med J. 1968;61(8):813–6.
19. Blanton FM. Anterior chamber angle recession and secondary glaucoma, a study of the after effects of traumatic hyphemas. Arch Ophthalmol. 1964;72:39–43.
20. Walton W, Von Hagen S, Grigorian R, et al. Management of traumatic hyphema. Surv Ophthalmol. 2002;47(4):297–334.
21. Kaufman JH, Tolpin DW. Glaucoma after traumatic angle recession. A ten-year prospective study. Am J Ophthalmol. 1974;78(4):648–54.
22. Mooney D. Angle recession and secondary glaucoma. Br J Ophthalmol. 1973;57(8):608–12.
23. Sihota R, Sood NN, Agarwal HC. Traumatic glaucoma. Acta Ophthalmol Scand. 1995;73(3):252–4.
24. Tesluk GC, Spaeth GL. The occurrence of primary open-angle glaucoma in the fellow eye of patients with unilateral angle-cleavage glaucoma. Ophthalmology. 1985;92(7):904–11.
25. Fukuchi T, Iwata K, Sawaguchi S, et al. Nd: YAG laser trabeculopuncture (YLT) for glaucoma with traumatic angle recession. Graefes Arch Clin Exp Ophthalmol. 1993;231(10):571–6.
26. Goldberg I. Argon laser trabeculoplasty and the open-angle glaucomas. Austral N Z J Ophthalmol. 1985;13(3):243–8.
27. Manners T, Salmon JF, Barron A, et al. Trabeculectomy with mitomycin C in the treatment of post-traumatic angle recession glaucoma. Br J Ophthalmol. 2001;85(2):159–63.
28. Mermoud A, Salmon JF, Barron A, et al. Surgical management of post-traumatic angle recession glaucoma. Ophthalmology. 1993;100(5):634–42.
29. Campbell DG. Ghost cell glaucoma following trauma. Ophthalmology. 1981;88(11):1151–8.
30. Cameron JD, Havener VR. Histologic confirmation of ghost cell glaucoma by routine light microscopy. Am J Ophthalmol. 1983;96(2):251–2.
31. Maumenee AE, Paton D, Morse PH, et al. Review of 40 histologically proven cases of epithelial downgrowth following cataract extraction and suggested surgical management. Am J Ophthalmol. 1970;69(4):598–603.
32. Paterson CA, Pfister RR. Intraocular pressure changes after alkali burns. Arch Ophthalmol. 1974;91(3):211–8.
33. Green K, Paterson CA, Siddiqui A. Ocular blood flow after experimental alkali burns and prostaglandin administration. Arch Ophthalmol. 1985;103(4):569–71.
34. Donshik PC, Berman MB, Dohlman CH, et al. Effect of topical corticosteroids on ulceration in alkali-burned corneas. Arch Ophthalmol. 1978;96(11):2117–20.

8 Posterior Segment Manifestations of Ocular Trauma and Their Management

Devesh Kumawat and Pradeep Venkatesh

Posterior segment injuries are an important cause of visual morbidity following ocular trauma during armed conflicts. Being more explosive and fragmentary in nature, improvised modern warfare is likely to produce more severe posterior segment injuries than trauma from civilian accidents. Though blasts and gunshots injuries to the eye are very common, these are often first evaluated by trauma surgeons and later referred to ophthalmologist for definitive management. Hence, it is important for trauma surgeons and ophthalmologists to work as a team in the identification of the extent and severity of overall injuries, regular monitoring, and the initiation of prompt treatment. Given the potential blindness that may result from these posterior segment injuries despite aggressive intervention, as with other injuries, prevention of ocular war injuries cannot be overemphasised.

8.1 Blast Injuries

The commonly used weaponry for blasts includes conventional bombs, improvised explosive devices (IEDs), rocket-propelled grenades (RPG), land mines, thermobaric explosives, and explosively formed projectiles (EFPs). Blasts generate a huge amount of kinetic energy within a fraction of second at very high temperature and pressure, leading to the formation of a blast wave [1]. The sudden pressure change induced by the blast wave damages cellular tissues it comes in contact with. Multiple mechanisms, such as spalling (fragmentation), implosion, acceleration-deceleration, and pressure differentials, are involved in the genesis of tissue damage [2].

Following the explosion of modern-day ammunition, overall injury may evolve through five different phases [3]. The primary phase is due to the initial blast propagation; the secondary phase due to exploding fragments and debris; the tertiary phase due to propelling of the body against objects or walls; the quaternary phase is due to inhalational asphyxia and thermal burns; and the last, quinary is due to the absorption of toxic substances by inhalation or through wounds [1, 3, 4].

The type of posterior segment injury varies with the blast phase [1]. Injuries from the primary phase of the blast result from contact of the blast wave with the upper-mid third of the facial skeleton and include conditions such as scleral rupture, commotio retinae, macular holes, retinal dialysis and detachment, and optic neuropathy. Injuries sustained during the secondary phase are much more common than the primary phase. These include penetrating trauma such as scleral

D. Kumawat
Department of Ophthalmology, Lady Hardinge Medical College, New Delhi, India

P. Venkatesh (✉)
Diseases of the Retina, Vitreous and Uvea, AIIMS, New Delhi, India

S. Waikar (ed.), *Ocular Trauma in Armed Conflicts*, https://doi.org/10.1007/978-981-19-4021-7_8

lacerations or rupture with retained intraocular foreign bodies [RIOFB, discussed in a different chapter]. Penetrating wounds and intraocular foreign bodies are often multiple, of varying sizes, and bilateral in combat settings than the usual civilian injuries. Common penetrating fragments during warfare include shell fragments from grenades, rockets, and mines, which are usually non-magnetic particles [5, 6]. On the contrary, in civilian settings, glass fragments from shattered windows are the most common penetrating object. During the tertiary phase of injury, a combination of both blunt and penetrating trauma occurs as the person is propelled and falls on surrounding blunt or sharp objects. Injury from toxins during the quaternary phase, is usually limited to the anterior segment only, while in the quinary phase, ophthalmic and central retinal vascular occlusions can occur due to a hyperinflammatory state and hypercoagulability [secondary to the absorption of toxins into the circulation] [7, 8].

8.2 Gunshot Injuries

The majority of firearms include handguns, followed by shotguns, hunting rifles, and military guns [9]. Facial and cranial gunshot victims often have ocular injuries. Apart from these, ball-bearing guns, airsoft guns, and paintball guns, although of lower projectile mass and velocity, may also cause globe rupture, vitreous hemorrhage, and other posterior segment injuries [10].

The wounding potential from gunshot bullets depends upon the distance from the face, the entrance angle, the "yaw" or deviation of the bullet after exiting the barrel, and the distance travelled within the tissue [11, 12]. Close-range injuries are more destructive [12]. While military guns propel the bullet at high velocity, civilian handgun bullets often have low velocity. Correspondingly, military gun related injuries may pass through and through ocular tissues, while civilian handgun injuries result in disruptive ocular tissue destruction to the extent that the globe may not be salvaged [10, 11].

The common presentation in gunshot ocular injuries may be either a penetrating wound with a retained foreign body in the vitreous, retina, and choroid, or a perforating wound with entry and exit. Clinical manifestations would include vitreous hemorrhage, vitreous incarceration, retinal detachment, endophthalmitis, and optic nerve injury. Apart from penetrating trauma, contusion injuries in the form of commotio retinae may also be observed. Rarely, intraocular damage may occur from a bullet that passes through the orbit without direct contact with the globe. The high kinetic energy of the bullet gets transmitted to the ocular coats, resulting in rupture of the choroid and sometimes the retina, producing a clinical condition called retinitis sclopetaria [13]. Direct trauma from a bullet lodged in the orbit and indirect trauma from shock waves may crush and shear the orbital blood vessels, leading to orbital hemorrhage [14]. In severe cases, compartment syndrome may occur and compromise the optic nerve and retinal perfusion [10].

During tissue injury by a bullet, a temporary cavity forms perpendicular to the path of the bullet. This creates a vacuum and draws contaminants into the wound, thereby increasing the risk of post-traumatic endophthalmitis [10, 14].

8.3 Manifestations of Blunt Trauma

Blunt ocular trauma cases need a thorough dilated examination since myriad posterior segment injuries may result, involving one or several ocular structures. Manifestations include commotio retinae, macular hole, vitreous hemorrhage, vitreous base avulsion, retinal tear or dialysis, retinal detachment, traumatic optic neuropathy, choroidal rupture, retinitis sclopetaria and scleral rupture.

Commotio Retinae or Berlin's Edema Commotio retinae is a transient opacification of the neurosensory retina after a contusion injury to the eye (Fig. 8.1). It is reported to account for 15% of the military eye injuries, far greater than civilian injuries [8]. The retina becomes grayish-white in the area of impact (coup injury) or in the area diagonally opposite

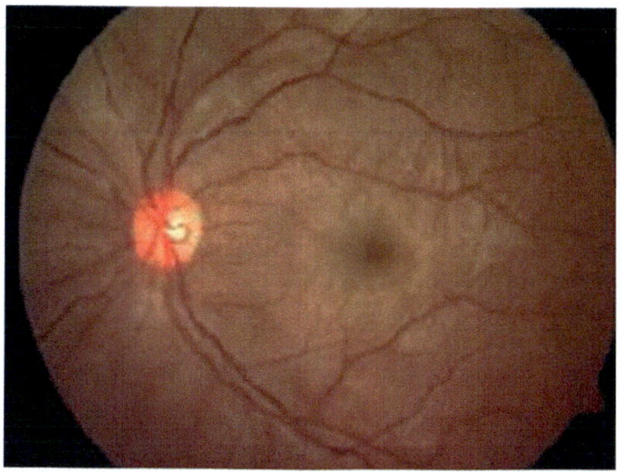

Fig. 8.1 Opacified (grayish-white) retina at the posterior pole (commotio retinae or Berlin edema) following contusion injury to the eye

to the impact site (countercoup injury). The most common site of involvement is the macula in military eye injuries, while in civilian injuries, extramacular commotio is seen more frequently [8, 15].

Commotio retinae at the macula is associated with a sudden, profound, temporary loss of vision. In blast injuries, there exists a positive correlation between the dose effect of the blast wave propagation and the extent of macular injury [1]. Extramacular commotio, mostly in the temporal retina, is associated with visual field disturbances instead of visual loss [15]. The universal histopathological feature, also seen on optical coherence tomography at the site of opacification, is disruption at the level of photoreceptor outer segments [16]. Coexistent is the edema of Muller cells and ganglion cell axons, which causes the retinal whitening [17]. In extensive injuries, the retinal pigment epithelium (RPE) may also be involved.

The retinal opacification settles spontaneously in 4–6 weeks' time with some RPE alteration. Visual recovery is the norm, but the extent of recovery depends on the level of injury [18]. If extensive RPE and photoreceptor outer segment loss are present at the macula, then permanent visual acuity loss and field defects (paracentral scotomas) occur due to macular atrophy [15]. Apart from observation, there is no treatment available for commotio retinae.

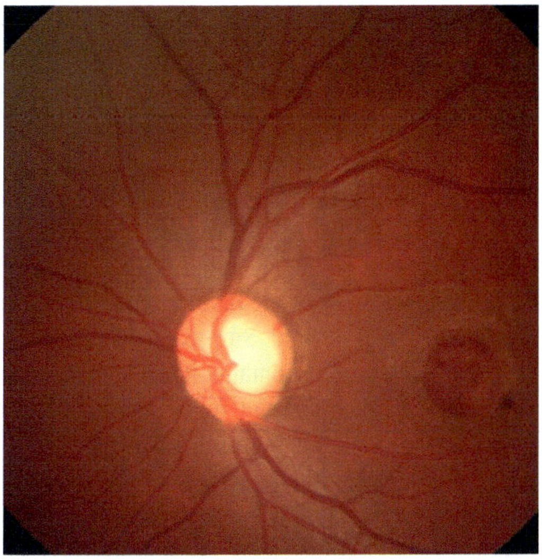

Fig. 8.2 Large full-thickness macular hole following closed globe injury. Note the prominence of pigment alteration at the base and margins of macular hole

Traumatic Macular Hole TMH can occur in both closed and open globe combat trauma, although it is more commonly reported following closed globe injuries. In contrast to their idiopathic counterparts, TMH often presents immediately after the insult [19]. With blunt trauma, there is anteroposterior compression of the globe. The subsequent rebound countercoup leads to anteroposterior vitreous traction. In addition, there also occurs equatorial globe expansion and transmission of tangential vitreoretinal forces onto the macula. Both anteroposterior and tangential vitreous traction are responsible for TMH formation.

Sometimes, TMH develops after several days of trauma. This usually occurs in the setting of extensive commotio retinae, where mechanical disruption of the photoreceptor leads to a full-thickness tissue defect at the fovea (Fig. 8.2) [19]. Rarely, cystic degeneration may also lead to TMH formation [20].

Visual acuity is often variable due to coexistent Berlin edema, subretinal haemorrhage, RPE damage, vitreous haemorrhage, choroidal rupture, and traumatic optic neuropathy (TON). Retinal detachment may also occur from a TMH, but this is uncommon, and so a concurrent peripheral tear or dialysis should always be considered.

Spontaneous closure and visual recovery may often occur in TMH up to six months after trauma [21]. This happens due to glial cell proliferation, which exerts centripetal force on the edges of the hole and fills up the defect. Spontaneous closure often occurs in young patients with a smaller TMH (less than 1/3 of the disc diameter) and no surrounding cuff of fluid. Surgical treatment may be considered when spontaneous closure fails to occur. The anatomical and functional outcomes of vitrectomy, internal limiting membrane peeling, and internal gas tamponade depend not only on the hole characteristics but also on coexistent macular (e.g., submacular haemorrhage) and traumatic optic nerve damage. An issue that may be faced in military settings is that, if gas tamponade is used, the patient may not be fit for further aeromedical transport unless ground altitude air pressures are set. Tamponade with air alone may suffice in a majority of these patients, unless there is concurrent retinal detachment, whence silicone oil should be preferred over expansile gas.

Choroidal Rupture choroidal rupture is a breach in the inner layers of the choroid, Bruch's membrane, and RPE following blunt trauma to the eye. Rupture could be partial or full thickness. With antero-posterior compression and equatorial expansion of the globe, the relatively inelastic choriocapillaris, Bruch's membrane, and RPE rupture, while the elastic neurosensory retina and collagenous sclera escape the injury [22]. These can be either direct (ruptures occurring parallel to the ora serrata, anterior to the equator, at the site of impact) or more commonly indirect (crescent shaped tears due to compressive injury occurring in the posterior pole, usually concentric to the optic disc).

The majority of the indirect choroidal ruptures involve the macula (Fig. 8.3). These may be associated with choroidal, subretinal, or intraretinal hemorrhage. When associated with superficial haemorrhage, these may be concealed, only to be noted 2-3 months later when the bleed clears.

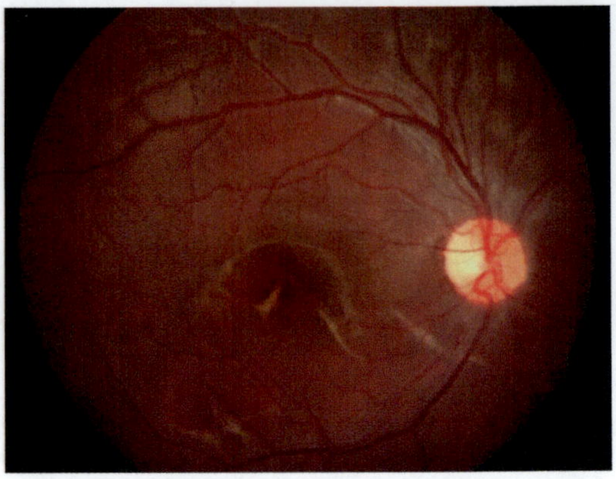

Fig. 8.3 Multiple crescent shaped choroidal ruptures concentric to the optic disc (indirect ruptures). Foveal region is also involved

Visual loss from choroidal rupture may occur immediately if the fovea is involved or later when the choroidal neovascular membrane (CNVM) develops [23]. CNVM develops in around 5–10% of such eyes, with risk factors being older age, macular rupture, and greater length of rupture [23, 24]. Close monitoring is advised in cases of macular choroidal rupture as CNVM can develop. If CNVM develops, treatment with an intravitreal anti-vascular endothelial growth factor injection is advisable. In prognosticating patients with choroidal rupture, one must also factor in the possibility of concurrent traumatic optic neuropathy. As a general rule, in all patients with blunt ocular injuries, in spite of the presence of an obvious feature like choroidal rupture, it is mandatory to undertake a thorough peripheral examination of the retina to rule out retinal dialysis or tears. In addition, damage to other ocular rings, like the trabecular meshwork and angle recession, must also be assessed.

Retinal Breaks and Detachment Blunt ocular trauma may lead to the development of different types of retinal breaks: retinal dialysis (the most common), horse-shoe tears, and necrotic irregular atrophic breaks [25]. Retinal dialysis is segmental, circumferential disinsertion of the retina from the ora serrata. Equatorial expansion and vitreous base traction cause mechanical separation of the retina from the ora. While the most common site of retinal dialysis is the inferotemporal quadrant, superonasal dialysis is pathognomonic of blunt trauma [26]. Vitreous base avulsion with its characteristic 'clothes line' or 'hammock' appearance may accompany retinal dialysis.

Retinal dialysis may vary from small and inconspicuous to a very obvious separation. To detect the former, one may need to perform a meticulous indirect ophthalmoscopic examination with scleral indentation [with or without a drop of topical anesthesia]. A useful indicator for confirming the presence of a small retinal dialysis is the identification of a 'bifurcation' of the margin of the ora serrata, at both ends of the dialysis. Retinal detachment may develop secondary to undetected retinal dialysis, and in young individuals, these may present several months after the trauma and oftentimes show features of a longstanding retinal detachment, particularly when the dialysis is inferior [26].

Retinal breaks may also develop immediately after trauma at the site of impact from contusion necrosis or later when posterior vitreous detachment occurs [27]. These breaks are often located in the region of the vitreous base. Similar to retinal dialysis, retinal detachment develops weeks to months later when the vitreous gel liquefies. An exception occurs in cases of giant retinal tears (tears extending circumferentially for more than 3 contiguous clock hours), where retinal detachment may develop rapidly [28].

Isolated traumatic retinal breaks are amenable to cryotherapy or LIO with indentation, as most of these are located anterior to the equator. Posterior breaks may be treated with single- spot or multi-spot retinal laser photocoagulation using a conventional laser machine or PASCAL. When associated with retinal detachment, the type of treatment is governed by the extent of the detachment, the presence of proliferative vitreoretinopathy (PVR), the age of the patient, the status of the lens, and access to a vitreous surgery facility in the military setting. Most dialysis related retinal detachments can be managed with scleral buckling surgery. Vitrectomy is necessary in cases of giant retinal tears associated with retinal detachments, retinal detachments with vitreous hemorrhage, posterior breaks, and significant PVR.

Vitreous Hemorrhage The source of vitreous hemorrhage in blunt trauma settings may be either ciliary body vessels or retinal vessels. If media permits, a thorough retinal examination needs to be performed as soon as possible, as retinal breaks may be coexistent. If examination of the visible retina is postponed to a later time, hemorrhage may disperse into the entire vitreous cavity, making subsequent visualisation difficult (Fig. 8.4). Scleral depression may only be performed if scleral rupture has been ruled out. In case the fundus could not be visualised with indirect ophthalmoscopy, an ultrasonography of the posterior segment needs to be performed. The key details that need to be looked at are posterior vitreous detachment, vitreous incarceration, retinal tear, localized retinal detachment, giant retinal tear, and choroidal detachment (serous or hemorrhagic).

Observation is generally advised for vitreous hemorrhage in blunt trauma settings unless associated with retinal detachment or vitreous incarceration in occult scleral rupture, where immediate vitrectomy should be performed if a facility for vitreous surgery is available. In a conservative approach, indirect ophthalmoscopy and ultrasonography should be performed every 1–2

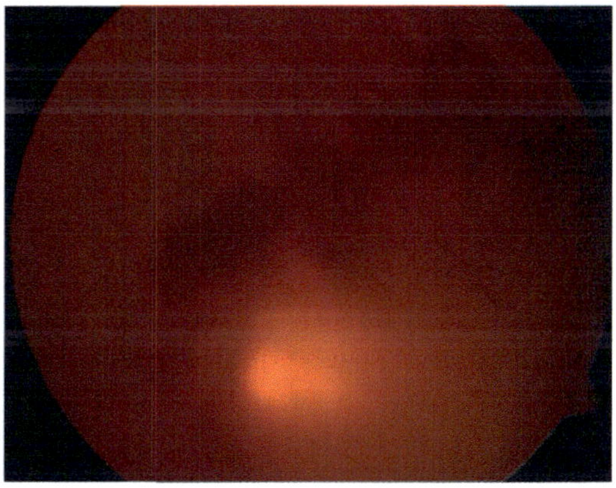

Fig. 8.4 Vitreous hemorrhage after severe blunt ocular trauma. The underlying retina is hazily visible

weeks till the bleed settles. In patients where the other eye has acceptable vision and the vitreous hemorrhage has not resolved over 12 weeks (and no RD is noted on a thoroughly performed USG), a vitrectomy may be performed as an elective procedure. The visual prognosis after resolution of hemorrhage depends upon the presence of coexistent macular damage, optic neuropathy, and retinal detachment.

Vitreous hemorrhage may also occur in head trauma patients without clear evidence of ocular injury. This type of bleed occurs secondary to subarachnoid or subdural hemorrhage and is termed as Terson syndrome [29]. Whether this occurs due to extension of intracranial bleed to the sub-arachnoid space around the optic nerve and subsequent escape into the vitreous cavity along the perivascular spaces, or due to decrease in venous return from high intracranial pressure and subsequent retinal venous stasis and hemorrhage, is not clear [30, 31]. Intraocular hemorrhage in Terson syndrome is characteristic as it occurs at multiple levels in the posterior segment: subretinal, intraretinal, sub-internal limiting membrane, sub-hyaloid, and vitreous. The approach to treatment remains the same as discussed above. In contrast to vitreous hemorrhage occurring from ocular trauma, the visual improvement is considerable in Terson syndrome [32].

Chorioretinitis Sclopetaria This is a rare and unusual pattern of chorioretinal rupture that happens when a high-velocity missile or gun pellet settles in the orbit adjacent to the globe without direct contact with the globe [13]. The kinetic energy transferred and the shock waves delivered to the globe rupture the retina and choroid and spare the densely fibrous sclera (Fig. 8.5). The ruptured tissue retracts, exposing the overlying sclera. The rupture is typically radially oriented. With time, chorioretinal inflammation settles and produces intense scarring and pigment proliferation around the rupture [33]. The typical picture in the late stages may be a chorioretinal defect exposing bare white sclera with pigmentation and scarring at the margin. The scarring at the margin causes firm attachment of the retinochoroidal tissue to the sclera, and therefore the chance of developing retinal detachment is very low [33]. Treatment may be required for associated vitreous hemorrhage or complications from intra-orbital foreign bodies.

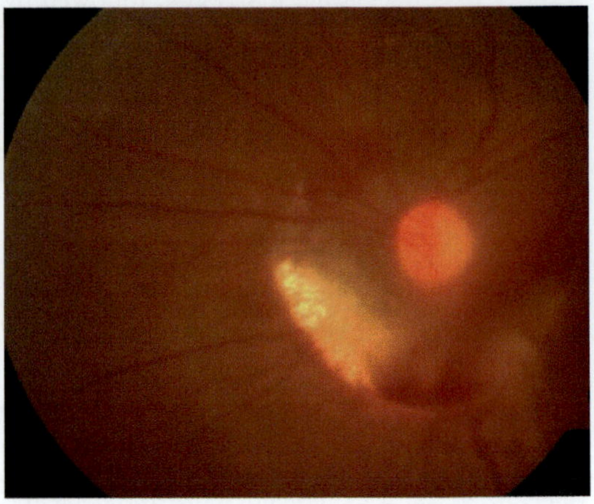

Fig. 8.5 Chorioretinal rupture infero-nasal to the optic disc, with visible sclera in the area of rupture and overlying dispersed preretinal hemorrhage

Traumatic Optic Neuropathy (TON) TON is reported to occur in up to 20% of combat ocular injuries [8]. Direct injury occurs from physical disruption of the ganglion cell axons in the optic nerve [34]. In very severe forms, the optic nerve may avulse from the globe, a feature that is not very common (Fig. 8.6). Indirect injury occurs for several reasons: vasoconstriction of the pial vessels from primary blast injury, compressive neuropathy from retrobulbar hemorrhage, and shearing of the pial vessels at the level of the optic canal where the optic nerve sheath is tethered to the surrounding bone [34, 35].

Clinical examination may reveal a relative or absolute afferent pupillary defect, severe vision loss and dyschromatopsia, normal optic disc appearance (early stage), or disc pallor (late stage). Excavation in the area of optic disc with overlying hemorrhage may be noted in case of complete optic nerve avulsion [34]. In cases with dense vitreous hemorrhage, ultrasonography may show a hypoechoic defect in the area of the optic nerve head shadow suggestive of avulsion. A

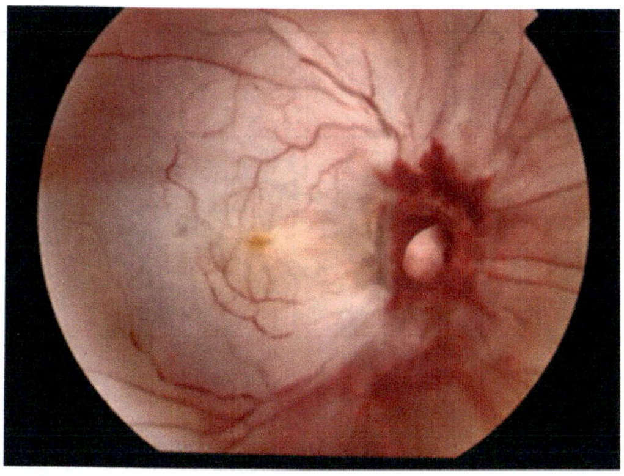

Fig. 8.6 Traumatic optic nerve avulsion with excavation in the area of optic disc, overlying retinal hemorrhages and surrounding retinal opacification from ischemia

computed tomography of the orbit is often advised to rule out bony impingement or compression of the optic nerve, which may otherwise be surgically relieved or decompressed by a team of an ophthalmologist and a neurosurgeon.

There is no effective medical treatment for TON [36]. High-dose corticosteroids have often been used, but with no definitive evidence of benefit [37]. In addition, there is an increased risk of death in patients with clinically significant head injury with the use of high dose steroids [38]. The visual prognosis is often dismal, and spontaneous resolution with visual improvement occurs only infrequently.

Scleral Rupture Globe rupture occurs from an inside-out force following blunt trauma at sites where the ocular coat is weakest, i.e., in the limbus, just posterior to the insertion of extraocular muscles, and at the equator where vortex veins penetrate the sclera. The orientation of ruptures follows the direction of collagen fibers running at that place, i.e., circumferential at the limbus and radial/meridional at the equator [39].

Overt scleral rupture is easily identified by a deformed globe, localised or diffuse subconjunctival hemorrhage and uveal tissue prolapse. Sometimes, s scleral rupture can be occult, often hidden under the extraocular muscles. Indicators of occult scleral rupture include diffuse subconjunctival hemorrhage, slightly lower intraocular pressure (tested cautiously with gentleness), an irregular pupil, a displaced lens, and the presence of vitreous hemorrhage. Incarceration may be noted on ultrasonography, while CT orbit may reveal a flat posterior contour of the sclera (the flat tire sign). The development of endophthalmitis is highly possible and may manifest with severe ocular pain, chemosis, hypopyon, and vitreous exudation.

A protective Cartella eye shield should be applied in case of overt scleral rupture. Undue manipulation of the globe or ultrasonography should be avoided in the presence of an open wound to prevent or worsen prolapse of intraocular contents. Wherever suspected, a radiograph of the orbit or CT orbit (preferred) [40] should be performed for ruling out intraocular foreign bodies since the secondary blast phase may cause penetrative ocular injuries as well. Tetanus toxoid should be administered if required. Prophylactic systemic broad-spectrum antibiotics should be started after admission to prevent endophthalmitis.

Surgical exploration and primary repair of the scleral defect with 8.0 non-absorbable suture should promptly be performed under general anaesthesia (mandatory in severe intraocular injury). The wound edges should be properly exposed and visible before suturing. Prolapsed uveal, retinal tissue, and vitreous should either be gently reposted or abscised without traction, as the case may be. The wound is closed from anterior to posterior. When the rupture extends underneath a muscle, the muscle may be gently retracted with muscle hook or temporarily disinserted to close the defect. In the event that one is unable to trace the posterior limit of the rupture with gentle but adequate dissection, it is best to leave without attempts at forcible tissue closure. This is because, attempts at forcibly retracting the globe would result in additional damage and prolapse of the intraocular contents. Cryotherapy at the margin of a scleral rupture has been traditionally advocated for sealing any retinal breaks that may have occurred [41]. However, this may be counterproductive as it increases intraocular inflammation and fibrosis. Instead, retinal laser photocoagulation around the retinal breaks may be performed during follow up, if possible, using LIO. Treatment options for coexistent endophthalmitis include intravitreal antibiotic injection or media clearing vitrectomy at the end of repair. In extensive globe injuries with a dismal visual prognosis, enucleation or evisceration may be performed after informed consent to prevent sympathetic ophthalmia. However, it is advisable to repair the globe primarily, as enucleation or evisceration may also be performed within 2 weeks of trauma, to minimize the risk of developing sympathetic ophthalmia.

8.4 Manifestations of Penetrating Trauma

Scleral Laceration Unlike scleral rupture, scleral lacerations occur from an outside-in force with a sharp object. Usually these objects are shrapnel propelled during the secondary blast phase or gunshot pellets. Penetrating injuries have a single entry wound. The clinical features are usually obvious with an entry wound, distortion of the globe, vitreous and uveal tissue prolapsing through the wound, and vitreous hemorrhage. Intraocular foreign bodies occur in around 15 to 17% of combat ocular trauma (Fig. 8.7) [4, 6]. The foreign body injuries are different in combat settings than civilian settings [42]. Often, both eyes are involved with multiple foreign bodies. The extent of damage depends upon the size, shape, number, composition, speed, trajectory within the ocular tissues, and final location of the foreign body. Reactive metallic foreign bodies such as copper, iron, and zinc and organic matter such as wood can cause fulminant intraocular inflammation. Intraocular foreign bodies in the posterior segment are removed by the pars plana vitrectomy approach with the help of foreign body forceps or intravitreal magnets. Unfortunately, most of the intraocular foreign bodies in combat settings are pebbles and grit that are non-ferromagnetic and cannot be removed with the help of magnets [42]. An in-depth discussion on intraocular foreign bodies and their management is provided in a separate chapter. Perforating injuries are among the less common eye injuries in war [43]. These have entrance as well as exit wounds. The posterior exit wounds have a tendency to allow the ingrowth of fibrovascular tissues, which leads to complex tractional and rhegmatogenous retinal detachment with severe PVR [43].

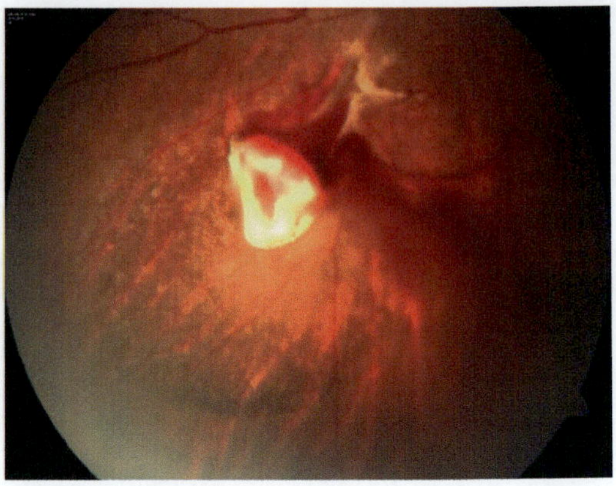

Fig. 8.7 Intraocular foreign body in the vitreous cavity with ricochet injury to the retina and localized vitreous hemorrhage

The principles of managing scleral lacerations are similar to those of managing scleral ruptures.

The exit wound in perforating injuries is usually difficult to approach. The majority of the posterior scleral wounds self-seal by day 7 of injury [44]. The transvitreal proliferation of fibrovascular tissue can however be prevented by early vitrectomy (after this initial 7-10 day wait period for spontaneous closure of the posterior unsutured wound) and thorough cortical vitreous removal in the area of defect [45]. If a stump of proliferation through the exit wound is noted, it should be trimmed but not completely removed in order to prevent reopening of the defect. Recently, chorioretinectomy has been advocated for the removal of necrotic incarcerated retinal and choroidal tissue using diathermy and a vitreous cutter [46]. Retinal detachment, if present, is managed with fluid-air exchange, laser photocoagulation, and oil endotamponade. An encircling silicone element is difficult to pass in these cases and may be considered at a secondary stage if external support for the vitreous base is felt to be necessary during follow-up.

Vitreous Hemorrhage Vitreous hemorrhage can occur for similar reasons as those mentioned in the section on blunt trauma. The prognosis for penetrating ocular injuries worsens with the presence of vitreous hemorrhage. There is prominent intravitreal fibrovascular and fibroglial proliferation, which exerts traction on the retina, optic nerve, and ciliary body. Unlike its blunt trauma counterpart, vitreous hemorrhage in penetrating ocular injuries requires early vitrectomy to minimize the proliferation, and to visualise the retina for the identification of retinal breaks and retinal incarceration. However, the appropriate timing of early surgery is not clear. While some surgeons advocate early vitreous surgery within 48-72 h, sometimes along with primary repair, to prevent the above-mentioned complications [47], others suggest waiting for up to 7–10 days to allow for better diagnostic evaluation of the injury and spontaneous separation of the posterior hyaloid phase [48]. The site of entry for vitrectomy may either be pars plana or limbal, depending upon factors such as the presence of hyphema, ruptured crystalline lens, and retinal detachment with an anteriorly drawn up retina.

Retinal Detachments Retinal detachments in penetrating ocular injuries occur due to retinal incarceration in the scleral laceration site. The detachments are often complex and carry a poor prognosis even when managed aggressively with surgery [49]. Scleral buckling, though difficult to perform under these circumstances, may suffice in a minority of cases with anterior incarceration and minimal PVR. In a majority of cases, a vitrectomy with retinotomy or retinectomy circumscribing the laceration site is required to release the traction [50]. Intraoperative hemorrhage needs to be prevented or minimized with adequate diathermy before retinotomy or retinectomy.

Endophthalmitis Endophthalmitis occurs in around 1-11% of open-globe injuries [51–53]. The risk factors for development include lens capsule rupture, large scleral rupture or laceration, delayed wound closure (beyond 24 h), vitreous and uveal tissue prolapse, and a retained intraocular foreign body [53]. The prophylactic use of intravitreal antibiotics to prevent endophthalmitis following penetrating ocular injuries is not well supported. The clinical signs and symptoms are similar to those of post-operative endophthalmitis, but it may be difficult to diagnose affirmatively early as intraocular inflammation and ocular pain from trauma itself may obscure the presentation. The microorganisms commonly isolated include Bacillus cereus, Gram-negative bacteria, and Streptococcus [53]. The principles of management remain the same as in post-operative endophthalmitis. Aqueous or vitreous samples should be obtained for Gram stain and culture. Antibiotic therapy should include topical, intraocular, and oral and intravenous medications. Systemic broad-spectrum antibiotics are strongly recommended for empirical treatment, such as a third or fourth-generation fluoroquinolone (levofloxacin or moxifloxacin); vancomycin for gram-positive organisms, including Bacillus; and ceftazidime for gram-negative organisms. Definitive intraocular and systemic treatment may later be delivered based on smear or culture results. A low threshold for early vitrectomy should be kept, especially in cases with retained foreign bodies and coexistent retinal detachment [53].

Sympathetic Ophthalmia Sympathetic ophthalmia is a bilateral granulomatous panuveitis occurring following penetrating ocular trauma and is reported to occur in 0.3–1.9% of ocular trauma cases [10, 54]. The majority of cases occur within the first 3 months after trauma [55]. The clinical features may be difficult to identify in the injured (exciting) eye. The sympathizing eye develops mild-moderate anterior uveitis, vitritis, disc edema, multifocal whitish choroidal nodules (Dalen-Fuchs nodules), and exudative retinal detachment in severe cases. The risk for sympathetic ophthalmia is significantly reduced if the exciting eye is removed by enucleation or evisceration within 2 weeks of trauma [55]. Enucleation is preferred over evisceration due to the theoretical advantage of complete removal of uveal tissue. Once the inflammation sets in, secondary enucleation of the eye does not help in reducing the severity of the disease. High-dose systemic corticosteroids remain the initial treatment of choice for sympathetic ophthalmia. Thereafter, immunomodulator therapy is often required for a period of 3–6 months.

8.5 Conclusion

Posterior segment injuries in armed conflicts are often bilateral and extensive. Blunt trauma patients need to be closely followed closely to detect complications that may occur later, such as retinal detachment and choroidal neovascular membrane formation. Penetrating injuries should always be ruled out, even in blunt ocular combat trauma. Timely surgical intervention is important in open-globe injuries to preserve the globe and prevent permanent visual loss. However, the importance of preventing such injuries with protective eye gear cannot be overemphasized, especially since these injuries often do not have a favorable visual prognosis despite timely treatment.

References

1. Phillips BN, Chun D. Ocular blast injuries in modern warfare. Expert Rev Ophthalmol. 2014;9(1):17–23.
2. Shuker ST. Mechanism and emergency management of blast eye/orbital injuries. Expert Rev Ophthalmol. 2008;3(2):229–46.
3. Nakagawa A, Manley GT, Gean AD, Ohtani K, Armonda R, Tsukamoto A, et al. Mechanisms of primary blast-induced traumatic brain injury: insights from shock-wave research. J Neurotrauma. 2011;28(6):1101–19.
4. Mader TH, Carroll RD, Slade CS, George RK, Ritchey JP, Neville SP. Ocular war injuries of the Iraqi insurgency, January-September 2004. Ophthalmology. 2006;113(1):97–104.
5. Wong TY, Seet MB, Ang CL. Eye injuries in twentieth century warfare: a historical perspective. Surv Ophthalmol. 1997;41(6):433–59.
6. Thach AB, Johnson AJ, Carroll RB, Huchun A, Ainbinder DJ, Stutzman RD, et al. Severe eye injuries in the war in Iraq, 2003-2005. Ophthalmology. 2008;115(2):377–82.
7. Kluger Y, Nimrod A, Biderman P, Mayo A, Sorkin P. The quinary pattern of blast injury. Am J Disaster Med. 2007;2(1):21–5.
8. Weichel ED, Colyer MH, Ludlow SE, Bower KS, Eiseman AS. Combat ocular trauma visual outcomes during operations Iraqi and enduring freedom. Ophthalmology. 2008;115(12):2235–45.
9. Cook A, Osler T, Hosmer D, Glance L, Rogers F, Gross B, et al. Gunshot wounds resulting in hospitalization in the United States: 2004-2013. Injury. 2017;48(3):621–7.
10. Erickson BP, Feng PW, Ko MJ, Modi YS, Johnson TE. Gun-related eye injuries: a primer. Surv Ophthalmol. 2020;65(1):67–78.
11. Lichte P, Oberbeck R, Binnebösel M, Wildenauer R, Pape H-C, Kobbe P. A civilian perspective on ballistic trauma and gunshot injuries. Scand J Trauma Resusc Emerg Med. 2010;18:35.
12. Stefanopoulos PK, Filippakis K, Soupiou OT, Pazarakiotis VC. Wound ballistics of firearm-related injuries–part 1: missile characteristics and mechanisms of soft tissue wounding. Int J Oral Maxillofac Surg. 2014;43(12):1445–58.
13. Ahmadabadi MN, Karkhaneh R, Roohipoor R, Tabatabai A, Alimardani A. Clinical presentation and outcome of chorioretinitis sclopetaria: a case series study. Injury. 2010;41(1):82–5.
14. Cunningham LL, Haug RH, Ford J. Firearm injuries to the maxillofacial region: an overview of current thoughts regarding demographics, pathophysiology, and management. J Oral Maxillofac Surg. 2003;61(8):932–42.
15. Scott RA, Blanch RJ, Morgan-Warren PJ. Aspects of ocular war injuries. Trauma. 2015;17(2):83–92.
16. Mendes S, Campos A, Campos J, Neves A, Beselga D, Fernandes C, et al. Cutting edge of traumatic maculopathy with spectral-domain optical coherence tomography - a review. Med Hypothesis Discov Innov Ophthalmol J. 2015;4(2):56–63.
17. Blanch RJ, Ahmed Z, Sik A, Snead DRJ, Good PA, O'Neill J, et al. Neuroretinal cell death in a murine model of closed globe injury: pathological and functional characterization. Invest Ophthalmol Vis Sci. 2012;53(11):7220–6.
18. Eagling EM. Ocular damage after blunt trauma to the eye. Its relationship to the nature of the injury. Br J Ophthalmol. 1974;58(2):126–40.
19. Yanagiya N, Akiba J, Takahashi M, Shimizu A, Kakehashi A, Kado M, et al. Clinical characteristics of traumatic macular holes. Jpn J Ophthalmol. 1996;40(4):544–7.
20. Oehrens AM, Stalmans P. Optical coherence tomographic documentation of the formation of a traumatic macular hole. Am J Ophthalmol. 2006;142(5):866–9.
21. Yamashita T, Uemara A, Uchino E, Doi N, Ohba N. Spontaneous closure of traumatic macular hole. Am J Ophthalmol. 2002;133(2):230–5.
22. Aguilar JP, Green WR. Choroidal rupture. A histopathologic study of 47 cases. Retina. 1984;4(4):269–75.

23. Ament CS, Zacks DN, Lane AM, Krzystolik M, D'Amico DJ, Mukai S, et al. Predictors of visual outcome and choroidal neovascular membrane formation after traumatic choroidal rupture. Arch Ophthalmol. 2006;124(7):957–66.
24. Carrim ZI, Simmons IG. Traumatic choroidal rupture. Emerg Med J. 2009;26(12):880.
25. Dolan BJ. Traumatic retinal detachment. Optom Clin. 1993;3(2):67–80.
26. Hollander DA, Irvine AR, Poothullil AM, Bhisitkul RB. Distinguishing features of nontraumatic and traumatic retinal dialyses. Retina. 2004;24(5):669–75.
27. Youssri AI, Young LHY. Closed-globe contusion injuries of the posterior segment. Int Ophthalmol Clin. 2002;42(3):79–86.
28. Nacef L, Daghfous F, Chaabini M, Azaiez A, Ayed S. Ocular contusions and giant retinal tears. J Fr Ophtalmol. 1997;20(3):170–4.
29. De Terson A. l'hemorrhagie dans le corps vitre au cours de l'hemorrhagie cerebrale. Clin Ophthalmol. 1900;6:309–12.
30. Sakamoto M, Nakamura K, Shibata M, Yokoyama K, Matsuki M, Ikeda T. Magnetic resonance imaging findings of Terson's syndrome suggesting a possible vitreous hemorrhage mechanism. Jpn J Ophthalmol. 2010;54(2):135–9.
31. McCarron MO, Alberts MJ, McCarron P. A systematic review of Terson's syndrome: frequency and prognosis after subarachnoid haemorrhage. J Neurol Neurosurg Psychiatry. 2004;75(3):491–3.
32. Murjaneh S, Hale JE, Mishra S, Ling RH, Simcock PR. Terson's syndrome: surgical outcome in relation to entry site pathology. Br J Ophthalmol. 2006;90(4):512–3.
33. Martin DF, Awh CC, McCuen BW, Jaffe GJ, Slott JH, Machemer R. Treatment and pathogenesis of traumatic chorioretinal rupture (sclopetaria). Am J Ophthalmol. 1994;117(2):190–200.
34. Warner N, Eggenberger E. Traumatic optic neuropathy: a review of the current literature. Curr Opin Ophthalmol. 2010;21(6):459–62.
35. Steinsapir KD, Goldberg RA. Traumatic optic neuropathy: an evolving understanding. Am J Ophthalmol. 2011;151(6):928–33.
36. Levin LA, Beck RW, Joseph MP, Seiff S, Kraker R. The treatment of traumatic optic neuropathy: the International Optic Nerve Trauma Study. Ophthalmology. 1999;106(7):1268–77.
37. Yu-Wai-Man P, Griffiths PG. Steroids for traumatic optic neuropathy. Cochrane Database Syst Rev. 2013;6:CD006032.
38. Roberts I, Yates D, Sandercock P, Farrell B, Wasserberg J, Lomas G, et al. Effect of intravenous corticosteroids on death within 14 days in 10008 adults with clinically significant head injury (MRC CRASH trial): randomised placebo-controlled trial. Lancet Lond Engl. 2004;364(9442):1321–8.
39. Meek KM, Newton RH. Organization of collagen fibrils in the corneal stroma in relation to mechanical properties and surgical practice. J Refract Surg. 1999;15(6):695–9.
40. Dass AB, Ferrone PJ, Chu YR, Esposito M, Gray L. Sensitivity of spiral computed tomography scanning for detecting intraocular foreign bodies. Ophthalmology. 2001;108(12):2326–8.
41. Mittra RA, Mieler WF. Controversies in the management of open-globe injuries involving the posterior segment. Surv Ophthalmol. 1999;44(3):215–25.
42. Blanch RJ, Scott R, a. H. Military ocular injury: presentation, assessment and management. J R Army Med Corps. 2009;155(4):279–84.
43. Colyer MH, Chun DW, Bower KS, Dick JSB, Weichel ED. Perforating globe injuries during operation Iraqi Freedom. Ophthalmology. 2008;115(11):2087–93.
44. Topping TM, Abrams GW, Machemer R. Experimental double-perforating injury of the posterior segment in rabbit eyes: the natural history of intraocular proliferation. Arch Ophthalmol. 1979;97(4):735–42.
45. Mohamed AAEA. Vitrectomy in double-perforation gunshot injury. Clin Ophthalmol. 2013;7:2219–24.
46. Weichel ED, Bower KS, Colyer MH. Chorioretinectomy for perforating or severe intraocular foreign body injuries. Graefes Arch Clin Exp Ophthalmol Albrecht Von Graefes Arch Klin Exp Ophthalmol. 2010;248(3):319–30.
47. Coleman DJ. Early vitrectomy in the management of the severely traumatized eye. Am J Ophthalmol. 1982;93(5):543–51.
48. Yu H, Li J, Yu Y, Li G, Li D, Guan M, et al. Optimal timing of vitrectomy for severe mechanical ocular trauma: a retrospective observational study. Sci Rep. 2019;9:4543. Available from https://www.ncbi.nlm.nih.gov/pmc/articles/PMC6884543.
49. Han DP, Mieler WF, Abrams GW, Williams GA. Vitrectomy for traumatic retinal incarceration. Arch Ophthalmol. 1988;106(5):640–5.
50. Wei Y, Zhou R, Xu K, Wang J, Zu Z. Retinectomy vs vitrectomy combined with scleral buckling in repair of posterior segment open-globe injuries with retinal incarceration. Eye. 2016;30(5):726–30.
51. Ahmed Y, Schimel AM, Pathengay A, Colyer MH, Flynn HW. Endophthalmitis following open-globe injuries. Eye. 2012;26(2):212–7.
52. Andreoli CM, Andreoli MT, Kloek CE, Ahuero AE, Vavvas D, Durand ML. Low rate of endophthalmitis in a large series of open globe injuries. Am J Ophthalmol. 2009;147(4):601–8.
53. Bhagat N, Nagori S, Zarbin M. Post-traumatic infectious endophthalmitis. Surv Ophthalmol. 2011;56(3):214–51.
54. Gasch AT, Foster CS, Grosskreutz CL, Pasquale LR. Postoperative sympathetic ophthalmia. Int Ophthalmol Clin. 2000;40(1):69–84.
55. Arevalo JF, Garcia RA, Al-Dhibi HA, Sanchez JG, Suarez-Tata L. Update on sympathetic ophthalmia. Middle East Afr J Ophthalmol. 2012;19(1):13–21.

9 Intraocular Foreign Body: Approach to Management

S. Natarajan, Sneha Makhija, and Aishwarya B. Iyer

9.1 Introduction

Birmingham Eye Trauma Terminology System (BETTS) classification [1] (Fig. 9.1) refers to Intraocular Foreign bodies(IOFBs) as a "difficult to classify entity," considering the possibility of a sharp object, such as a glass particle, or a blunt object, such as a pellet, resulting in injury to the eye. They advise to either describe the injury as 'mixed' (i.e., a rupture due to IOFB) or select the most serious type of the mechanisms involved [1].

9.2 Epidemiology and IOFB Features

18–41% of all open globe injuries show the presence of intraocular foreign bodies [2–4]. Most IOFB patients are male, and most are between 21 and 40 years old [5]. The most common location of injury is the workplace [5]. The majority of IOFBs are small projectiles resulting from hammering on metal or stone, machine tool use, firing of weapons, explosions, motor vehicle accidents, and lawn mower accidents [6–8]. Up to 90% of

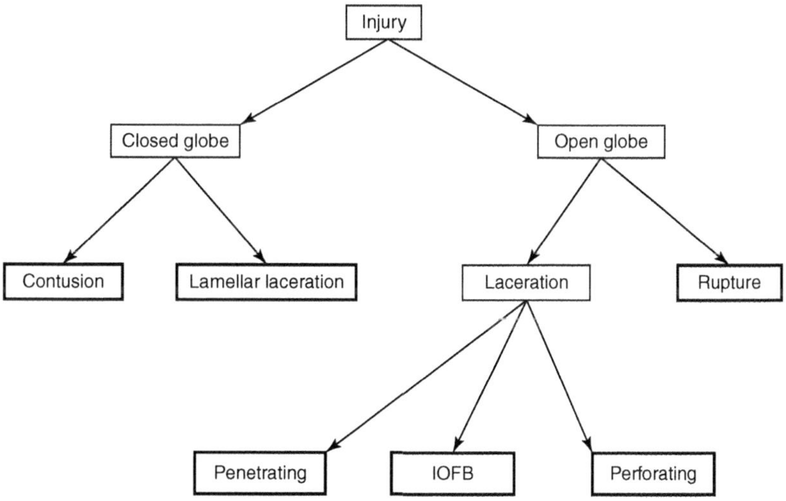

Fig. 9.1 BETTS classification

S. Natarajan (✉) · S. Makhija · A. B. Iyer
Aditya Jyot Eye Hospital (AJEH), Mumbai, India

S. Waikar (ed.), *Ocular Trauma in Armed Conflicts*, https://doi.org/10.1007/978-981-19-4021-7_9

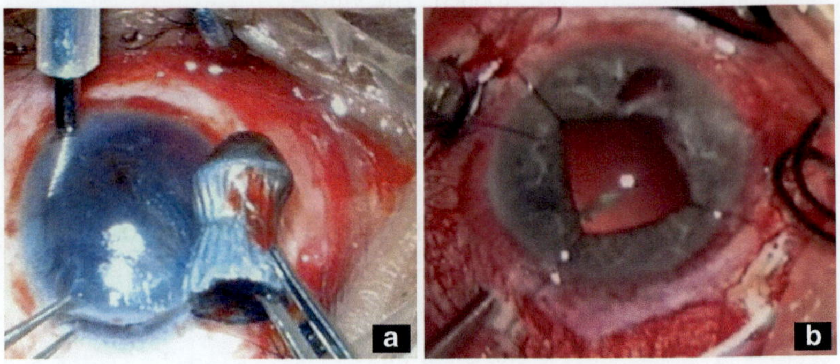

Fig. 9.2 (**a**) An unusually large metallic IOFB (firearm injury) is removed via a limbal incision. (**b**) A thorn seen within the pupil being removed via a scleral tunnel. (Courtesy: Aditya Jyot Eye Hospital, Mumbai)

IOFBs are metallic, followed by organic materials and nonmetallic inorganic materials [5, 7, 9] (Fig. 9.2).

9.3 Location of Foreign Body

An IOFB can be localized in the cornea, iris, ciliary body, crystalline lens, or posterior segment, or if an exit wound is present, an intraorbital foreign body may be present. There have even been reports of intracranial foreign bodies that have gained access through orbital route [10]. The Ocular Trauma Classification Group provided "zones of open globe injury" that help to prognosticate the injury: zone 1 (the whole cornea, including corneoscleral limbus), zone 2 (corneoscleral limbus to a point 5 mm posterior into the sclera), and zone 3 (posterior to the anterior 5 mm of the sclera) [11]. The location of the foreign body and the associated structural damage help to plan the surgical approach and to determine the prognosis.

9.4 Pathophysiology

Depending on the size, shape, and composition of the foreign body and the momentum at the time of impact [12], the foreign body can cause damage to the structures of the eye by the following mechanisms:

- Direct mechanical trauma: at the site of the entry wound, throughout the intraocular tract of the projectile, and at the site of impaction of a foreign body. Projectiles can also ricochet within the eye to cause further damage.
- Composition of foreign bodies: copper or iron foreign bodies resulting in chalcosis or siderosis bulbi, respectively. Inert substances (i.e., glass or plastic) are better tolerated.
- Infection and severe tissue reactions: organic IOFBs such as vegetative material or cilia pose a significant risk of endophthalmitis.
- Site of entry: The scleral site of entry is far more damaging than the corneal site.

As a golden rule, one can remember that a small, high-speed foreign body will cause significantly less damage than a large irregular IOFB causing blunt trauma.

9.5 Approach to a Patient with Intraocular Foreign Body

The diagnosis of an IOFB begins with a thorough history and a high degree of suspicion about its presence in a case of ocular injury.

9.5.1 History Taking

It is extremely necessary to inquire about the elements associated with the ocular injury. One must inquire about, but is not limited to, the following:

- The circumstances of trauma,
- Time has elapsed since the injury.

- Use of safety glasses if associated with industrial work,
- Type of activity at the time of injury-whether hammering, grinding, or drilling
- Any explosion or gunshots
- Use of spectacles at the time of injury; if yes, then whether spectacles were broken
- Any ongoing or past medical or surgical treatment taken for the injury
- Nature of foreign body if known to the patient (pellet injury, firecracker injury)
- unilateral or bilateral injury
- Systemic history must be considered in all cases.
- History of last meal must be asked in cases of children as the surgery will have to be done under general anesthesia
- A very important question not to be missed is the history of tetanus toxoid prophylaxis. IOFBs of any composition, inert or metallic, classify as injuries prone to tetanus [12].

History taking and proper documentation of the same are of prime value in these cases for medicolegal as well as workers compensation purposes in the case of a workplace injury.

Patients with an injury of this nature usually present with diminution of vision, pain, redness, watering, flashes, or floaters. Patients will oftentimes present with no symptoms or external signs, resulting in the diagnosis being missed initially. In some cases, a patient with no symptoms or external changes may show on exam a small entry wound that warrants further investigation. It is hence very important to thoroughly examine a patient presenting to our clinic with a history of a projectile to the eye with no symptoms or a mild foreign body sensation.

9.5.2 Examination

It is prudent to recognize and treat any other injuries, such as head injuries, that pose a risk to health or life before commencing the examination of the eye. A complete examination of the supposedly uninvolved eye must also be done.

It must be borne in mind while examining a patient with a possible open globe injury that procedures causing inadvertent pressure, such as eyelid retraction or intraocular pressure measurement, must be avoided.

In pediatric who are mentally challenged or uncooperative, examination under anesthesia is indicated.

The following must be done in all patients with a history of injury by a projectile object, irrespective of the presence or absence of ocular symptoms.

- Assessment of Visual Acuity: It must always be checked monocularly. A standard Snellen's visual acuity chart can be used at a distance of 6 m. If the vision is not adequate to read from an eye chart, the ability to count fingers, detect hand motions, or the presence of light perception versus no light perception should be noted. Visual acuity is usually decreased, it may be normal in some cases only to deteriorate later after the onset of inflammation or flare-up of infection.
- Pupillary examination: size, shape, presence of anisocoria, and reaction to light must be noted. In advanced cases, a relative afferent pupillary defect is often present.
- Torch-light examination: careful examination of the eyelids and anterior segment. Any lacerations, canalicular injuries or small foreign bodies must be inspected.
- Slit-lamp examination: a comprehensive examination to look for the entry site, whether scleral or corneal; a scleral entry site is seen with an area of conjunctival congestion or chemosis, and that of a corneal entry site is seen with surrounding corneal edema. To differentiate a lamellar corneal tear from a full thickness tear, a Siedel's test is done; however, this may be falsely negative in self-sealing wounds. A note here is that fluorescein staining or the use of topical medications such as anesthetic agents must never be resorted to in the case of an obvious or highly likely open globe injury (gross deformity of the eye, obvious volume loss, corneal/corneo-scleral tears, etc.).

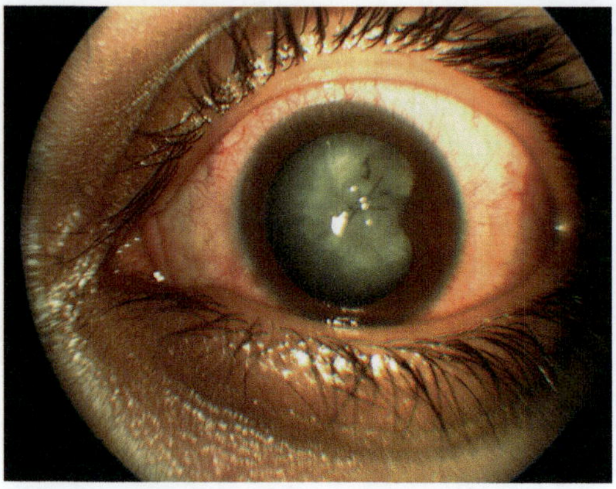

Fig. 9.3 A traumatic cataract is seen in a patient post corneal tear repair with sutures in situ. Posterior synechia is seen at 3 o clock position. (Courtesy: Aditya Jyot Eye Hospital, Mumbai)

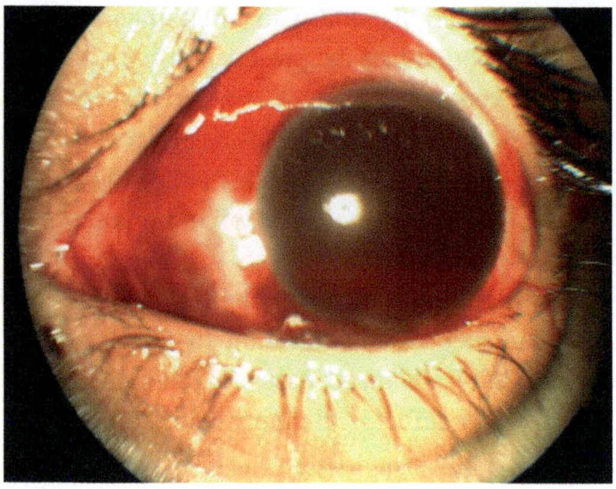

Fig. 9.4 Traumatic hyphema. (Courtesy: Aditya Jyot Eye Hospital, Mumbai)

The iris is best examined in its undilated state, and the crystalline lens is the best examined with the pupil dilated. An obvious traumatic cataract (Fig. 9.3) or a small focal lenticular opacity may be seen. A small foreign body can sometimes be lodged within the lens itself. Based on the entry site and injury to the ocular structures, a trajectory of the foreign body can be imagined to localize the site of foreign body impaction. Inflammatory reactions should be looked for in the anterior chamber.

Extrusion of vitreous and/or uveal tissue must be noted.

In some cases, diffuse corneal edema or hyphema (Fig. 9.4) may preclude one from

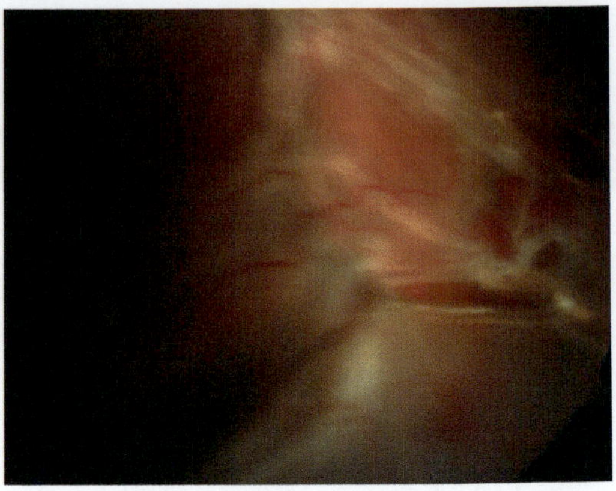

Fig. 9.5 Traumatic retinal detachment with multiple retinal tears. (Courtesy: Aditya Jyot Eye Hospital, Mumbai)

examining the anterior segment; one must solely rely on imaging to quantify the damage and localize the foreign body in these cases.

- Gonioscopy: To look for small foreign bodies in the intestine if suspected. However, it should be done carefully, and it is best deferred if deemed inappropriate with regards to the injury.
- Dilated Fundus Examination: A dilated fundus examination of both eyes is sine qua non in all cases of suspected intraocular foreign bodies with or without symptoms, unless uveal incarceration is present in the wound. Uveal incarceration is a relative contraindication to pupillary dilation, and a decision must be made in the best interest of the patient by the clinician after reviewing the eye condition. The presence of traumatic retinal detachment (Fig. 9.5), dialysis, retinal tears, choroidal detachment, or partial or complete vitreous haemorrhage may be noted. A careful peripheral examination to look for foreign bodies must be done without scleral depression if the foreign body is not visualized near the posterior pole. In late cases, an encapsulated foreign body may be visualized.

9.5.3 Investigations

Investigations in a case of IOFB play an important role in localizing a difficult-to-visualize foreign body to strategize the management, especially when the view is obscured due to hyphema, corneal edema, or vitreous haemorrhage. Several imaging modalities are available and must be chosen wisely based on an individualistic approach.

- X-ray

  In the pre-CT era, a standard X-ray was used to localize the foreign bodies. Water's view, Caldwell's view, and lateral views form the "foreign body X-ray series'. Plain X-ray is rarely used now for IOFBs, but it is an option in cases where CT is not available. Many IOFB materials are identifiable using X-rays, including metal, glass, slate, and polyvinyl chloride [13] (Fig. 9.6).

  "The Sweet localization technique" includes frontal and lateral projections. A foreign body within the globe can be localized to anterior or posterior segment with a bone-free examination by eye movement. The IOFB moves with the movement of the eye if located in the anterior segment and against the movement of the eye if located in the posterior segment [14].

  Contact lens-assisted or sutured metal locators may also be used. The various metal locators are Berman, Roper-Hall, and Bronson-Turner.

- Computed Tomography Scan

  Computed tomography has become the method of choice for demonstrating an IOFB. It is a reliable investigation to describe the size, shape, and localization of the foreign body and is the preferred imaging modality. Thin (1-mm) cuts with coronal, axial, and sagittal views are ideal to identify IOFBs and to assess the globe contour, site of posterior rupture, and any other cranial (e.g., subarachnoid haemorrhage) or ophthalmic traumatic sequelae (e.g., orbital fractures or retrobulbar hemorrhage) (Fig. 9.7). Although CT is able to detect most IOFBs well, wood IOFBs are usually hypodense and may be mistaken for air or fat [15]. The presence of linear-appearing air should raise suspicion for a wood IOFB.

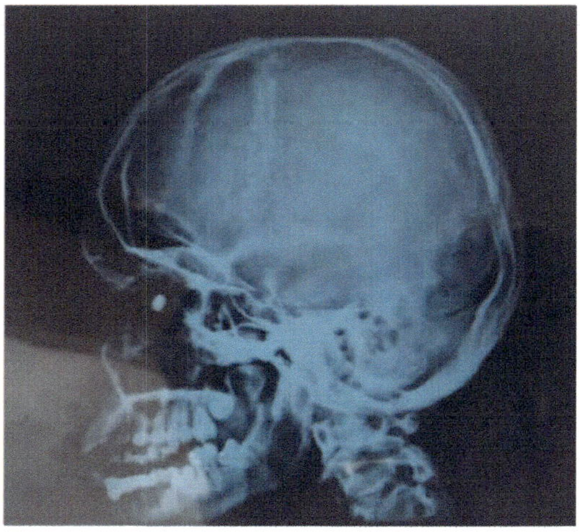

Fig. 9.6 X-ray showing an unusually large metallic intraocular foreign body (as seen in Fig. 9.2a). (Courtesy: Aditya Jyot Eye Hospital, Mumbai)

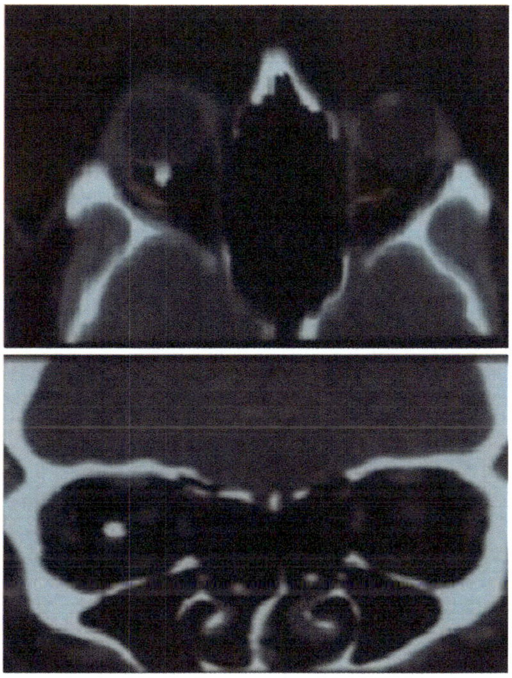

Fig. 9.7 CT scan showing IOFB in the right orbit. (Courtesy: Aditya Jyot Eye Hospital, Mumbai)

- The advantages of CT include high sensitivity, little need for patient cooperation, and the ability to localize accurately, even multiple or anteriorly located IOFBs. Furthermore, measuring the Hounsfield units of an IOFB identified on CT may provide some insight into its composition [13]. The disadvantages are that a foreign body less than 0.7 mm [16], one composed of wood [17], or lying next to the sclera may not be detected. It may also have difficulty differentiating motor vehicle glass from crystalline lenses as their radiodensities are similar [18]. Helical CTs are known to be more sensitive than axial CT scanners using 1–3 mm cuts [19]. It is also advisable to scan the paranasal sinuses and brain to rule out intracranial foreign bodies [10].

- Magnetic Resonance Imaging

  It is contraindicated in cases of metallic IOFB since dislodgement of the foreign body can occur and can cause further destruction [20]. MRI is the preferred modality to localize nonmetallic IOFB, such as wood or plastic [21]. It should only be used if CT has excluded metallic IOFB.
- Echography (Bscan)

  It is a valuable tool for IOFB detection. It can be used in the office by the ophthalmologist and can detect radiolucent as well as radiopaque IOFBs. In one series of 46 eyes, echography identified and localized all IOFBs, including a cilium [22]. It also has the advantage of being able to detect foreign bodies located next to the sclera, unlike a CT scan. It can also detect retinal and choroidal detachment, the presence of vitreous hemorrhage and an exit wound [22]. (Fig. 9.8)

  However, it should be performed cautiously and gently in cases of an open globe injury, and care must be taken to avoid prolapse of intra—orbital tissues.
- Ultrasound biomicroscopy

  It can be used to localize IOFB in the suspected angle, lens, or ciliary body. It some cases, It can also help to evaluate the status of the posterior capsule of the lens..

9.5.4 Medical Management

The treatment approach is based on the localization of the foreign body.

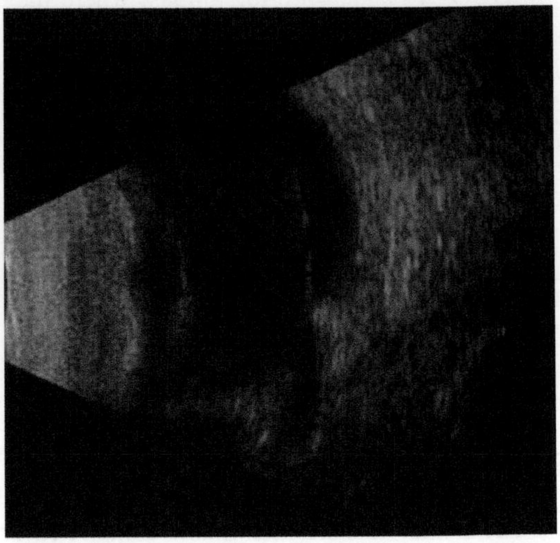

Fig. 9.8 Bscan of eye demonstrating a scleral tear at the equator and vitreous haemorrhage. (Courtesy: Aditya Jyot Eye Hospital, Mumbai)

Superficial foreign bodies should be removed, but it is best deferred if they are likely to cause further damage to the eye.

The following are the objectives of the initial treatment given to the patient:

- Prevent further damage. Avoid pressure on the eyeball and any procedures that would result in the same. A fox shield can be taped to the patient's eye to prevent further damage after the initial examination.
- Prevent infection: The lids and surrounding area are cleaned and cleared of any foreign bodies, especially in cases of explosives.
- Tetanus prophylaxis is given in all cases of IOFB.
- Antibiotics: Broad-spectrum intravenous or oral antibiotics are started especially to cover virulent organisms like Bacillus and Clostridium.
- Medical-legal case: Of utmost importance is to alert the local police about such injuries.
- Systemic workup for anesthesia should be initiated.
- Counseling: Once the presence of IOFB is confirmed, the management plan and the visual prognosis must be discussed with the patient and close family members. Patients

with better-presenting vision are more likely to have better visual outcomes than those with worse-presenting vision [23]. Anterior chamber IOFBs are associated with better visual outcomes than posterior segment IOFBs [24]. However, all patients must be informed about the unpredictable visual prognosis in cases of IOFB. The patient must be informed about the possible need for multiple surgeries and the complications of the surgery.

9.5.5 Surgical Management

Ideally, all IOFBs must be removed within 24 h of injury. However, certain foreign bodies like glass, graphite, stone, plastic, aluminum, or gold can be tolerated when left within the eye. A two-step procedure is adopted, where the primary repair should be done immediately, the second surgery must be done within a maximum of six days.

9.5.5.1 Indications for Removal of Foreign Bodies

1. Toxicity: Metallic objects consisting of copper or iron and their alloys are known to damage the tissue of the eye due to their toxic effects.
   (a) Siderosis bulbi: Ionized iron is known to cause rust-colored corneal stroma, iris heterochromia, orange deposits on the lens epithelium, and retinal degeneration [25]. The time since injury and degree of tissue destruction are determined by the iron content and location of the foreign body. Classic electroretinographic changes consist of an initial supernormal signal followed by a progressive decrease in the b-wave amplitude. The implicit time usually remains normal [26]. These changes may be progressive and irreversible despite IOFB removal [25].
   (b) Chalcosis: Toxicity with from foreign bodies containing copper depends on the concentration of copper. Foreign bodies with 100% copper cause rapid vision loss and severe, purulent endophthalmitis. Foreign bodies with more than 85% copper produce vision loss by depositing in Descemet's membrane, forming a Kayser-Fleischer ring, and greenish refractile deposits in the internal limiting membrane, anterior subcapsular sunflower cataracts, and greenish discoloration of the iris and vitreous. Vision loss is usually mild in these cases. IOFBs containing less than 85% copper typically produce no discernible copper deposition and no vision loss [27].
2. Contamination: vegetative foreign bodies are especially notorious for causing infection within the eye, leading to endophthalmitis. Post-traumatic endophthalmitis occurs in 8–13% of cases with a retained IOFB [3, 7]. In a retrospective study of 589 eyes with a retained IOFB, 7.5% were found to have endophthalmitis [24].

   In post-traumatic endophthalmitis, gram-positive organisms (including coagulase-negative staphylococci and streptococci species) are more common. Bacillus cereus, a gram-positive organism, presents with an aggressive and rather fulminant type of endophthalmitis that needs prompt treatment, or there is a risk of completely losing the eye [28–30].
3. For visual recovery in cases of traumatic retinal detachment.

9.5.5.2 Patient Consent

It is of utmost importance to be aware of the traumatic and difficult mental space the patient is in. One must take time to explain the condition and set realistic expectations in terms of the visual prognosis and long-term outcome if surgery is opted for. The consent-taking process must be well documented for legal purposes. One can also take a video consent of the patient and have a close relative be a witness during the process.

9.5.5.3 Surgical Procedure

The surgical treatment varies based on the *location* of the foreign body–in front of the iris plane or behind the iris plane. We will discuss the approach to each of these scenarios separately. Any hyphema, cataract, or vitreous hemorrhage that obscures the view of the retina should be removed [4].

1. Foreign bodies in front of iris plane
   (a) Anterior intraocular foreign body with no lens involvement:

   If the lens is not involved, it is best not to use any mydriatics or miotics to dilate or constrict the pupil, as that may result in further damage to the lens. A careful examination to look for the entry wound is done. A watertight suturing of the entry wound is done. Corneal wounds should be closed with 10-0 nylon sutures and sclera can be closed with 9-0 or 8-0 nylon sutures. The foreign body can be approached through a shelved limbal incision or a scleral tunnel, depending on the size of the foreign body or the surgeon's preference. The anterior segment is filled and maintained with the help of a viscoelastic substance. The entry wound should never be used to inject OVDs into the AC. A thorough AC wash is necessary to prevent a spike in intraocular pressure post-operatively. A rare-earth magnet can be used for metallic foreign bodies, whereas intraocular forceps are used for non-metallic ones. Samples of AC aspirate may also be sent for microbiological testing.

   (b) Anterior intraocular foreign body with lens involvement

   The integrity of the posterior capsule guides one towards the surgical procedure of choice. If the posterior capsule is intact, phacoemulsification with IOFB removal is performed. However, if the posterior capsule is compromised or there is marked instability or zonular dialysis, a pars plana approach to lensectomy and vitrectomy is preferred. Due to the increased risk of endophthalmitis with primary IOL placement, the authors recommend leaving the patient aphakic initially [31]. Additionally, lens calculations may be inaccurate due to the difficulty in measuring axial length and keratometry measurements at the time of an open globe injury.

2. Foreign bodies behind the iris plane

Treatment of the posterior segment IOFB varies based on the visibility of the foreign body (Fig. 9.9).

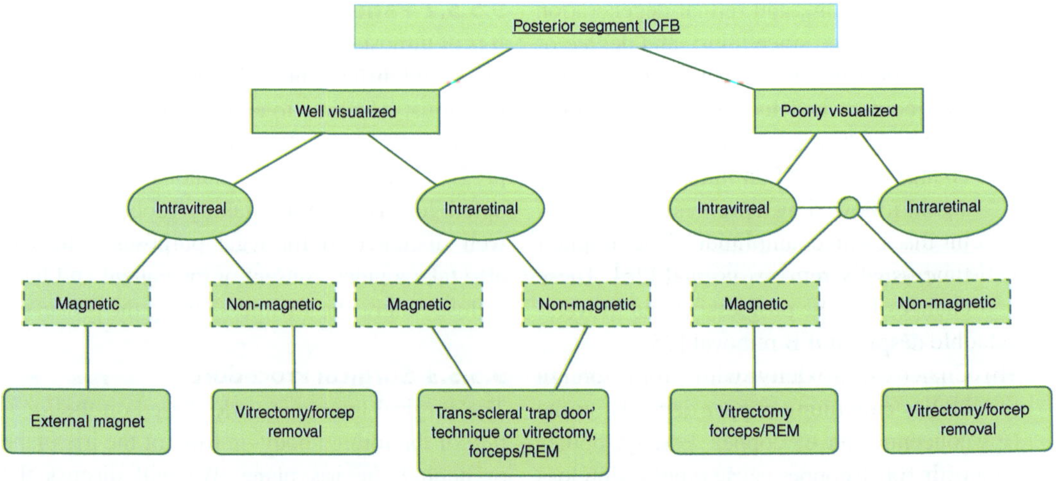

Fig. 9.9 Approach to a patient with posterior segment IOFB based on visualization of a foreign body (REM = Rare Earth Magent). (Reproduced in flowchart form from Textbook of Surgical Oncology, Ryan Stephen [32])

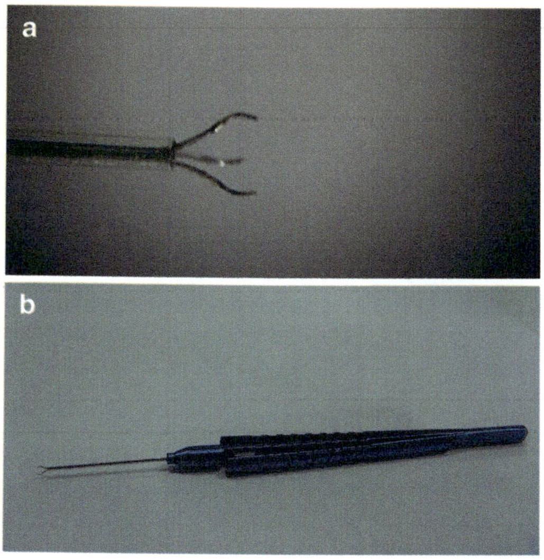

Fig. 9.10 The claw—a unique IOFB forceps. (**a**) The claw forceps showing the widest extent of the prongs and (**b**) shaft with open prongs

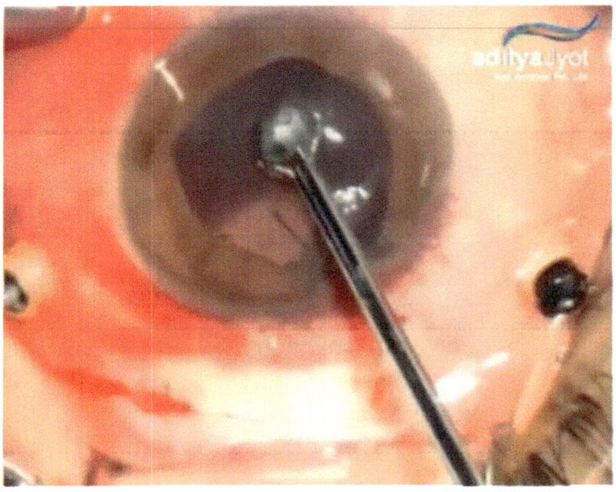

Fig. 9.11 A pellet foreign body is removed using the claw. (Courtesy: SMHS Hospital, Kashmir)

- External approach: best for a small magnetic foreign body in the region of the pars plana. The conjunctiva is carefully incised, the rectus muscles are tagged if necessary, and a partial thickness scleral flap or a sclerotomy is performed. Diathermy to the choroid is applied. A pre-placed mattress suture is placed, and the IOFB is removed using an external electromagnet. The site is closed, and indirect ophthalmoscopy is performed to look for and laser-barrage any retinal tears. The complications of the external approach are hemorrhage and extrusion of intraocular tissue with, possible retinal incarceration. AC paracentesis and external pressure on the globe at the time of IOFB removal to reduce the intraocular pressure reduce the chances of this complication.
- Internal approach: An internal approach is used in cases with opaque media and nonmagnetic, large, or subretinal IOFB that must be approached through an internal approach. A standard 3-port pars plana vitrectomy, followed by removal of IOFB by IOFB forceps [33] (Figs. 9.10 and 9.11) or an IOFB magnet (Fig. 9.12) is done. The ILM is peeled and, the area of impaction is laser barraged. A retinectomy can be done to relieve any traction (Fig. 9.13). PFCL is used to float the foreign

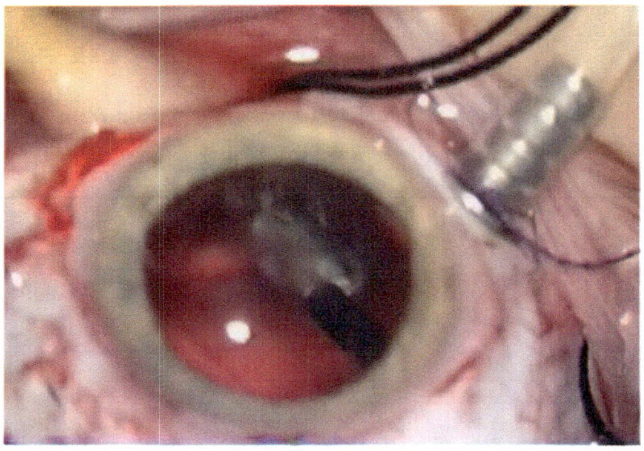

Fig. 9.12 Use of an intraocular foreign body magnet to remove metallic foreign body. (Courtesy: Aditya Jyot Eye Hospital, Mumbai)

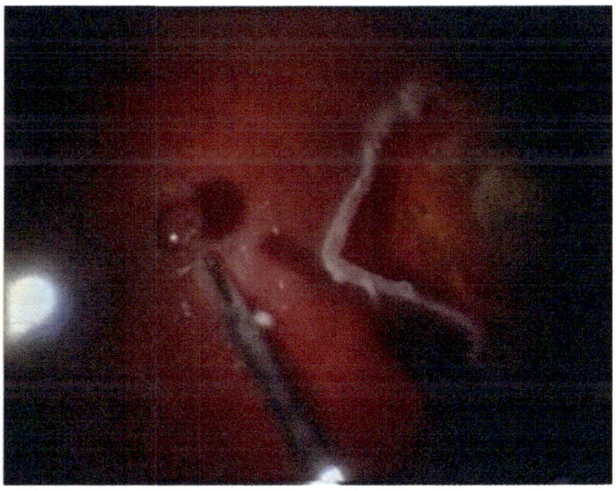

Fig. 9.13 Retinectomy done between area of impaction and healthy retina. (Courtesy: Aditya Jyot Eye Hospital, Mumbai)

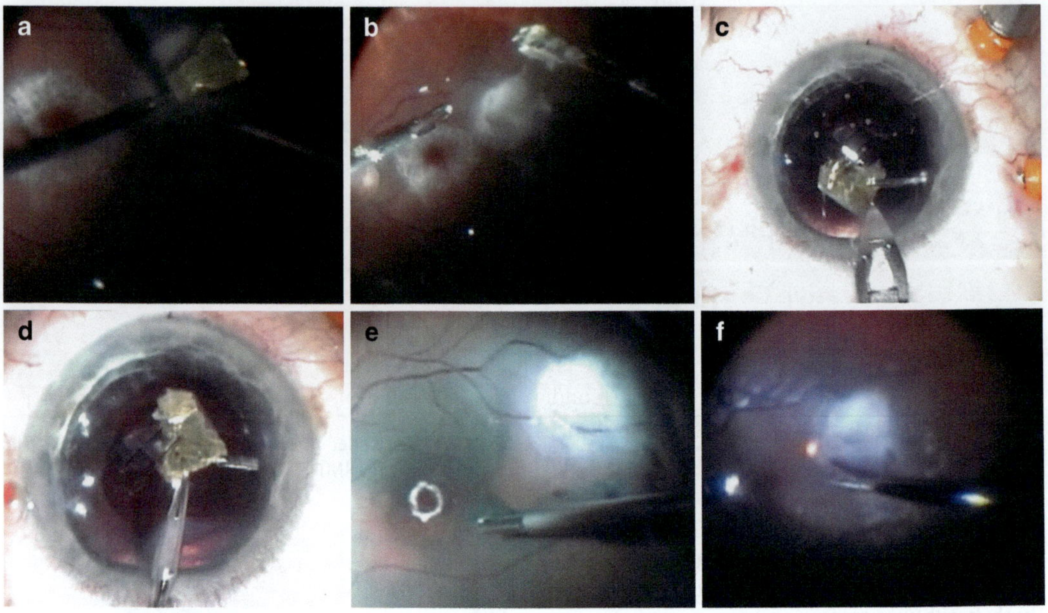

Fig. 9.14 Some surgical steps for the internal approach of posterior segment IOFB removal. (**a**) Identification of impacted glass foreign body, (**b**) grasping of the IOFB with intraocular foreign body forceps, (**c**) shelved limbal incision being fashioned for removal of foreign body, (**d**) removal of foreign body using handshake technique, (**e**) ILM peeling being done, (**f**) endo-laser barrage of the site of impaction. (Courtesy: Aditya Jyot Eye Hospital, Mumbai)

Fig. 9.15 Advantages of PPV

Advantages of PPV

- Increases retinal oxygenation
- Reduces load of inflammatory debris hence decreases its harmful effects on retina
- Allows direct visualization of retina for assessing status, aiding further management
- Reduces severity of retinal complications

body and protect the macula. Figure 9.14 summarizes the steps of IOFB removal, and Fig. 9.15 lists the advantages of PPV.

9.5.5.4 A Word for Eyes with No Perception of Light

Boucenna et al. [34] in their study of 15 patients who presented with ocular injury and no perception of light, that six patients experienced an improvement in their visual acuity. They believe functional recovery of vision is possible if there is no irreversible anatomical damage. Soni et al. [35] in their study of 73 patients reported an improvement in visual acuity from no perception of light to hand movements or better in 17 patients.

The authors thus believe that irrespective of the presenting vision, every eye should be given a chance to see again. One must do everything possible to achieve anatomic success in all cases.

Do's	*Don'ts*
- Take a detailed history *- Always speak to the patient alone to get the whole story* *- Clean wounds thoroughly* *- Intimate the local police if not done* *- Give tetanus prophylaxis*	*- Use any stain or topical anesthetics in open globe injuries* *- Put external pressure or perform procedures that do so* *- Don't start surgery before accurate localization of foreign body*

Fig. 9.16 Approach to management of a patient with an intraocular foreign body

9.5.5.5 Do's and Don't's for Intraocular Foreign Bodies (Fig. 9.16)

Prevention

Most of the ocular injuries causing intraocular foreign bodies are preventable. Protective glasses must be used for industrial work, the use of helmets while driving two-wheelers, and the use of polycarbonate lenses for spectacles can be fruitful in cases of accidents. A patient with one useful eye must at all costs protect it by using of protective goggles.

9.6 Summary

In conclusion, IOFB is an ophthalmic emergency. It must be catered to with the utmost urgency. Hence, the author, Prof. Dr. S. Natarajan, has labeled any ocular trauma as 'Code Orange' or 'Code O.' Once generated in the EMR at the reception or optometry room of the hospital, it alerts the staff and doctors alike to deal with these patients on a priority basis with vigilance. All eyes must be treated with equal care and conviction. Every eye has a right to light.

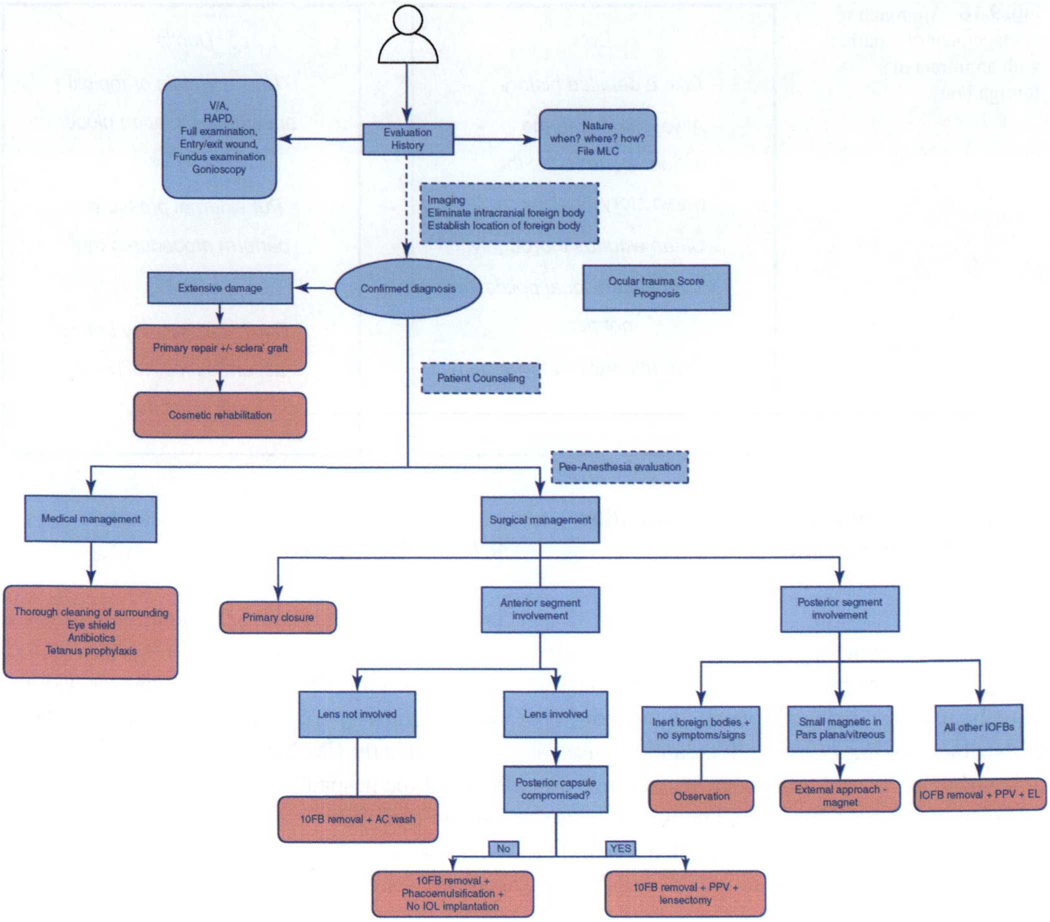

Fig. 9.17 Intraocular foreign body: approach to management

To summarize, refer to the flowchart given in Fig. 9.17 on 'Intraocular Foreign Body: Approach to Management."

Acknowledgement We would like to thank the Head of the Department of Ophthalmology, at the SMHS Hospital in Srinagar, Jammu and Kashmir, and the Chief Secretary and Chief Minister of the Government of Jammu and Kashmir for their support.

References

1. International Society of Ocular Trauma. 2020. BETTS. Available https://isotonline.org/betts/. Accessed 1 November 2020.
2. De Juan E, Sternberg P, Michels RG. Penetrating ocular injuries. Types of injuries and visual results. Ophthalmology. 1983;90:1318.
3. Thompson WS, Rubsamen PE, Flynn HW Jr, et al. Endophthalmitis after penetrating trauma. Risk factors and visual acuity outcomes. Ophthalmology. 1995;102:1696.
4. American Academy of Ophthalmology. Management of intraocular foreign bodies. 2020. Available https://www.aao.org/eyenet/article/management-of-intraocular-foreign-bodies. Accessed 1 November 2020.
5. Loporchio D, Mukkamala L, Gorukanti K, Zarbin M, Langer P, Bhagat N. Intraocular foreign bodies: a review. Surv Ophthalmol. 2016;61:582–96.
6. Blomdahl S, Norell S. Perforating eye injury in the Stockholm population. An epidemiological study. Acta Ophthalmol. 1984;62:378.
7. Williams DF, Mieler WF, Abrams GW, Lewis H. Results and prognostic factors in penetrating ocular injuries with retained intraocular foreign bodies. Ophthalmology. 1988;95:911.
8. Khani SC, Mukai S. Posterior segment intraocular foreign bodies. Int Ophthalmol Clin. 1995;35:151.

9. Fulcher TP, McNab AA, Sullivan TJ. Clinical features and management of intraorbital foreign bodies. Ophthalmology. 2002;109:494–500.
10. Chowdhary S, Garg P, Sawhney V, Pandya A, Sambhav K, Gupta S. Unusual missed diagnosis of foreign body: a case report. Int Med Case Rep J. 2020;13:187–90. https://doi.org/10.2147/IMCRJ.S246924.
11. Pieramici DJ, Sternberg P, Aaberg TM, et al. A system for classifying mechanical injuries of the eye (globe). Am J Ophthalmol. 1997;123(6):820–31. https://doi.org/10.1016/s0002-9394(14)71132-8.
12. Albert D, Miller J, Azar D, Young L. Albert and Jakobiec's principles and practice of ophthalmology. 3rd ed. Berlin: Springer; 2008. p. 5089–144.
13. Modjtahedi BS, Rong A, Bobinski M, McGahan J, Morse LS. Imaging characteristics of intraocular foreign bodies: a comparative study of plain film X-ray, computed tomography, ultrasound, and magnetic resonance imaging. Retina. 2015;35:95–104.
14. Ahlbom H. A new method of localizing foreign bodies in the eye. Teleradiography with visualization of the cornea. Acta Radiol. 1931;12(3):212–35. https://doi.org/10.3109/00016923109132245.
15. Pinto A, Brunese L, Daniele S, et al. Role of computed tomography in the assessment of intraorbital foreign bodies. Semin Ultrasound. 2012;33:392–5.
16. Zinreich SJ, Miller NR, Aguayo JB, et al. Computed tomographic three dimensional localization and compositional evaluation of intraocular and orbital foreign bodies. Arch Ophthalmol. 1986;104:515–9.
17. Specht CS, Varga JH, Jalali MM, Edelstein JP. Orbitocranial wooden foreign body diagnosed by magnetic resonance imaging. Dry wood can be isodense with air and orbital fat by computed tomography. Surv Ophthalmol. 1992;36:341–4.
18. Hagedorn CL, Tauber S, Adelman RA. Bilateral intraocular foreign bodies simulating crystalline lens. Am J Ophthalmol. 2004;138:146–7.
19. Dass AB, Ferrone PJ, Chu YR, et al. Sensitivity of spiral computed tomography scanning for detecting intraocular foreign bodies. Ophthalmology. 2001;108:2326–8.
20. LoBue TD, Deutsch TA, Lobick J, Turner DA. Detection and localization of nonmetallic intraocular foreign bodies by magnetic resonance imaging. Arch Ophthalmol. 1988;106(260–261):19.
21. Kelly WM, Paglen PG, Pearson JA, et al. Ferromagnetism of intraocular foreign body causes unilateral blindness after MR study. AJNR. 1986;7:243–5.
22. Rubsamen PE, Cousins SW, Windward KE, Byrne SF. Diagnostic ultrasound and pars plana vitrectomy in penetrating ocular trauma. Ophthalmology. 1994;101:809–14.
23. Ehlers JP, Kunimoto DY, Ittoop S, Maguire JI, Ho AC, Regillo CD. Metallic intraocular foreign bodies: characteristics, interventions, and prognostic factors for visual outcome and globe survival. Am J Ophthalmol. 2008;146:427–33.
24. Chaudhry IA, Shamsi FA, Al-Harthi E, Al-Theeb A, Elzaridi E, Riley FC. Incidence and visual outcome of endophthalmitis associated with intraocular foreign bodies. Graefes Arch Clin Exp Ophthalmol. 2008;246:181–6.
25. Hope-Ross M, Mahon GJ, Johnston PB. Ocular siderosis. Eye. 1993;7:419–25.
26. Good P, Gross K. Electrophysiology and metallosis: support for an oxidative (free radical) mechanism in the human eye. Ophthalmologica. 1988;196:204–9.
27. Rosenthal AR, Marmor MF, Leuenberger P, Hopkins JL. Chalcosis: a study of natural history. Ophthalmology. 1979;86:1956–72.
28. Thompson JT, Parver LM, Enger CL, et al. Infectious endophthalmitis after penetrating injuries with retained intraocular foreign bodies. Ophthalmology. 1993;100:1468–74.
29. Mieler WF, Ellis MK, William DF, Han DP. Retained intraocular foreign bodies and endophthalmitis. Ophthalmology. 1990;97:1532–8.
30. Alfaro DV, Roth D, Liggett PEP. Posttraumatic endophthalmitis: causative organisms, treatment, and prevention. Retina. 1994;14:206–11.
31. Andreoli CM, Andreoli MT, Kloek CE, Ahuero AE, Vavvas D, Durand ML. Low rate of endophthalmitis in a large series of open globe injuries. Am J Ophthalmol. 2009;147:601–8.
32. Stephen R. Textbook of surgical ophthalmology, vol. 3. 3rd ed. New York: Springer; 2017. p. 2358–77.
33. Bapaye M, Shanmugam MP, Sundaram N. The claw: a novel intraocular foreign body removal forceps. Indian J Ophthalmol. 2018;66(12):1845–8. https://doi.org/10.4103/ijo.IJO_759_18.
34. Boucenna W, Taright N, Delbarre M, et al. Functional results and prognostic factors in open-globe ocular trauma with presenting visual acuity of no-light perception. J Fr Ophtalmol. 2020;43(6):517–24. https://doi.org/10.1016/j.jfo.2019.11.006.
35. Soni NG, Bauza AM, Son JH, Langer PD, Zarbin MA, Bhagat N. Open globe ocular trauma: functional outcome of eyes with no light perception at initial presentation. Retina. 2013;33(2):380–6. https://doi.org/10.1097/IAE.0b013e318263cefb.

Traumatic Uveitis and Sympathetic Ophthalmia

10

Sudha K. Ganesh, Saurabh Mistry, and Deepali Velani

In modern warfare, ocular injuries are quite common. These injuries can carry high morbidity, which can in turn determine an injured person's future independence and employability. It has been observed that soldiers who sustain eye injuries during warfare often become unfit for further continuation of military service and also for many civilian occupations.

It is quite surprising to see that the ocular surface area comprises only 0.27% of the total body surface, 0.54% of the anterior body surface, and 4% of the face. Still, the preferential exposure of the face in modern warfare and the exceptional vulnerability of the eye to small particles result in a higher incidence of eye injuries of almost 20–50 times more [1]. Improvised explosive devices (IEDs) have now become the sine qua non of modern warfare. These devices are highly explosive and fragmentary with a large blast radius, thus leading to increased ocular injuries [2].

Birmingham Eye Trauma Terminology (BETT) categorised mechanical trauma to the eyes into open and closed globe injuries [3, 4]. The focus of this chapter is primarily on trauma affecting the uveal tract, the middle layer of the eye. Uvea is a vascular structure made up of the iris, the ciliary body, and the choroid. Inflammation of the uveal tract is termed uveitis, and ocular inflammation following trauma is termed traumatic uveitis.

10.1 Traumatic Uveitis

Traumatic uveitis is typically unilateral; however ocular warfare injuries are bilateral in 15–25% of cases [1]. Military ophthalmologists have also reported that eye injuries following blasts are often bilateral with multiple foreign bodies [5]. However, epidemiological information regarding this remains limited.

Traumatic uveitis may be iritis, limited to the iris, and/or iridocyclitis when the ciliary body is also involved [6]. Studies on blunt traumatic injury to the eye reveal that the incidence of uveitis is as high as 10%, however, in the context of penetrating eye injury, the incidence of uveitis is not well defined in the literature [7]. It is important to note that in any penetrating eye injury, there is a definite increase in ocular inflammation, and infection with or without the presence of intraocular foreign bodies [8, 9].

10.1.1 Pathogenesis

Ocular trauma that leads to uveitis is a result of the disruption of the microvasculature within the

S. K. Ganesh (✉) · S. Mistry
Department of Uveitis, Medical Research Foundation, Sankara Nethralaya, Chennai, India
e-mail: drskg@snmail.org

D. Velani
Dr Agarwal's Eye Hospital, Chennai, India

S. Waikar (ed.), *Ocular Trauma in Armed Conflicts*, https://doi.org/10.1007/978-981-19-4021-7_10

uveal tissue. This results in the infiltration of leukocytes and other pro-inflammatory mediators into the uveal tissue and anterior chamber [6, 10]. It is believed that autoimmune diseases and other inflammatory disorders predispose to an increased risk of ocular inflammation following ocular trauma [11, 12].

10.1.2 Signs and Symptoms

Signs and symptoms of traumatic iritis usually occur within 24 hours of injury. Ocular pain, photophobia, tearing, perilimbal conjunctival hyperemia, and decreased vision are the common presenting symptoms [13].

Ocular pain is often caused by ciliary muscle spasms, which is a characteristically dull aching, or throbbing type of pain. Ocular pain can also be caused by raised intraocular pressure, which is much more severe in intensity as compared to the pain caused by ciliary muscle spasms.

Miosis and photophobia are the hallmark findings of traumatic iritis. Irritation of the iris and its attachment to the anterior ciliary body causes spasms of accommodation leading to sustained miosis. However, a larger mydriatic pupil can be seen with an iris sphincter muscle tear, called traumatic mydriasis.

Photophobia can be due to ciliary muscle spasms, anterior chamber cellular infiltration, and/or corneal epithelial edema. Consensual photophobia occurs when a light shone into the unaffected eye causes pain in the affected eye. The stimulus to the opposite eye causes both pupils to constrict (consensual response) and inflammation in the affected eye causes pain.

Perilimbal conjunctival hyperemia, called circumciliary congestion, is a red or purplish ring that surrounds the cornea and increases in intensity as it approaches the limbus. This is in contrast to the perilimbal sparing often seen in conjunctivitis.

The breakdown of the blood aqueous barrier following trauma leads to the entry of white blood cells and proteins in the anterior chamber, which can be rendered visible by slit lamp biomicroscopy examination as a result of the Tyndall effect of the bright beam. The grading of anterior chamber cells and flare helps in the assessment of the severity of anterior uveitis. Grading is also useful in determining the patient's response to therapy as well as long-term monitoring. In some cases, following eye trauma, the anterior chamber reaction can be surprisingly minimal. On the contrary, persistent or recurrent inflammation of the uveal tract can result in the formation of synechiae. Synechiae are adhesions that attach the iris to the lens capsule or the peripheral cornea.

Intraocular pressure (IOP) measurements may show a decrease or an increase. It is often found to be low when decreased aqueous production results from ciliary body shock, damage to the trabecular meshwork however clogging of the trabecular meshwork by inflammatory debris can result in elevated IOP.

Traumatic anterior uveitis may be associated with "commotio retinae," which represents damage to the outer retinal layers as a result of shock waves that traverse the eye from the site of impact following blunt trauma. On indirect ophthalmoscopic examination, a sheen like retinal whitening may appear a few hours after injury. It is commonly seen in the posterior pole (Berlin's edema) but may occur peripherally as well. Mechanisms proposed are extracellular edema, glial swelling, and photoreceptor outer segment disruption. A cherry-red spot may appear when fovea is involved, as the cells involved in the whitening are not present in the fovea. With foveal involvement, there is a decrease in visual acuity to as low as 20/200. However, visual recovery is good, with the condition improving in 3–4 weeks.

10.1.3 Ancillary Testing

Ancillary testing is not required unless the view of the fundus is limited by cataract or vitreous hemorrhage or when there is a concern about a ruptured globe, intraocular foreign body, or orbital fracture. In these cases, B scan ultrasonography or CT scan may be indicated to determine the extent or cause of ocular damage.

Optical coherence tomography may be useful for the assessment of disc, macular status, Berlin edema, and cystoid macular edema. Ultrasound biomicroscopy would be useful in cases with non-dilating pupils and ocular hypotony to assess the status of, the ciliary body, zonules supraciliary effusions, choroidal detachments, and the crystalline lens.

10.1.4 Differential Diagnosis

Infectious and non-infectious causes of anterior uveitis, traumatic corneal abrasion, traumatic hyphema, and traumatic retinal detachment all have a similar presentation to traumatic iritis [14]. A careful history and clinical examination will help differentiate these entities.

Traumatic hyphema presents with red blood cells in the anterior chamber and blurred vision, whereas iritis presents with photophobia and white blood cells in the anterior chamber. Hyphema presents earlier than traumatic iritis and may indicate injury to the iris, sphincter muscle, or ciliary body.

A patient with retinal detachment presents mainly with complaints of flashes of light and a decreased field of vision, and the condition is usually not painful. On slit lamp examination, the patient may present with an anterior chamber reaction and pigments in the anterior vitreous face.

10.1.5 Treatment

Traumatic anterior uveitis can generally be managed by medical therapy and requires surgical intervention only if structural complications such as secondary glaucoma or secondary cataract occur.

Traumatic iritis is a self-limiting entity and usually resolves within 7–14 days [13]. In most cases, practitioners choose to observe mild cases of traumatic iritis with close follow-ups. The treatment for moderate to severe cases includes cycloplegic agents (homatropine or cyclopentolate) and topical corticosteroids (prednisolone acetate) to avoid complications associated with prolonged inflammation.

The main aims of medical management are as follows:

- To provide relief from pain and photophobia
- Decrease inflammation
- To prevent structural complications such as secondary cataracts, synechiae, and glaucoma
- To preserve or restore good visual function.

10.1.6 Cycloplegics

Its main role is to paralyze the ciliary muscle and immobilize the iris. This allows it to rest and thus helps to reduce inflammation and pain by preventing adhesion of the iris to the anterior lens capsule and eliminating the frequent movement of the ciliary muscle as the pupil adapts to changing light conditions.

10.1.7 Corticosteroids

Corticosteroids are the drug of choice in the treatment of moderate to severe traumatic anterior uveitis. These act by inhibiting both the cycloxygenase pathways, thus modifying and decreasing the inflammatory response. Topical corticosteroids if administered in frequent doses, can achieve adequate therapeutic levels in the anterior chamber. However, one should be aware of potential side effects and long-term iatrogenic complications secondary to the use of steroid therapy.

Available topical corticosteroids are as follows:

- Prednisolone acetate 0.125% and 1%
- Betamethasone 1%
- Dexamethasone sodium phosphate 0.1%
- Fluorometholone 0.1% and 0.25%
- Loteprednol
- Rimexolone 1%

The choice of topical steroids should be based on the severity of uveitis; in cases of severe anterior chamber reactions, topical steroids with strong potencies such as prednisolone acetate should be preferred, whereas in cases of mild anterior uveitis, weak topical steroids such as betamethasone or dexamethasone can be used.

It is important to look for a steroid-induced rise in IOP when topical steroids are used for more than 2 weeks. In such cases, one should try to avoid steroids and can use alternatives such as topical non-steroidal anti-inflammatory drugs (NSAIDs) like flurbiprofen, weak steroids, or steroids with the least propensity to raise IOP, such as Rimexolone1%. Initially, topical beta-blockers (e.g. timolol maleate 0.5% bid) may be added to decrease IOP if secondary glaucoma is present.

In the presence of a corneal epithelial defect, topical steroids should be avoided. Steroids can delay healing, promote infection, and worsen already-existing corneal epithelial defects. Corneal infections should therefore be ruled out prior to starting steroid therapy.

The use of systemic corticosteroids is indicated when anterior uveitis does not respond to topical steroids and/or when the inflammation is bilateral or recurrent. The decision to use systemic corticosteroids must include consideration of the risks and benefits.

10.1.8 Follow-up

Ideally, the first recommended follow-up visit should occur 5–7 days after the initial traumatic event [14]. During this period, iritis resolves, cycloplegics can be discontinued, and steroids are to be tapered gradually over a period of a few weeks. The risk of rebound iritis is high if the steroid is not tapered. Follow-up should be done at the end of a 1 month [14]. It is important to perform a gonioscopy to rule out angle recession at this visit. Indirect ophthalmoscopy should also be performed using scleral depression to rule out peripheral retinal breaks, retinal dialysis, and retinal detachments.

10.1.9 Complications

Complications include traumatic cataracts, posterior synechiae, secondary glaucoma, band-shaped keratopathy, and cystoid macular edema. While these complications may be the result of prolonged inflammation, it is also important to note that cataracts and increased IOP can also be a result of the long-term use of topical corticosteroids. Secondary glaucoma in particular when unnoticed can lead to optic neuropathy and permanent vision loss. Hence, the judicious use of topical corticosteroids is advocated.

To conclude, traumatic uveitis, if detected early and treated on time, can be managed without any long-term sequelae or complications.

10.2 Phacoanaphylaxis/ Phacoantigenic Uveitis

Phacoanaphylaxis/Phacoantigenic or lens-induced uveitis (LIU) is an intraocular inflammation induced by lens protein, usually after a traumatic rupture of the lens capsule that exposes the antigenic lens proteins.

A penetrating injury to the globe may result in severe lens-induced uveitis. The incidence of LIU following penetrating injury is, however, unknown. On the contrary, the uveitis may remain undiagnosed clinically because of hyphema, decreased corneal clarity, and inflammation related to the trauma.

10.2.1 Pathogenesis

Lens proteins are the most immunologically privileged and may initiate an immunologic sensitization only after entering the aqueous humor. The term phacoanaphylaxis is a misnomer because no evidence exists in the literature of a classic type I immunoglobulin E (IgE)-mediated anaphylactic reaction. It is believed to be the result of autosensitization to lens proteins with type II, III, and IV hypersensitivity reactions that play a major role [15]. This immunologic reaction occurs only after a latent period during which sensitization takes place.

10.2.2 Signs and Symptoms

Patients with traumatic lens-induced uveitis present within 1–14 days, with a time range varying from hours to months. Typically, the inflammation is unilateral and involves only the traumatized eye.

In a less severe form of LIU, previously termed phacoantigenic uveitis, the patient may experience mild to moderate photophobia and a diminution of vision [16]. Slit lamp biomicroscopy reveals non-granulomatous uveitis with mild cells and flare. Rarely, vitreous cells may be found. The presence of a disrupted lens capsule or opacified lens material can be seen. If inflammation persists, posterior synechiae may form.

A severe form of LIU, termed phacoanaphylactic endophthalmitis, presents with a panophthalmitis-like picture and significant vision loss [16]. Slit lamp biomicroscopy reveals granulomatous uveitis manifesting as "mutton fat" keratic precipitates, iris nodules, a severe anterior chamber reaction with hypopyon, posterior synechiae, and vitreous cells.

Although the optic nerve, choroid, and retina are unaffected in LIU, retinal vasculitis affecting both the arteriole and venules has been reported, particularly in the area immediately surrounding a fragment of retained lens lying on the retina [17].

10.2.3 Ancillary Testing

Aqueous paracentesis in subtle or early cases may reveal inflammatory cells and particulate lens proteins without bacteria, although its utility is not well established [18].

Aqueous or vitreous biopsy in phacoanaphylactic reactions reveals a zonal type of granulomatous inflammation with lens remnants surrounded by a zone of neutrophils, which in turn is surrounded by a zone of macrophages, epithelioid cells, and giant cells; the outermost layer is composed of lymphocytes and plasma cells [19].

When posterior segment evaluation is not possible due to media opacities or in cases that simulate endophthalmitis, a B-scan ultrasonography reveals a posteriorly dislocated lens fragment. Also, it is important to diagnose posterior capsule rupture of the lens by imaging tests like ultrasonography, UBM, and AS-OCT. Such ruptures are characterized by the irregular extension of the highly reflective posterior capsule toward the vitreous with significantly increased thickness of the lens.

10.2.4 Differential Diagnosis

Differential diagnosis for mild to moderate cases of LIU includes uveitis associated with HLA-B27 disease and autoimmune conditions. Interestingly, Propionibacterium acnes infection is more likely to mimic mild to moderate cases of LIU. In such cases, slit lamp examination of the lens implant and or remnant capsule may reveal the presence of a whitish plaque [20]. An aqueous biopsy study helps in confirming the diagnosis.

Phacoanaphylactic endophthalmitis, representing the severe form of LIU, may mimic posttraumatic endophthalmitis or sympathetic ophthalmia. The incidence of posttraumatic endophthalmitis is higher when associated with intraocular foreign bodies. It can progress rapidly. Clinical signs include marked inflammation with fibrin, hypopyon, and retinal phlebitis. Additionally, the patient with infectious endophthalmitis will experience more pain than with severe LIU. Aqueous or vitreous biopsy is often diagnostic.

While LIU is usually unilateral, sympathetic ophthalmia is a rare condition and is typically bilateral. One differentiating feature is the presence of diffuse choroidal thickening observed in sympathetic ophthalmia on B-scan ultrasonography, which is quite minimal, even in severe forms of phacoanaphylactic endophthalmitis [21].

10.2.5 Treatment

Medical therapy includes topical/systemic corticosteroids and cycloplegics. Management should be tailored to the individual patient and adjusted according to the response. However, the only definitive treatment is the surgical removal of any inciting intraocular lens material.

10.2.6 Complications

If diagnosed and treated early, LIU has favourable outcomes. However, if left untreated, it can lead to sequelae like chronic cystoid macular edema, tractional retinal detachment, cyclitic membrane formation, and phthisis bulbi.

10.3 Sympathetic Ophthalmia

Sympathetic Ophthalmia (SO) is a rare, bilateral, diffuse granulomatous uveitis that presents insidiously after open globe injury or ocular surgery. The injured eye is known as the exciting eye and the fellow eye, which develops inflammation weeks to years later, is the sympathizing eye.

Perforating eye injuries with trauma to the uveal tissue, especially the ciliary body are known to incite SO. Incarceration of the uveal tissue is a common feature in almost all reported cases [22].

As SO is a rare disease, it is difficult to comment on the exact incidence of the disease. However, SO in general does not have any predilection for age, race, or gender [22]. More recently, epidemiological estimates have shown the incidence to be 0.2–0.5% after penetrating ocular injuries and 0.01% after intraocular surgery [23, 24].

Amongst military personnel, where penetrating eye injuries are quite common, the rate of reported SO cases decreased significantly throughout the last century. A very high incidence of SO was initially reported in the earlier wars of the nineteenth and early twentieth centuries, but this was noted to disappear in later wars. A review by Albert et al. asserts that very few well-documented cases of SO occurred during the two World Wars, and none in the Korean, Vietnam wars [22]. Wong et al. supported this data and cited four other twentieth century conflicts in the Middle East with no reported cases of SO [1]. A recent study by Colyer et al. wherein 65 eyes of 61 United States military soldiers deployed during Operation Iraqi Freedom who sustained perforating globe injuries showed no cases of endophthalmitis or SO. This reduction in the number of reported SO cases could probably be due to the provision of early medical care, and timely surgical intervention, and also due to fairly high rates of early enucleation of injured eyes. Of these, 39% were primary enucleation and 19% were secondary enucleation performed within 2 weeks of trauma [25].

10.3.1 Pathogenesis

The etiology of SO is not clearly understood. From the literature, it has been proposed that a T cell-mediated autoimmune response to an antigenic protein from the uvea to the retina, which mainly includes the tyrosinase family of proteins, is responsible for the pathogenesis of SO [26–29]. Penetrating injuries to the eye expose the regional lymphatic system to intraocular antigens, which leads to an autoimmune inflammatory response in both the traumatized and the fellow eye [30].

Immunohistochemical studies of SO reveal that CD4-positive T-helper cells predominate at an earlier stage of the disease and T cytotoxic cells at the latter part of the disease process. The chronic cellular infiltration has also been shown to generate proinflammatory cytokines such as IL-1, IL-2, and TNF-α [31]. Overall, the immunohistochemical features suggest that a T-cell-mediated response is involved in the pathogenesis of SO.

Penetrating injuries are considered a predisposing factor for the development of SO. However, all patients who have ocular injuries do not develop SO. This indicates a possible genetic predisposition to its development. HLA types reported in SO include HLA-11, HLA-DR4/DRw53, HLA-DR4/DQw3, HLA-DRB1*O4, DQA1*03, and DQB1*04 [23, 32].

A curious finding in SO is the lack of inflammation in the choriocapillaris. Wu and associates believed that the RPE may play a crucial role in the disease mechanism of SO by secreting anti-inflammatory agents, including TGF-β and "retinal pigment epithelium protective protein" that provides a relative protection for the choriocapillaris, the RPE, and the retina [33, 34].

10.3.2 Signs and Symptoms

SO begins after the latent period following an injury to the eye. The reported interval between ocular injury and the onset of SO ranges from 5 days to 66 years. Approximately, 65% of cases occur between 2 weeks and 2 months after injury, and 90% are diagnosed within the first year [34].

The exciting eye may show persistent inflammation, sometimes leading to phthisis bulbi, despite the resolution of damage from the initial injury. The sympathizing, non-injured eye presents with blurry vision, pain, epiphora, and photophobia. Transient hyperopia and difficulties with accommodation have been noticed in the early stages of the disease, presumably due to the involvement of the ciliary body (Fig. 10.1).

Initially in early SO, the anterior chamber reaction can be very mild, and the inflammation could be non-granulomatous, which is termed "sympathetic irritation". Without adequate treatment, the disease progresses to a granulomatous anterior chamber reaction with mutton-fat KPs on the corneal endothelium. Intraocular pressure may be elevated secondary to inflammatory cell blockage of the trabecular meshwork or it may be lower as a result of ciliary body shutdown (Fig. 10.2).

In the posterior segment, inflammation may present as vitritis, optic disc swelling or hyperae-

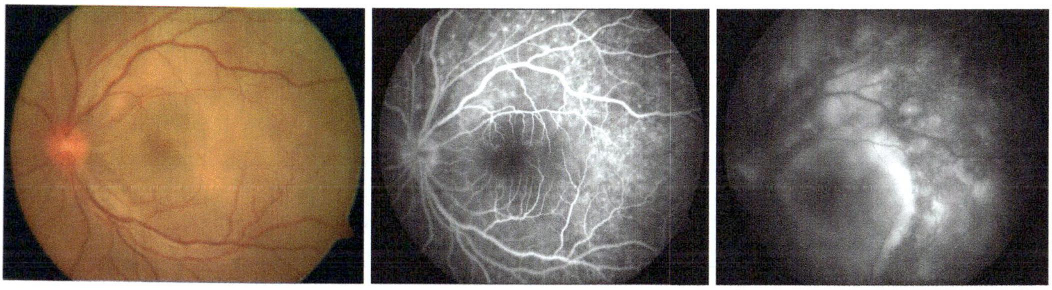

Fig. 10.1 Acute SO with early pinhead leaks and SRF pooling in late phases of FFA

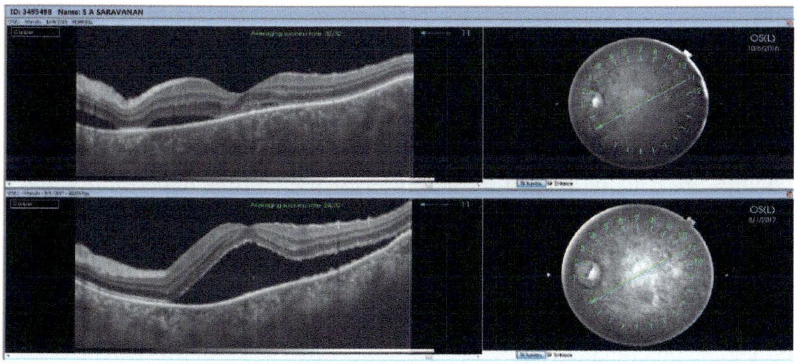

Fig. 10.2 OCT SRF noted Irregular and bumpy RPE, increased choroidal thickness noted

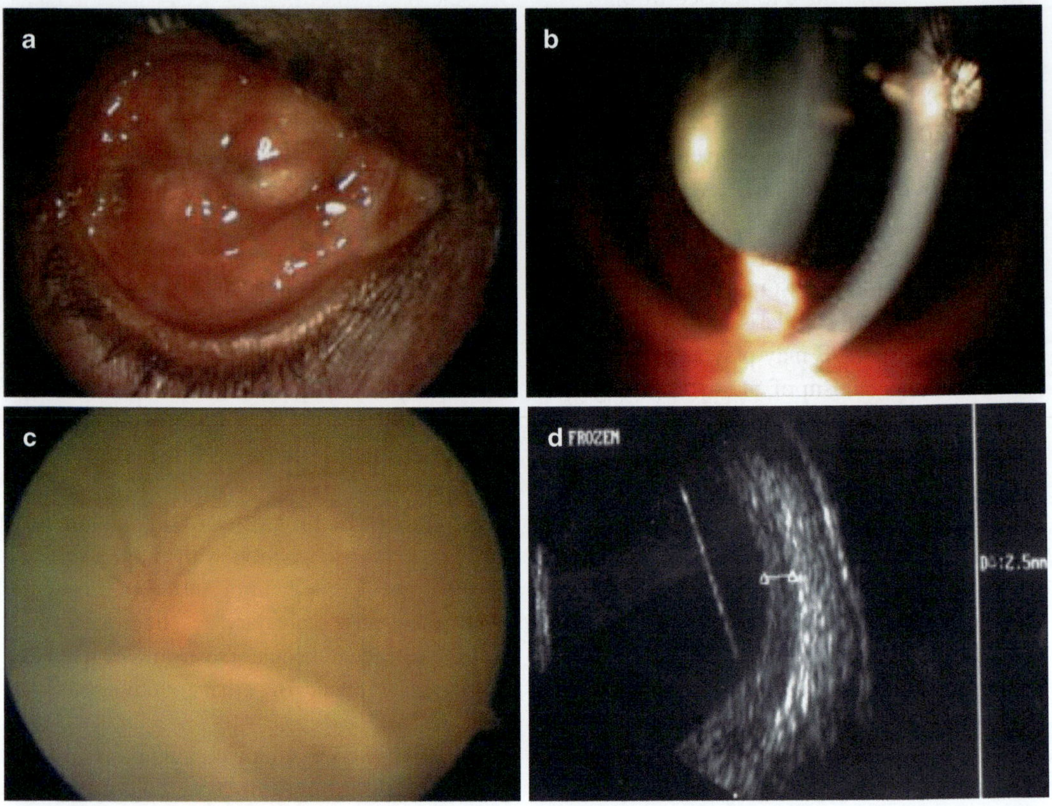

Fig. 10.3 (**a**) Penetrating injury in the right eye 5-year back following which enucleation was done. (**b**) Slit lamp examination of the left eye showed granulomatous anterior uveitis with mutton fat keratic precipitates. (**c**) Fundus left eye showed disc edema with exudative retinal detachment. (**d**) The ultrasound examination revealed marked choroidal thickening, confirming the diagnosis of sympathetic ophthalmia

mia, generalized retinal edema, and diffuse choroidal thickening. Multiple choroidal granulomas and exudative retinal detachment may also be noted (Fig. 10.3). In addition, in approximately one third of cases, multiple small yellow-white lesions known as Dalen-Fuchs nodules may be seen in the mid-periphery of the retina [34]. Initially, these nodules were considered to be characteristic of SO, but they are not pathognomonic, as these nodules are also found in conditions like Vogt-Koyanagi-Harada (VKH) disease and ocular sarcoidosis.

At the onset of the disease, the main clinical features are usually located in the posterior segment, such as optic nerve swelling and exudative retinal detachment, whereas severe and/or chronic recurrent cases present with granulomatous anterior segment inflammation with mutton-fat keratic precipitates [35].

Extraocular or systemic manifestations, though uncommon, are possible and include vitiligo (Fig. 10.4), poliosis, alopecia, dysacusis, and meningeal irritation. All these manifestations are also associated with VKH disease.

10.3.3 Diagnosis

Fluorescein angiography (FA) and indocyanine green angiography (ICG) are important diagnostic tools in the management of SO.

During the acute phase, FA demonstrates multiple hyperfluorescent early pinhead leakage sites at the level of RPE with late placoid pooling of dye (Fig. 10.1). Dalen-Fuchs nodules can sometimes be visualized as early areas of hypofluorescence with late staining. Less commonly, retinal vasculitis can be observed as late staining of reti-

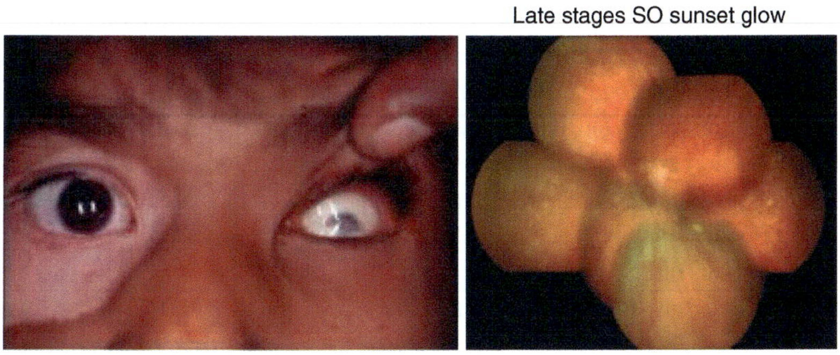

Fig. 10.4 Vitiligo in a patient with sympathetic ophthalmia

nal vessels, and the optic nerve head may also stain. Later in the disease, the FA may show multiple, peripheral spots of early hyperfluorescence that fade over time, and they represent window defects corresponding to mature Dalen-Fuchs nodules that have disrupted the RPE.

As the disease predominantly involves the choroid, ICG is found to be superior to FA for both diagnosis and evaluating the response to treatment. ICG studies show multiple hypofluorescent spots that became more prominent in later phases. These lesions are thought to be reflective of active choroidal lesions, as they resolve after long-term corticosteroid therapy.

SO shows peculiar findings on spectral domain optical coherence tomography (SD-OCT) during the whole course of the disease [36]. With recent advancements in technology, enhanced-depth imaging OCT (EDI-OCT) and swept-source OCT (SS-OCT) provide excellent high-resolution cross-sectional choroid morphology images, providing both qualitative and quantitative information that is almost comparable to the histopathological examination of the tissue.

In the acute phase, SD-OCT shows characteristic multiple serous neurosensory retinal detachments as seen in VKH disease. However, a more distinctive feature to be only reported in SO and VKH is the presence of hyperreflective septa crossing the detachment and dividing it into pockets. EDI-OCT shows choroidal thickening, subretinal choroidal folds, and loss of the physiologic choroidal vascular pattern. Choroidal thickness (CT) may be used as a marker to monitor disease activity as in VKH disease. Studies on EDI-OCT and SS-OCT have shown an increase in CT during the acute phase of the disease, with a subsequent reduction after systemic corticosteroid therapy [37, 38] (Fig. 10.2). During the chronic phase, atrophic changes are seen in the choroid, regardless of the inflammatory status of the patient.

SD-OCT is useful in imaging and monitoring the evolution of Dalen-Fuchs nodules [36, 39]. These lesions appear as round-shaped hyperreflective areas disrupting the retinal pigmented epithelium (RPE) and penetrating the outer retinal layers. With response to treatment, the lesions usually regress, but RPE disruption can persist.

When the media is hazy or in cases where EDI OCT is unavailable, an ultrasound B scan can be used to demonstrate diffuse choroidal thickening in the posterior pole with or without exudative retinal detachment.

10.3.4 Histopathology

Histopathological analysis of eyes with SO reveals uveal granulomatous inflammation comprised primarily of lymphocytes, surrounding macrophages, and some multinucleated giant cells [34]. The inflammation is comprised of T lymphocytes that switch from a predominant composition of CD4+ helper T cells in the early stage of the disease to a later predominance of CD8+ cytotoxic T cells. These findings suggest that type IV hypersensitivity plays an important role in the pathogenesis of SO [26, 27]. It has been classically described in the literature that the retina and choriocapillaris are spared in the disease process. However, few studies have suggested the involvement of the choriocapillaris, with one study reporting 40% of SO patients with choriocapillary involvement and another noting chorioretinal scarring in 25% of cases [21].

The Dalen-Fuchs nodules are small collections of epithelioid cells and lymphocytes covered by an intact dome of RPE in the peripheral retina, varying from focal RPE hyperplasia to disorganized nodules with degenerated RPE. These nodules consist of T lymphocytes of the helper/inducer or cytotoxic/suppressor type [40].

10.3.5 Differential Diagnosis

The differential diagnosis of SO includes any cause of bilateral granulomatous uveitis, especially bilateral lens-induced uveitis, VKH disease, sarcoidosis, and posterior scleritis.

Lens-induced uveitis (LIU) is a chronic granulomatous inflammation that occurs after traumatic or surgical lens capsule disruption and can closely mimic SO. Although LIU is a unilateral condition, a bilateral occurrence has been reported [41]. In such cases, the most important differentiating feature is the absence of choroidal thickening in the USG Scan, which is commonly seen in the SO. Also, in bilateral LIU, the first eye involved is usually quiet by the time the inflammation begins in the second eye, whereas in SO, the exciting eye is usually severely inflamed by the time the sympathizing eye becomes involved.

VKH disease is a bilateral, diffuse granulomatous uveitis with features strikingly similar to SO. Both entities have been associated with headache, tinnitus, alopecia, poliosis, and vitiligo. However, on detailed history taking, a prior penetrating ocular injury helps in confirming the diagnosis of SO. Ocular sarcoidosis is another disease with a clinical resemblance to SO. If systemic manifestations of sarcoidosis are present, such as erythema nodosum, lupus pernio, arthritis, etc. might help in the diagnosis. In its absence, the characteristic findings of SO seen in FA and USG B scan would help differentiate these two entities.

Both posterior scleritis and SO may present with exudative RD and optic disc edema. However, posterior scleritis most often presents as a unilateral condition associated with ocular pain, especially in ocular movement. USG B scans in both of these conditions show diffuse choroidal thickening and exudative retinal detachment, but in posterior scleritis, high internal reflectivity with evidence of retrobulbar edema known as the "T sign" is present on USG.

10.3.6 Prevention

The classic method for prevention of SO is enucleation of the injured eye, ideally performed within 14 days post-injury [22, 42]. Unfortunately, uncertainty exists regarding this time frame, as the onset of the disease has been reported as early as 5 days after injury [34, 43]. Also, few studies claim that early enucleation has no effect on the visual outcome and can be detrimental since vision in the injured eye with adequate treatment can ultimately be better than vision in the sympathetic eye [44].

With the advancements in surgical techniques, it appears that evisceration has a preference over enucleation and has greater benefits. In the past decade, only two cases of SO following evisceration have been reported, of which one was not confirmed through histopathology, and the other was believed to have resulted from residual uveal tissue left in the eye [35, 45]. This assumption that SO can occur after evisceration is largely theoretical and is supported only by a handful of single or small series of questionable cases.

A retrospective study on patients over a 10-year period from 1995 to 2004 showed that no cases of SO were found in 491 primary eviscerations and 11 secondary eviscerations [46]. In a recent study by Holmes et al., 20 eye removals were performed on 19 British military patients during the Iraq and Afghanistan wars. Of these, 4 (70%) were eviscerations, and 6 (30%) were enucleations [47]. They found no clear relationship between complication rates and time to procedure, and no cases of sympathetic uveitis were recorded in either group of enucleation and evisceration.

An important point to make note of here is that the surgical procedure of choice in ocular trauma should be based on the surgeon's preference and experience, given that minimal evidence exists in the literature to support either enucleation or evisceration in the prevention of SO. Thus, with a low incidence of SO supported by superior functional and cosmetic outcomes, evisceration may be a suitable alternative to enucleation [48].

10.3.7 Management

When there is doubt regarding the visual potential of an injured eye, then every effort should be made to preserve it. Meticulous surgical management of the wound with adequate closure of all penetrating wounds is an effective measure, though not an absolute, for the prevention of the development of SO. Uveal tissue incarceration in the wound must be avoided.

Once the diagnosis of SO is confirmed in the sympathizing eye, the systemic treatment of choice remains corticosteroids, and it usually responds rapidly. Secondary enucleation of the inciting eye is of little or no value at this point and may not be advisable, except when it is blinding or painful [49]. The recommended treatment is to immediately begin intravenous steroid (IVMP) or a large dose of oral corticosteroids, 1.5–2 mg/kg, during the first week, followed by gradual tapering to a minimum maintenance dose. Oral corticosteroids should be continued for at least 6 months or until the inflammation resolves completely. This could be supplemented with sub-tenon steroid injections. Useful adjuncts include mydriatic and cycloplegic agents.

Few studies have demonstrated the efficacy of intravitreal steroid implants in SO [50, 51]. This route has the potential to limit the systemic side effects of oral corticosteroids. However, local side effects of the implant, such as raised IOP, cataract, infectious endophthalmitis, and retinal detachment, must be considered. Moreover, the anti-inflammatory response is transient, requiring multiple intravitreal implant procedures.

Steroid-sparing immunosuppressive therapy (IMT) should be considered in severe SO. Immunosuppressive drugs like cyclosporine, methotrexate, azathioprine, mycophenolate mofetil, cyclophosphamide, and chlorambucil have shown considerable benefit in such patients [52–55]. The minimum duration of IMT therapy required to control inflammation is at least 1 year in most cases.

Serum and ocular TNFα levels are noted to be increased in SO; hence, therapy with TNFα antagonists may be effective in the treatment of SO [56]. Few cases of refractory SO that was successfully treated with TNFα antagonists have been reported in the literature [57–60]. Although experience is limited to case reports, the use of infliximab and adalimumab may be considered for refractory SO cases.

Without adequate treatment, the disease usually runs a chronic course with a marked tendency toward relapses, and the disease may culminate in a phthisical eye and blindness. Possible complications include rubeosis iridis, pupillary membranes, secondary glaucoma, cataracts, band keratopathy, corneal edema/bullous keratopathy, macular edema, exudative retinal detachments, choroidal/disc neovascularization, as well as chorioretinal scarring and depigmentation (Fig. 10.5). Surgical management of some of these complications must be done in order to visually rehabilitate the patient.

However, prior to any ocular surgery, adequate control of inflammation for at least 3–6 months with steroids and immunosuppressive therapy, or even triple immunosuppressive therapy may be necessary, failing which may result in a flare-up of the inflammation in both the inciting and sympathizing eyes with a high chance of surgical failure [61, 62]. Multiple studies report favourable outcomes of cataract surgery and penetrating keratoplasty in both sympathizing and exciting eyes of SO patients [61, 63–67]. Patients in all of these studies have tolerated surgical procedures well with favourable outcomes.

A recent large retrospective multicenter study of SO [68], amongst five tertiary centers in the United Kingdom, India, and Singapore reports that the most common cause of SO was trauma, and the majority of patients with SO were males. This study also revealed an increasing trend of vitreoretinal surgery as a surgically-induced cause of SO and hence the importance of includ-

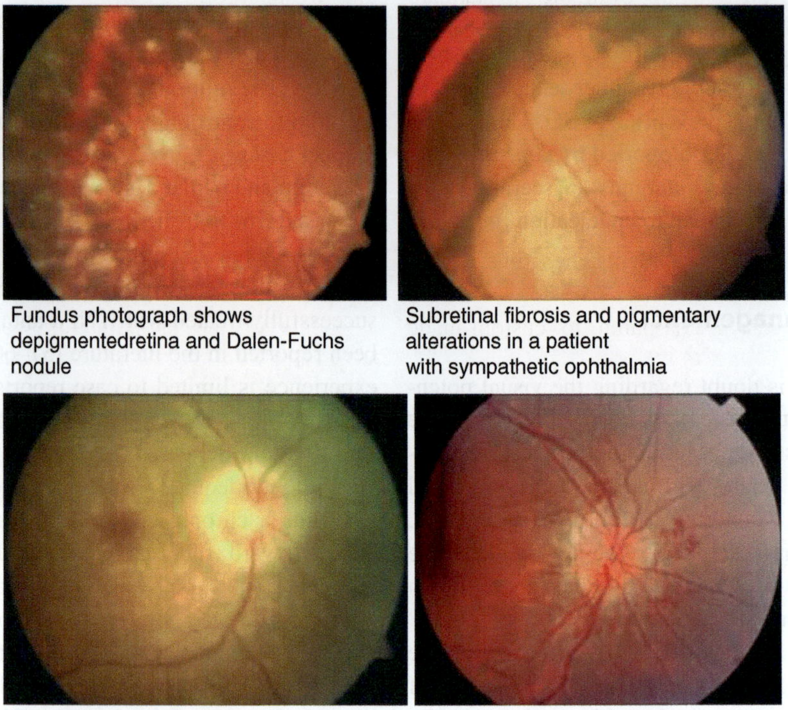

Fig. 10.5 Complications of sympathetic ophthalmia

ing the risk of sympathetic ophthalmia, especially in the consent for retinal surgery. A recent study [68] showed that patients who presented within 5 years of the inciting injury had better visual improvement than those who presented after 10 years. Azathioprine was the most commonly prescribed immunosuppressant in India and Singapore, as compared to mycophenolate mofetil (MMF) in the United Kingdom.

10.4 Conclusion

To conclude, SO is a rare but vision-threatening condition. For military personnel, in whom the rates of penetrating ocular injuries are quite high, the risk of SO does exist, though its rate of incidence has dramatically reduced in recent years. Soldiers with a history of ocular trauma or repeated retinal surgery should be counseled to visit an ophthalmologist early if they notice a loss of vision in the contralateral eye. Prompt and aggressive treatment with corticosteroids and immunosuppressive agents has led to a more favourable prognosis.

References

1. Wong TY, Seet MB, Ang C-L. Eye injuries in twentieth century warfare: a historical perspective. Surv Ophthalmol. 1997;41(6):433–59.
2. Phillips BN, Chun D. Ocular blast injuries in modern warfare. Expert Rev Ophthalmol. 2014;9(1):17–23.
3. Kuhn F, Morris R, Witherspoon CD, Heimann K, Jeffers JB, Treister G. A standardized classification of ocular trauma. Ophthalmology. 1996;103(2):240–3.
4. Kuhn F, Morris R, Witherspoon CD. Birmingham eye trauma terminology (BETT): terminology and classification of mechanical eye injuries. Ophthalmol Clin N Am. 2002;15(2):139–43, v.
5. Thach AB, Johnson AJ, Carroll RB, Huchun A, Ainbinder DJ, Stutzman RD, et al. Severe eye injuries in the war in Iraq, 2003-2005. Ophthalmology. 2008;115(2):377–82.
6. Rosenbaum JT, Tammaro J, Robertson JE. Uveitis precipitated by nonpenetrating ocular trauma. Am J Ophthalmol. 1991;112(4):392–5.

7. Eagling EM. Ocular damage after blunt trauma to the eye. Its relationship to the nature of the injury. Br J Ophthalmol. 1974;58(2):126–40.
8. Vemulakonda A, Sychev S, Verner-Cole SE. Occult nonmetallic intraocular foreign bodies presenting as fulminant uveitis: a case series and review of the literature. Clin Ophthalmol. 2013;7:1747.
9. Essex R, Yi Q, Charles P, Allen P. Post-traumatic endophthalmitis. Ophthalmology. 2004;111(11):2015–22.
10. Martin TM, Smith JR, Rosenbaum JT. Anterior uveitis: current concepts of pathogenesis and interactions with the spondyloarthropathies. Curr Opin Rheumatol. 2002;14(4):337–41.
11. Petrou P, Reddy MA. Unusually resistant post-traumatic uveitis with high serum ACE—an occult ocular sarcoidosis? Ocul Immunol Inflamm. 2008;16(3):117–8.
12. Seymour R, Ramsey MS. Unusually severe traumatic uveitis associated with occult ankylosing spondylitis. Can J Ophthalmol J Can Ophtalmol. 1991;26(3):156–8.
13. Reidy JJ. Section 08: External disease and cornea. In: Basic and clinical science course. San Francisco: American Academy of Ophthalmology; 2015. p. 363.
14. Bagheri N, Wajda BN. Chapter 3: trauma. In: The Wills eye manual: office and emergency room diagnosis and treatment of eye disease. 7th ed. Philadelphia: Wolter Kluwer; 2017.
15. Graham R. Phacoanaphylaxis: background, pathophysiology, epidemiology. 2016. Emedicine.medscape.com. Available https://emedicine.medscape.com/article/1211403-overview. Accessed 4 April 2020.
16. Federici TJ, Tsai JH. Lens-induced uveitis. In: Zierhut M, Pavesio C, Ohno S, Orefice F, Rao NA, editors. Intraocular inflammation. Berlin: Springer; 2016. p. 985–90. https://doi.org/10.1007/978-3-540-75387-2_89.
17. Besen G, Freeman WR. Intraoperative recognition of retinal vasculitis in a patient with early lens-induced uveitis. Ophthalmic Surg Lasers. 1997;28(1):67–8.
18. Hochman M, Sugino IK, Lesko C, Friedman AH, Zarbin MA. Diagnosis of phacoanaphylactic endophthalmitis by fine needle aspiration biopsy. Ophthalmic Surg Lasers. 1999;30(2):152–4.
19. Marak GE. Phacoanaphylactic endophthalmitis. Surv Ophthalmol. 1992;36(5):325–39.
20. Samson CM, Foster CS. Chronic postoperative endophthalmitis. Int Ophthalmol Clin. 2000;40(1):57–67.
21. Croxatto JO, Rao NA, McLean IW, Marak GE. Atypical histopathologic features in sympathetic ophthalmia. A study of a hundred cases. Int Ophthalmol. 1982;4(3):129–35.
22. Albert DM, Diaz-Rohena R. A historical review of sympathetic ophthalmia and its epidemiology. Surv Ophthalmol. 1989;34(1):1–14.
23. Marak GE. Recent advances in sympathetic ophthalmia. Surv Ophthalmol. 1979;24(3):141–56.
24. Makley TA. Sympathetic ophthalmia: a long-term follow-up. Arch Ophthalmol. 1978;96(2):257.
25. Colyer MH, Chun DW, Bower KS, Dick JSB, Weichel ED. Perforating globe injuries during operation Iraqi freedom. Ophthalmology. 2008;115(11):2087–93.
26. Jakobiec FA, Marboe CC, Knowles DM, Iwamoto T, Harrison W, Chang S, et al. Human sympathetic ophthalmia. Ophthalmology. 1983;90(1):76–95.
27. Chan C-C, Benezra D, Rodrigues MM, Palestine AC, Hsu S-M, Murphree AL, et al. Immunohistochemistry and electron microscopy of choroidal infiltrates and Dalen-Fuchs nodules in sympathetic ophthalmic. Ophthalmology. 1985;92(4):580–90.
28. Rao NA. Experimental allergic uveitis: clinicopathologic features associated with varying doses of S antigen. Arch Ophthalmol. 1979;97(10):1954.
29. Yamaki K, Gocho K, Hayakawa K, Kondo I, Sakuragi S. Tyrosinase family proteins are antigens specific to Vogt-Koyanagi-Harada disease. J Immunol. 2000;165(12):7323–9.
30. Rao NA. The role of the penetrating wound in the development of sympathetic ophthalmia: experimental observations. Arch Ophthalmol. 1983;101(1):102.
31. Boyd SR, Young S, Lightman S. Immunopathology of the noninfectious posterior and intermediate uveitides. Surv Ophthalmol. 2001;46(3):209–33.
32. Shindo Y, Ohno S, Usui M, Ideta H, Harada K, Masuda H, et al. Immunogenetic study of sympathetic ophthalmia. Tissue Antigens. 1997;49(2):111–5.
33. Wu G-S, Swiderek KM, Rao NA. A novel retinal pigment epithelial protein suppresses neutrophil superoxide generation. II. Purification and microsequencing analysis. Exp Eye Res. 1996;63(6):727–37.
34. Gasch AT, Foster SC, Grosskreutz CL, Pasquale LR. Postoperative sympathetic ophthalmia. Int Ophthalmol Clin. 2000;40(1):69–84.
35. Chu XK, Chan C-C. Sympathetic ophthalmia: to the twenty-first century and beyond. J Ophthal Inflamm Infect. 2013;3(1):49.
36. Mahajan S, Invernizzi A, Agrawal R, Biswas J, Rao NA, Gupta V. Multimodal imaging in sympathetic ophthalmia. Ocul Immunol Inflamm. 2017;25(2):152–9.
37. Behdad B, Rahmani S, Montahaei T, Soheilian R, Soheilian M. Enhanced depth imaging OCT (EDI-OCT) findings in acute phase of sympathetic ophthalmia. Int Ophthalmol. 2015;35(3):433–9.
38. Agrawal R, Jain M, Khan R, Jaisankar D, Xin W, Ding J, et al. Choroidal structural changes in sympathetic ophthalmia on swept-source optical coherence tomography. Ocul Immunol Inflamm. 2019;2019:1–6.
39. Correnti AJ, Read RW, Kimble JA, Morris R. Imaging of Dalen–Fuchs nodules in a likely case of sympathetic ophthalmia by fluorescein angiography and OCT. Ophthalmic Surg Lasers Imaging. 2010;9:1–3. https://doi.org/10.3928/15428877-20100215-56.
40. Arevalo JF, Garcia R, Al-Dhibi H, Sanchez J, Suarez-Tata L. Update on sympathetic ophthalmia. Middle East Afr J Ophthalmol. 2012;19(1):13.
41. Easom HA. Sympathetic ophthalmia and bilateral phacoanaphylaxis: a clinicopathologic correlation of the sympathogenic and sympathizing eyes. Arch Ophthalmol. 1964;72(1):9.

42. Bilyk JR. Enucleation, evisceration, and sympathetic ophthalmia. Curr Opin Opthalmol. 2000;11(5):372–86.
43. Lubin JR, Albert DM, Weinstein M. Sixty-five years of sympathetic ophthalmia. Ophthalmology. 1980;87(2):109–21.
44. Galor A, Davis JL, Flynn HW, Feuer WJ, Dubovy SR, Setlur V, et al. Sympathetic ophthalmia: incidence of ocular complications and vision loss in the sympathizing eye. Am J Ophthalmol. 2009;148(5):704–10.
45. McCulley T, Phan L, Hwang T. Evisceration in the modern age. Middle East Afr J Ophthalmol. 2012;19(1):24.
46. du Toit N, Motala MI, Richards J, Murray ADN, Maitra S. The risk of sympathetic ophthalmia following evisceration for penetrating eye injuries at Groote Schuur Hospital. Br J Ophthalmol. 2008;92(1):61–3.
47. Holmes CJ, McLaughlin A, Farooq T, Awad J, Murray A, Scott R. Outcomes of ocular evisceration and enucleation in the British Armed Forces from Iraq and Afghanistan. Eye. 2019;33(11):1748–55.
48. Migliori ME. Enucleation versus evisceration. Curr Opin Ophthalmol. 2002;13(5):298–302.
49. Kilmartin DJ, Dick AD, Forrester JV. Prospective surveillance of sympathetic ophthalmia in the UK and Republic of Ireland. Br J Ophthalmol. 2000;84(3):259–63.
50. Mahajan VB, Gehrs KM, Goldstein DA, Fischer DH, Lopez JS, Folk JC. Management of sympathetic ophthalmia with the fluocinolone acetonide implant. Ophthalmology. 2009;116(3):552–7.
51. Mansour AM. Dexamethasone implant as sole therapy in sympathetic ophthalmia. Case Rep Ophthalmol. 2018;9(2):257–63.
52. Hrarat L, Fardeau C, Lehoang P. Immunosuppressive treatment in sympathetic ophthalmia long-term visual outcome. Acta Ophthalmol. 2014;92:253.
53. Nussenblatt RB, Palestine AG, Chan C-C. Cyclosporin a therapy in the treatment of intraocular inflammatory disease resistant to systemic corticosteroids and cytotoxic agents. Am J Ophthalmol. 1983;96(3):275–82.
54. Tessler HH, Jennings T. High-dose short-term chlorambucil for intractable sympathetic ophthalmia and Behcet's disease. Br J Ophthalmol. 1990;74(6):353–7.
55. Lau CH, Comer M, Lightman S. Long-term efficacy of mycophenolate mofetil in the control of severe intraocular inflammation. Clin Exp Ophthalmol. 2003;31(6):487–91.
56. Santos Lacomba M, Marcos Martín C, Gallardo Galera JM, Gómez Vidal MA, Collantes Estévez E, Ramírez Chamond R, et al. Aqueous humor and serum tumor necrosis factor-α in clinical uveitis. Ophthalmic Res. 2001;33(5):251–5.
57. Gupta SR. Successful treatment of refractory sympathetic ophthalmia in a child with infliximab. Arch Ophthalmol. 2011;129(2):250.
58. Soheilian M, Jabbarpourbonyadi M, Soheilian R, Peyman GA. Bilateral uveitis after phakic intraocular lens implantation and management with adalimumab. J Cataract Refract Surg. 2012;38(6):1094–6.
59. Kim J-B, Jeroudi A, Angeles-Han ST, Grossniklaus HE, Yeh S. Adalimumab for pediatric sympathetic ophthalmia. JAMA Ophthalmol. 2014;132(8):1022–4.
60. Hiyama T, Harada Y, Kiuchi Y. Effective treatment of refractory sympathetic ophthalmia with glaucoma using adalimumab. Am J Ophthalmol Case Rep. 2019;14:1–4.
61. Dogra M, Samanta R, Singh P, Singh SR, Bajgai P, Sharma A, et al. Surgical intervention in inciting eyes of patients with sympathetic ophthalmia: a case series and review of literature. Ocul Immunol Inflamm. 2019;27(7):1154–9.
62. Ganesh SK, Narayana KM, Biswas J. Peripapillary choroidal atrophy in sympathetic ophthalmia and management with triple-agent immunosuppression. J Ocular Immunol Inflamm. 2003;11(1):61–5.
63. Ganesh SK, Sundaram PM, Biswas J, Babu K. Cataract surgery in sympathetic ophthalmia. J Cataract Refract Surg. 2004;30(11):2371–6.
64. Ramamurthi S, Obi EE, Dutton GN, Ramaesh K. Management and clinical outcome of penetrating keratoplasty for long-term corneal changes in sympathetic ophthalmia. J Ophthalmol. 2011;2011:1–5.
65. Ramamurthi S, Cornish KS, Steeples L, Ramaesh K. Penetrating keratoplasty for the exciting eye in sympathetic ophthalmia. Cornea. 2008;27(9):1080–1.
66. Reynard M, Minckler DS. Cataract extraction in the sympathizing eye. Arch Ophthalmol. 1983;101(11):1701–3.
67. Henkind P, Wise GN. Cataract extraction in a sympathizing eye. Am J Ophthalmol. 1974;77(1):112–4.
68. Tan XL, Seen S, Majumder PD, Ganesh SK, Agarwal M, Soni A, Biswas J, Aggarwal K, Mahendradas P, Gupta V, Ling HS, Teoh S, Agrawal CPR. Analysis of 130 cases of sympathetic ophthalmia a retrospective multicenter case series. Ocul Immunol Inflamm. 2019;27(8):1259–66. https://doi.org/10.1080/09273948.2018.1517894.

11 Endophthalmitis Following Ocular Trauma in Armed Conflicts

R P Gupta

11.1 Introduction

Endophthalmitis is the most devastating condition of the eye. In all cases of ocular trauma affecting the continuity of the cornea or sclera, the chances of infection getting introduced inside the eye are enhanced. Various studies reveal that 2.4–7.4% of eyes with penetrating ocular trauma develop endophthalmitis [1, 2]. The type of injury, the type of weapon causing the injury, and the nature of infecting organism greatly influence the prognosis in these eyes [2, 3]. Increasing risk factors include:

1. Mine blast injury in which, in addition to gunpowder, mud, plastic, stone, and organic matter enters the eyes [3].
2. Delay in primary repair [2, 4–6].
3. Presence of other retained intraocular foreign bodies (IOFB) [1]. Incidences of endophthalmitis as high as 35% have been reported when an IOFB is present [4].
4. Visual prognosis depends upon early antimicrobial therapy and early surgical intervention wherever needed.

11.2 Etiopathogenesis

Staphylococcus epidermidis is the commonest organism isolated from the vitreous aspirate and vitrectomy fluid of eyes with endophthalmitis. Bacillus cereus and Streptococcus are common organisms isolated from cases of endophthalmitis with retained IOFB. Bacillus cereus infection is more often associated with organic foreign bodies (FBs). It rapidly spreads and destroys the eye within 12–48 h [1]. Other species include Propionibacterium acne, Pseudomonas pyocyaneous, Gram-negative organisms, fungi, and mixed pathogens [5]. Pseudomonas pyocyaneous is also a fulminating infection and, if not treated early, leads to endophthalmitis and panophthalmitis. Infection with multiple organisms is more common in armed conflicts. Most fungal infections are caused by filamentous fungi [5].

11.3 Clinical Features

Following trauma to the eye in armed conflicts, endophthalmitis may occur within a few hours to a few days afterward, depending upon the virulence of the causative organism. Due to trauma, the normal anatomical configuration of the eye structures may get distorted.

R P Gupta (✉)
Department of Ophthalmology, MIMER Medical College, Talegaon, Dabhade, Pune, India

S. Waikar (ed.), *Ocular Trauma in Armed Conflicts*, https://doi.org/10.1007/978-981-19-4021-7_11

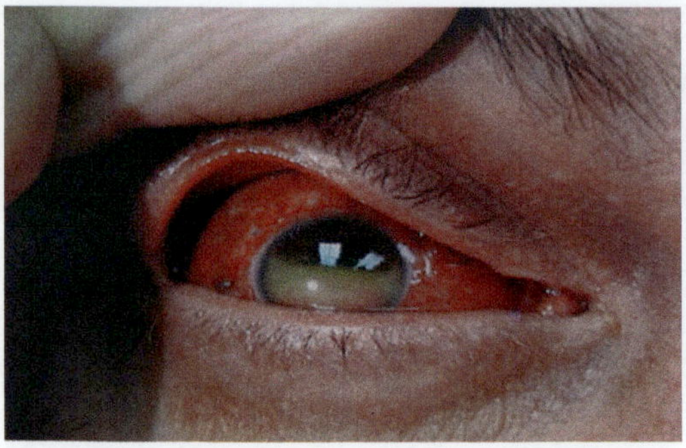

Fig. 11.1 Open globe injury with hypopyon (endophthalmitis)

11.3.1 Symptoms

Severe ocular pain and discomfort out of proportion to the degree of trauma is the most important symptom [4]. Along with pain, the patient may get lid swelling, redness, and a diminution of vision.

11.3.2 Signs

We may find wounds of penetrating injury, conjunctival tears, sub-conjunctival hemorrhage, corneal or scleral tears, traumatic lens capsule rupture [4, 6], and chemosis. Many a time we may find localized chemosis over a scleral perforation or tear. Periorbital swelling, corneal abscess, hypopyon in the anterior chamber, cells, and flare in the aqueous humour, and vitritis are other signs of endophthalmitis (Fig. 11.1). Development of a corneal ring abscess is a classic clinical sign of Bacillus cereus endophthalmitis [1, 6]. Proptosis of the globe is another important sign noticed in some cases [7].

11.4 Diagnosis

In the presence of injury-induced symptoms, the diagnosis of post-traumatic endophthalmitis may be more challenging. The presence of hypopyon, vitritis, and ocular pain should be considered probable signs of infection [8]. Many a time, the whole of the cornea is studded with multiple foreign bodies in cases of mine blast injuries [3]. In these cases, ultrasonography (USG) for assessment of the state of the posterior segment is helpful [3]. The USG, computed tomography (CT) scan, and MRI also reveal the presence of IOFB, which may be a nidus of infection.

11.5 Management

Management of ocular trauma in armed conflicts is usually in three phases:

1. Initial management at forward medical center
2. Management in an eye center of a hospital
3. Management at advanced ophthalmic center or eye center of tertiary care hospital

11.5.1 Management at Forward Medical Center

In armed conflicts or in war, casualties reach the forward medical establishment/Regimental Aid Post/Advanced Dressing Station within a few hours of the injury. Following norms is followed to prevent the spread of infection.

- Assume all eye injuries harbour a ruptured globe. Do not put any pressure on an eye that may cause rupture or increase the already existing corneoscleral tear, which may increase the chances of infection [9].
- Do not apply a patch or bandage to the eye. Use a convex plastic or metal shield and tape it properly to the surrounding bones to protect the eyes [9].
- If the globe is intact, a sterile saline wash should be given to remove particles of dirt.
- Start broad-spectrum antibiotic 0.5% Moxifloxacin eye drops topically 2 hourly.
- Do not put any ointment in a ruptured globe.
- Do not try to remove impaled foreign bodies from the conjunctiva or cornea.
- Administer tetanus toxoid 0.5 cc Intramuscular [9].
- Administer intravenous broad-spectrum antibiotics, particularly if globe perforation or rupture is suspected [3, 6, 9, 10]. Suggested

antibiotics presently include vancomycin/ceftazidime [9]. I/V antibiotics should be started as early as possible. Initiation of I/V antibiotics therapy later than 24 h after trauma is a high-risk factor for endophthalmitis [11]. Consider I/V clindamycin for mine blast injuries, dirty soil/organic material contaminated wounds [9].

- Administer anti-emetics to reduce nausea and vomiting; which in turn may increase tears and prolapse of eye tissue out of the wound.

  Above measures can be taken by a medical officer in a forward medical center where an ophthalmologist may not be available. Patients with ocular injuries should be evacuated as early as possible to an eye center in a Civil/Military Hospital.

11.5.2 Management at an Eye Center of Civil/Military Hospital by Ophthalmologist

11.5.2.1 Diagnostic

1. If any sticky or purulent discharge is sticking to the eyelids or lying in the conjunctival fornices, a swab should be taken for Gram staining, culture, and sensitivity. Gram staining can reveal whether the infection is caused by Gram-positive or Gram-negative organisms. In recent years, molecular techniques such as polymerase chain reaction (PCR) have gained clinical acceptance for the identification of microbes from ocular infections, particularly in culture-negative cases [1].
2. USG (Vector A-B Scan) to check for IOFB [12], particularly in localization of radiolucent IOFB [3], and also to see any evidence of vitritis, infection, exudates in the vitreous cavity, or underlying retinal detachment (Fig. 11.2).
3. CT scan to identify the presence of any IOFB (Fig. 11.3).
4. MRI is contraindicated in a case of magnetic FB and is hence usually avoided. It is helpful only in localizing non-metallic FBs.

If there is evidence of IOFB or infective exudates in the vitreous cavity, the patient must be promptly transferred to a vitreoretinal center for further management.

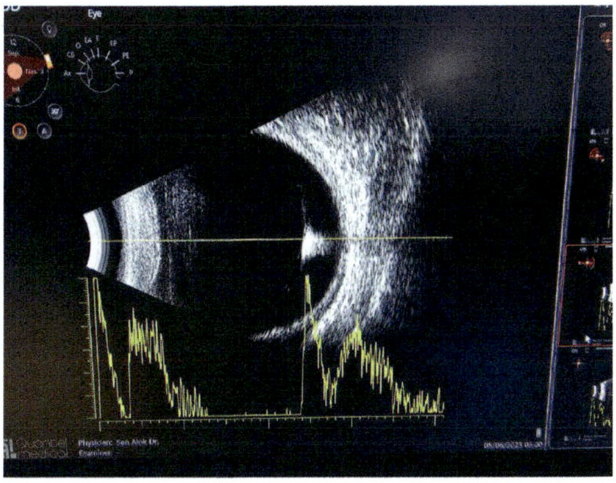

Fig. 11.2 USG (A-B Scan) revealing IOFB with retinal detachment

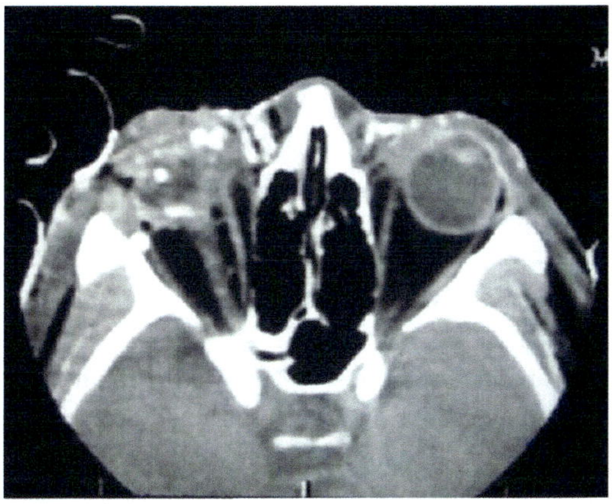

Fig. 11.3 CT Scan revealing IOFBs

11.5.2.2 Preventive

1. Lid wounds are cleaned and repaired.
2. If the eyeball is intact, a sterile saline wash should be given to remove all dirt.
3. Remove conjunctival and superficial corneal foreign bodies. If foreign bodies are located deep in the corneal stroma, these should be removed in the operation theatre (OT) under a microscope.
4. We must look for corneal or scleral tears, which must be repaired. Many a time, scleral tears are not visualized, and there may be localized chemosis over a scleral tear. In such cases, cut the conjunctiva and look for a scleral tear underneath. The same should be

repaired. Early closure of the corneoscleral tear prevents the spread of infection inside the eye. In cases of a scleral tear with exposed uveal tissue, lightly heated platinum-tipped cautery is applied to the uveal tissue which stops the oozing of the blood and causes uveal tissue retraction. Thereafter, it may be easy to approximate the margins of the scleral tear.

5. In cases of corneal tears, if any portion of the iris is prolapsing out (Fig. 11.4) and is dirty; it is abscised. If it is fresh and not contaminated, it is cleaned with sterile Ringer lactate or balanced salt solution and reposited. But if the prolapse is of 24 h or more; it is better to do an abscission of the iris.

All the above steps are taken to prevent endophthalmitis. However, if there are already clinical features suggestive of endophthalmitis, a swab from the lid and conjunctival fornices are taken for a smear, culture, and sensitivity. Treatment is continued for endophthalmitis as below.

11.5.2.3 Therapeutic

1. Topical antibiotics 0.5% Moxifloxacin/fortified eye drops are to be continued every 2 h.
2. Systemic I/V antibiotics are to be continued.
3. Subconjunctival antibiotics Gentamicin 20 mg in 0.5 ml may be given.
4. It is advocated to give intravitreal injections of Vancomycin 1 mg and Ceftazidime 2.25 mg, which are effective against most Gram-positive and Gram-negative organisms, including Bacillus cereus.

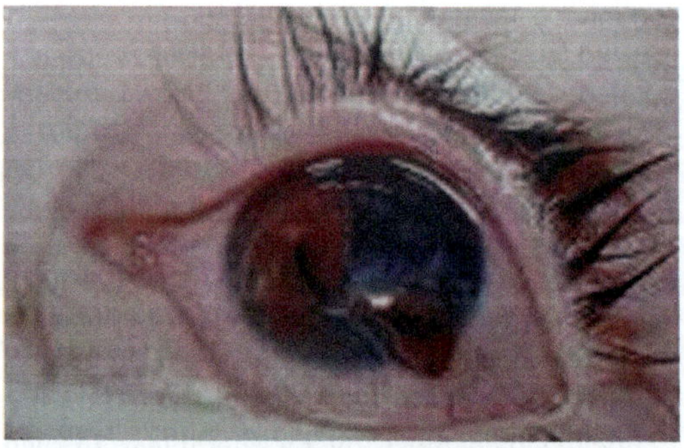

Fig. 11.4 Corneal tear with Iris prolapse

5. The patient should be evacuated to a tertiary care hospital or advanced ophthalmic center where vitreoretinal surgery facilities exist.

11.5.3 Management at Advanced Ophthalmic Center

In armed conflicts, it is not always possible to evacuate cases directly to an advanced ophthalmic center or a specialized vitreoretinal center. The chain of evacuation in armed conflicts certainly causes delay in specialized treatment, thereby affecting the prognosis to a great extent in cases of post-traumatic endophthalmitis [13].

Steps

1. Reassess the case from the documents and the clinical condition and compare it with the clinical condition at the Military/Civil Hospital.
2. If on examination, there is improvement in clinical condition with the first intravitreal injection given at Military/Civil Hospital, then the same intravitreal injection of Vancomycin 1 mg and Ceftazidime 2.25 mg may be repeated at an interval of 48 h.
3. Continue with I/V and subconjunctival antibiotics.
4. In the following situations, we should directly plan for an immediate vitrectomy.
   (a) If with strong light of indirect ophthalmoscope; there is no view of the fundus, even the optic disc is also not visualized.
   (b) Presence of IOFB.
   (c) If no improvement is noticed within 24 h of giving the intravitreal injection.
   (d) Fungal Endophthalmitis—but remember it takes time for fungal endophthalmitis to develop.

In a case of obviously severe endophthalmitis with gross lid oedema and early restriction of extraocular movements, it is wise to perform an immediate vitrectomy rather than waiting for 24 h for conservative treatment; especially in post-traumatic endophthalmitis, where Bacillus cereus infection can progress very rapidly [1].

11.5.4 Vitrectomy in Post-Traumatic Endophthalmitis

Vitrectomy allows the reduction of the bulk of the organisms and removes bacterial toxins [10]. After vitrectomy, penetration of antibiotics to ocular tissues is better and helps in sterilizing the eye [10]. Antibiotics administered after vitrectomy must be effective to cure the endophthalmitis.

11.5.5 Steps of Vitrectomy

1. Vitreous Specimen Collection

A 30° long bent cannula connected to an infusion line is introduced inside the anterior vitreous cavity through a superior nasal/temporal sclerotomy, keeping the infusion off. Another sclerotomy is made in the opposite superior quadrant, and a vitrectomy cutter is introduced. The suction outlet of the vitrectomy cutter is connected to a syringe via silicon tubing. Without turning the infusion on, the vitrectomy cutter is activated to cut the vitreous, and suction is done by the assistant through the connected syringe. 0.5 ml of the specimen is collected and then suction and cutting are stopped. The vitrectomy cutter is withdrawn [14]. Sclerotomy is closed with a scleral plug. Now infusion can be turned on so as to correct the hypotony created by the suction.

2. We should proceed with anterior vitrectomy with a vitrectomy cutter, suction, and infusion cannula in the other ports.
3. Now proceed with mid and post vitrectomy. Place a 6 mm infusion cannula in inferior temporal quadrant. As choroidal thickening is present in cases of endophthalmitis and if a 4mm cannula is placed, it can cause suprachoroidal effusion.
4. Proceed with posterior vitrectomy by using a vitreous cutter and light pipe. Clear the mid-vitreous cavity.
5. While doing a posterior vitrectomy, be careful that there should be a high cutting rate and low suction rate. If suction is more; it may cause a retinal tear.
6. If there are exudates on the surface of the retina, one should avoid suction evacuation, because there may be an inflamed and necrotic retina underneath. Removal of these exudates may leave behind a retinal hole which in turn can cause rhegmatogenous retinal detachment.
7. Peripheral vitreous should not be trimmed as it can lead to tear in the periphery of the retina.
8. We should not try to do a complete or total vitrectomy; rather a subtotal vitrectomy will be ideal.
9. Following the closure of sclerotomies, intravitreal injection of antibiotics (depending upon the Gram staining result of the smear of the vitreous specimen collected at the beginning of surgery) should be administered.
10. On the 1st or 2nd postoperative day if we detect mild exudates in the vitreous cavity; fluid gas exchange with a 27 gauge needle can be carried out in the outpatient department. If there is extensive exudation due to severe infection, then the patient has to be taken to OT. Revitrectomy should be done and intravitreal injection of antibiotics should be given at the conclusion of surgery.

11.6 Concurrent Associations

11.6.1 Endophthalmitis with Cornea Involvement

- The cornea may be steamy due to corneal oedema [14]. Corneal oedema may be epithelial, or stromal, or the cornea may have descemet's folds due to endophthalmitis.
- There may be corneal infiltration. It may be in the form of a ring, which is characteristic of a Bacillus cereus infection.
- In cases of epithelial oedema, scraping of the epithelium by knife may improve visualization.

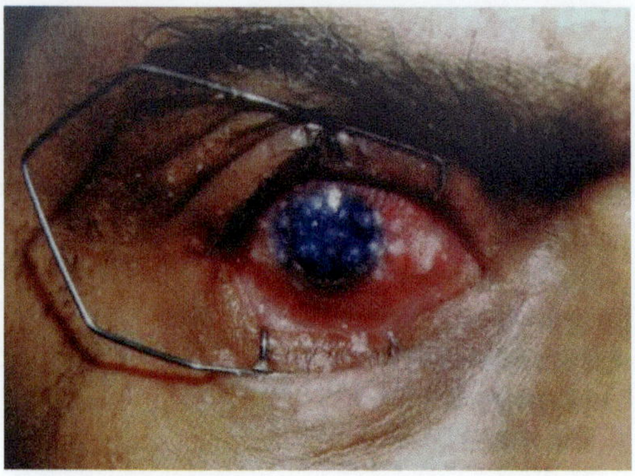

Fig. 11.5 Multiple FBs in deep corneal stroma

- In stromal oedema by scraping the epithelium and using viscoelastic, a vitrectomy can be performed.
- In armed conflicts, particularly mine blast injuries, the whole cornea may be studded with multiple foreign bodies, and it may not be possible to do a vitrectomy due to improper visualization (Fig. 11.5). In this situation, the corneal button is removed and a keratoprosthesis is used temporarily to do a vitrectomy. At the conclusion of the vitrectomy operation, the temporary keratoprosthesis is removed and replaced with a donor corneal graft. A team of vitreoretinal surgeons and keratoplasty surgeons is needed to perform such a heroic procedure. The availability of corneal donor material also has to be ensured.

11.6.2 Endophthalmitis with Scleral Tear

If the scleral tear has been repaired at the secondary level at the Military/Civil Hospital and vitrectomy for endophthalmitis is performed at the tertiary level; before proceeding with the vitrectomy, we should ensure that the scleral sutures are not loose. If loose; resuture the scleral tear with big bites to approximate the wound [14].

11.6.3 Endophthalmitis with Retinal Detachment

- While doing a vitrectomy, retinal detachment may occur as an iatrogenic complication. In these cases, fluid gas exchange, retinopexy, and tamponade with octafluoropropane (C3F8) gas are advised.
- It is also possible that retinal detachment might be due to necrosis of the retina due to infection in endophthalmitis.
- Preoperatively, retinal detachment should be ruled out by USG.
- Retinal detachment might be noticed postoperatively due to iatrogenic retinal breaks near the vitreous base.

11.6.4 Endophthalmitis with Retained IOFB

When there is the presence of IOFB with endophthalmitis, early vitrectomy with IOFB removal is indicated, as the IOFB is a nidus for infection. If a foreign body is lying in subretinal space or embedded in choroidal tissue, then it is better to do an initial vitrectomy and then remove the IOFB; otherwise, many a time, IOFB removal will lead to a retinal break which, may not be sealed properly in an inflamed and necrotic retina and lead to rhegmatogenous retinal detachment.

11.6.5 Hypotony

In a few cases of penetrating injury with endophthalmitis after vitrectomy, the author has been confronted with extreme hypotony leading subsequently to phthisis bulbi. This may be due to concurrent ciliary body shutdown in ocular trauma patients along with infection.

Vitrectomy facilities may not be there at the base hospital level, and it may take time for the casualty to reach the vitreoretinal center; hence, few of these cases may reach the stage of no perception of light in the affected eye or early panophthalmitis. In such badly traumatized unsalvageable eyes, the option is to do frill excision by leaving 2–3 mm of sclera all around the optic nerve and removing all other tissues [15]. When infection is fully controlled and the socket is well healed, then only artificial prosthesis is fitted in these patients [3]

11.7 Conclusion

In armed conflicts and war scenarios, there is generally a delay in primary repair, which can be carried out only when the patient reaches an ophthalmologist or specialist eye care centre. However, correct management at a forward medical centre can delay the progression of endophthalmitis. It is vital to recognize the variation in clinical presentation and stages of endophthalmitis at all echelons of treatment. Timely institution of treatment as detailed above may save vision in many patients.

References

1. Mursalin MH, Livingston ET, Callegan MC. The cereus matter of Bacillus endophthalmitis. Exp Eye Res. 2020;193:107959.
2. Kresloff MS, Castellarin AA, Zarbin MA. Endophthalmitis. Surv Ophthalmol. 1998;43(3):193–224.
3. Singh NB, Madan VK, Deshpande M, Gupta RP, Srivastava SK. Ocular injuries in IPKF in Sri Lanka. Med J Armed Forces India. 1990;46(3):159–64.
4. Vaziri K, Schwartz SG, Kishor K, Flynn HW. Endophthalmitis: state of the art. Ophthalmology. 2015;9:95–108. https://doi.org/10.2147/OPTH.S76406.
5. Mehta DK, Mathur DG. Post-traumatic endophthalmitis. In: Mehta DK, editor. Ocular trauma, vol. 7. Chennai: CBS Publishers; 2015. p. 193–6.
6. Bhagat N, Nagori S, Zarbin M. Post-traumatic infectious endophthalmitis. Surv Ophthalmol. 2011;56:214–51. https://doi.org/10.1016/j.survophthal.2010.09.002.
7. Pan Q, Liu Y, Wang R, Chen T, Yang Z, Deng Y, Zhao Z, Hu X, Chen X, Wei W, Zhang Z, Wang Y, Zheng J, Ke Z. Treatment of Bacillus cereus endophthalmitis with endoscopy-assisted vitrectomy. Medicine. 2017;96:e8701. https://doi.org/10.1097/MD.0000000000008701.
8. Ahmed Y, Schimel AM, Pathengay A, Colyer MH, Flynn HW. Endophthalmitis following open-globe injuries. Eye. 2012;26:212–7. https://doi.org/10.1038/eye.2011.313.
9. Gupta RP, Baranwal VK. Ocular trauma in war and insurgency. In: Mehta DK, editor. Ocular trauma, vol. 11. Chennai: CBS Publishers; 2015. p. 224–31.
10. Alfaro DV, Roth D, Liggett PE. Post traumatic endophthalmitis, causative organisms. treatment and prevention. Retina. 1994;14:206–11.
11. Schmidseder E, Kapsar HMD, Klauss V, Kampic A. Post traumatic endophthalmitis after penetrating injuries. Risk factors, microbiological diagnosis and functional outcome. Ophthalmology. 1998;95:153–7. https://doi.org/10.1007/5003470050254.
12. Baranwal VK, Gupta RP, Vats DP. Comparative evaluation of real time B-scan ultra-sound and computed tomography in management of penetrating ocular and orbital trauma. All India Ophthalmic Proc. 2004;5:516–8.
13. Boparai MS, Sharma RC. Ocular war injuries. Indian J Ophthalmol. 1984;32:277–9.
14. Gopal L. Endophthalmitis. In: Gupta AK, Krishna V, editors. Current topics in ophthalmology – VII, vol. 25. Amsterdam: Elsevier; 2004. p. 286–99.
15. Gupta RP, Baranwal VK, Pannu SS. Ocular trauma in war and peace: an experience. All India Ophthalmic Proc. 2002;5:482–3.

12 Stem Cell Transplantation for Ocular Surface Chemical Injuries: Techniques and Outcomes

Virender Sangwan and Aastha Singh

12.1 Anatomic Location and Limbal Stem Cell Characteristics

The healthy ocular surface is characterised by a non-keratinised, stratified, squamous (cornea) or columnar (conjunctiva) epithelium. The anatomic barrier between these contiguous epithelia is the limbus, which is Greek for "border" [1]. The limbal barrier, which is 1.5–2 mm in span, is both an anatomical and a functional divide. The palisades of Vogt at the limbus are radial projections of fibrovascular tissue that house the progenitor limbal stem cells. These palisades are more abundant in the superior and inferior limbus, where they are well protected by the eyelids and have undulations that increase their surface area. The first evidence of the exact anatomical location of stem cells in the corneal epithelium was given by Schermer, Galvin, and Sun [2].

The limbal "niche," located in the palisades of Vogt, is the natural habitat of LESCs. It is a micro-environment, naturally designed to protect the cells from injury and maintain their health. The niche is rich in melanocytes, which provide protection from ultraviolet ray damage, and has a sufficient blood supply from the adjacent conjunctival vasculature, which provides nutrition. Additionally, the stem cells are in contact with the limbal stroma, which provide various growth factors and cytokines essential for their survival [3].

The unique limbal epithelial stem cells (LESCs) have been described as basal limbal epithelial cells. Clonogenic cells can be either proliferative (stem cells and transiently amplifying cells) or non-proliferative/differentiative (post-mitotic or terminally-differentiated cells) (Fig 12.1). Stem cells undergo both self-replication to maintain their pool and mitosis to give rise to terminally differentiated cells. They are the only cells thus capable of self-renewal and are characterised by slow cycling, error-free proliferation, and poor differentiation [4]. In normal physiological processes or following traumatic insult, there is both centripetal movement of cells from the periphery as well as proliferation of basal epithelial cells to fill the gap as per the X, Y, and Z hypothesis described by Thoft and Fiend [5]. The stem cells thus maintain a healthy ocular surface through their unique dynamics.

V. Sangwan (✉) · A. Singh
Department of Cornea and Stem Cell Research,
Dr. Shroff's Charity Eye Hospital, New Delhi, India
e-mail: virender.sangwan@sceh.net

S. Waikar (ed.), *Ocular Trauma in Armed Conflicts*, https://doi.org/10.1007/978-981-19-4021-7_12

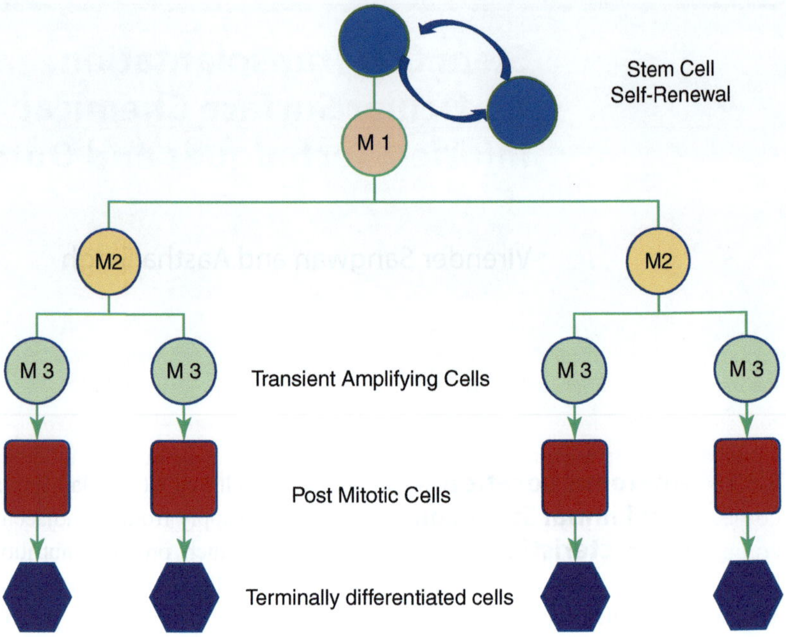

Fig. 12.1 Replication hierarchy of stem cells, M1, M2, M3 represent mitotic cycle

12.2 Etiological Subtypes and Demography of Limbal Stem Cell Deficiency (LSCD) Secondary to Injury

Chemical injury is the commonest identifiable cause of unilateral and bilateral LSCD (73–85%) [6]. Further, Lime injury is the most common implicating agent (62–70%) among cases of ocular surface burns [6, 7]. Alkali burns have been shown to cause more severe tissue damage than acid burns as they cause saponification of cellular membranes with deeper penetration in the limbal tissue. Thermal injury, commonly seen in industrial settings, results in LSCD, which is often severe in nature and a challenge to manage [8]. Sulfur mustard, a potent chemical warfare vesicating agent, has been shown to cause delayed onset LSCD [9]. Additionally, ocular burns associated with scleral ischemia have been shown to cause relatively greater damage and hence a poorer prognosis in the affected eye [10].

Demographically, a large case series from India reports unilateral LSCD to be more common than bilateral LSCD. Young males have been shown to be afflicted more commonly as compared to females, and total LSCD is more common than partial LSCD [6].

12.3 Mechanism of Development of LSCD

The basal epithelial cells of the palisades of Vogt are believed to be the driving force in epithelial regeneration. Stem cell transporter proteins ABCG2 and P63 (ΔNp63α) have been shown to be present in limbal epithelial stem cells. Additionally, expression of Connexin 43, a gap junction protein, is seen to be increased in niche cells during proliferation of stem cells. The basal limbal epithelium lacks cytokeratin 3, a differentiation keratin, while retaining cytokeratin 19, which in fetal life is present in all layers [11].

In response to injury, at first, the cells adjacent to the site of injury migrate to the injured site initiated by the epidermal growth factor. This is followed by the stage of proliferation wherein the limbal stem cells activated by various cytokines and growth factors, proliferate and give rise to the transient amplifying cells (TAC) which undergo cell division to generate supra-basal wing cells and superficial cells. In a partial insult to the limbus, there is circumferential migration from surviving cells to cover the defect until they are halted by conjunctival growth [12].

When the limbal barrier is breached and stem cells are damaged, the condition is termed LSCD wherein conjunctival epithelium together with blood vessels and fibrous tissue encroach onto the cornea leading to diminution of vision and ocular surface inflammation.

12.4 Classification of LSCD

Limbal stem cell deficiency has been classified as type 2 ocular surface failure in which normal corneal epithelial phenotype is replaced by the conjunctival epithelial phenotype identified on impression cytology [13]. LSCD can be classified on the basis of etiology and extent of the damage. Conditions leading to deficiency of limbal stem cells can be either primary or secondary. Primary conditions are characterised by the absence of identifiable external factors causing deficiency while secondary conditions are characterised by the destruction of limbal stem cells by external factors. LSCD caused by chemical injury thus falls in the group of secondary causes. Depending on the extent of damage LSCD may be either partial or total. In partial LSCD only a part of the limbus is damaged (expressed in clock hours of involvement) whereas in total LSCD there is 360° damage involving most to all of the limbal stem cells.

12.5 Clinical Features

12.5.1 Symptoms

LSCD is a gradually progressive disease entity wherein the patient may be asymptomatic initially but develops ocular discomfort, foreign body sensation, irritation, grittiness, dryness, redness, watering, pain, photophobia, and diminution of vision with disease progression. Ocular discomfort/pain due to recurrent epithelial breakdown and blepharospasm are particularly debilitating and significantly affect the quality of life of such patients [14].

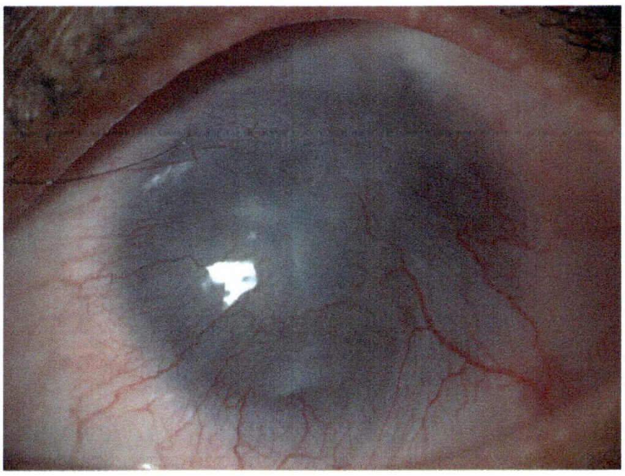

Fig. 12.2 Total limbal stem cell deficiency in a 24 year old, male, post lime injury depicting classic triad of conjunctival overgrowth on the cornea, vascularization and ocular surface inflammation

12.5.2 Signs

The hallmark triad of LSCD comprises of conjunctival overgrowth, neovascularisation, and chronic inflammation (Fig. 12.2). The condition is characterised by recurrent and persistent epithelial defects, stippled appearance on fluorescein-staining and corneal scarring. The de-epithelised areas can predispose to secondary microbial keratitis and corneal perforation. The palisades of Vogts are indistinct and the fibrovascular pannus tends to cover the cornea. The pannus being irregular in contour causes tear film disturbance and subsequently dry eye [14]. Persistent inflammation of the ocular surface in severe cases can lead to corneal melt [12].

12.6 Laboratory Work Up and Role of Investigational Modalities

While clinical diagnosis is often accurate and sufficient, various diagnostic modalities namely conjunctival impression cytology (CIC), in vivo confocal microscopy (IVCM), and anterior segment optical coherence tomography (AS-OCT) aid in the diagnosis of LSCD.

CIC performed by pressing nitrocellulose paper for a few seconds on the suspected area is considered the gold standard diagnostic modality. Conventional histopathology (haematoxylin and eosin/periodic acid schiff) detects goblet cells which is characteristic of conjunctival epithelium while immunohistochemistry detects specific conjunctival markers such as CK19, CK13, MUC 1, and MUC5AC [15]. Additionally, reverse transcriptase PCR (RT-PCR) can detect m RNA specific for conjunctiva [16, 17].

IVCM is a sensitive, predictable, non-invasive tool in the diagnosis of LSCD [18]. In the normal cornea, deep basal epithelial cells are small in size with well-defined borders and no nuclei. In early-stage LSCD, an average of 35–40% reduction in basal epithelial cell density and a 55–60% reduction in subbasal nerve density has been reported. The absence of palisades of Vogt and basal epithelial cells with less distinct borders and prominent nuclei have been found in patients with LSCD. Epithelial cells in the deeper layers have been shown to be affected in more advanced stages of LSCD. In the late stage, epithelial cells have been demonstrated to have metaplasia and neovascularization [19].

AS-OCT is a non-invasive modality that aids in measuring epithelial and stromal thickness, pannus depth as well as the architecture of the palisades of Vogt. Parallel, perpendicular, and en-face sections on spectral domain optical coherence tomography can demonstrate the absence of palisades of Vogt, thin limbal epithelium, loss of clear transition between the hyporeflective corneal epithelium and hyperreflective conjunctival epithelium [20]. The average limbal epithelial thicknesses in eyes with limbal stem cell deficiency have been shown to be 13–20% less than normal controls in literature [21]. Additionally, OCT- Angiography can give useful information, pertaining to ocular perfusion in cases of ocular burns.

12.7 Strategy of Managing LSCD

While management of LSCD is primarily surgical, topical steroid, interferon α-2b (IFN α-2b), and all-trans retinoic acid (ATRA) 0.01% application have been reported to be effective in alleviating symptoms in cases of partial LSCD [22, 23]. Y-27632 a ROCK (a Rho-associated protein kinase inhibitor) has also been reported to promote both ex vivo and in vitro proliferation of limbal epithelial cells [24].

The choice of surgical technique depends upon the extent and laterality of the disease (Fig. 12.3). Partial LSCD can be treated with amniotic membrane transplantation, while total LSCD is treated by limbal stem cell transplantation (LSCT) techniques such as conjunctival limbal autograft (CLAu), cultured limbal epithelial transplantation (CLET) and simple limbal epithelial transplantation (SLET). CLAu,

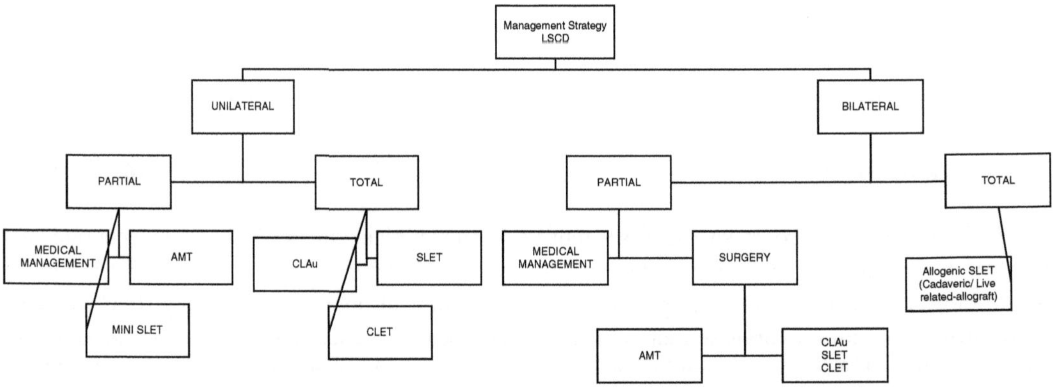

Fig. 12.3 Flowchart depicting management strategy for limbal stem cell deficiency. *LSCD* limbal stem cell deficiency, *AMT* amniotic membrane transplantation, *CLAU* conjunctival limbal autograft, *SLET* simple limbal epithelial transplantation, *CLET* cultivated limbal epithelial transplantation, *COMET* cultivated oral mucosal epithelial transplantation, *SOMET* simple oral mucosal epithelial transplantation

Table 12.1 Comparative analysis of various surgical techniques of limbal stem cell transplantation

Parameters	SLET	CLET	CLAU
Logistics			
• Cost	Inexpensive	Expensive	Inexpensive
• Sophisticated laboratory requirement	None	Required	None
• Regulatory control	Not required	Required	Not required
Surgical technique			
• Stages of procedure	1	2	1
• Donor tissue span in clock hours	<1	<1	~3
• AMG requirement	Yes	Yes	No
• Repeatability from same donor	Possible	Possible	Iatrogenic LSCD
• Reproducibility by other surgeons	Easy	Challenging	Easy
Results			
• Time to epithelialization	4–6 weeks	4–6 weeks	4–6 weeks
• Success rate in adults	65–80%	65–80%	60–80%
• Success rate in pediatric patients	75–85%	45–50%	60–70%

CLAU conjunctival limbal autograft, *SLET* simple limbal epithelial transplantation, *CLET* cultivated limbal epithelial transplantation, *AMG* amniotic membrane graft

which consists of transplantation of a conjunctival graft along with limbal tissue, was one of the earliest techniques of LSCT described in literature. More recently, transplantation of limbal stem cells either cultured in a laboratory (CLET) or grown directly (SLET) over the scaffold of an amniotic membrane from a minimal limbal tissue biopsy comprises the most commonly performed techniques. The limbal stem biopsy can be harvested either from the fellow eye (autograft), or from a donor (allograft), a living relative or a cadaver. A comparative analysis of the three surgical options is presented in Table 12.1.

12.8 Simple Limbal Epithelial Transplantation (SLET)

12.8.1 Pre-operative Considerations

Careful preoperative evaluation of the lid and adnexa of the patient must be done and conditions such as lagophthalmos, ectropion, entropion, trichiasis, irregular lid margin, lid margin keratinisation, and symblepharon must be addressed before performing LSCT.

Absolute contraindications of LSCT include a dry/keratinised ocular surface, blind eye, amblyopia, and disorganised anterior segment. Ocular factors such as the presence of stromal thinning, stromal opacification, raised intraocular pressure, glaucoma, previous failed penetrating keratoplasty or LSCT and history of multiple surgeries are poor prognostic factors [12].

A healthy donor site with ample viable tissue is critical for a successful LSCT. Typically, the superior limbus is the preferred site for donor tissue harvesting as the limbal palisades are more in number at this location. In the case of cadaveric SLET, fresh tissue, ideally harvested <48 h prior to surgery with visible intact limbal palisades, healthy epithelium, and preferably from a donor <60 years must be selected.

12.8.2 Surgical Technique of SLET

Depending on the age and systemic condition of the patient, surgery can be performed under peribulbar or general anaesthesia. For healthy adults, local anaesthesia is sufficient for performing surgery. Instillation of brimonidine tartrate 0.15% eyedrops 5–10 min before surgery in both donor and recipient is seen to reduce intraoperative bleeding.

Limbal biopsy (2–3 mm) from the donor 's eye is first harvested. The conjunctival flap is raised most commonly from the superior limbus, and sub-conjunctival dissection using surgical blade no. 15 on a Bard Parker (BP) handle is performed until the limbus is reached. Further dissection is then carried out 1 mm into the clear cornea. The limbal tissue is then excised with vannas scissors and placed in a balanced salt solution. In the recipient eye, symblephera if any are resected, a 360° peritomy is performed, and bleeders are cauterized. This is followed by pannus dissection, which is a crucial step, and meticulous dissection is recommended. The pannus is dissected using a surgical blade no. 15 on the BP handle or sharp vannas scissors. Care must be taken to avoid areas of thinning to prevent intraoperative perforation.

Human amniotic membrane (hAM) is then secured to the recipient bed with fibrin glue. The harvested donor tissue is divided into 8–10 smaller explants with vannas scissors and placed on the amniotic membrane in a circular fashion. Fibrin glue is then applied to each of the explants to ensure their adherence. A bandage contact lens is placed at the end of the procedure (Fig. 12.4).

12.8.3 Post Operative Management

Postoperatively, a topical broad-spectrum antibiotic is prescribed until the healing of epithelial defect in both the recipient and donor 's eye. Topical corticosteroids such as prednisolone acetate 1% eyedrop are prescribed 6 times a day and tapered slowly in the recipient 's eye over 6 weeks. Topical steroids in a low-maintenance dose are continued long-term in the recipient eye. In the donor eye topical steroids are prescribed 4 times a day and tapered over 4 weeks. Judicious use of preservative-free tear substitutes is recommended. In cases of allografts, immune suppression is prescribed as per standard protocols described in the literature.

In the immediate postoperative period, patients are kept under a close follow-up until the epithelium heals. A bandage contact lens can be removed after epithelisation is complete. In an in vivo study, the first clinical evidence of proliferation of the corneal epithelium from the limbal

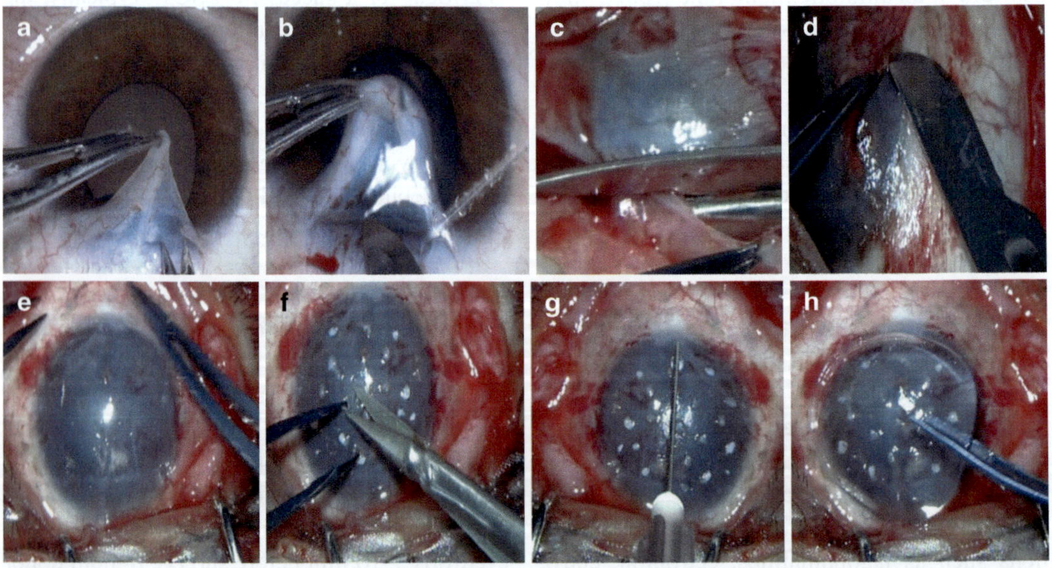

Fig. 12.4 Surgical Steps of Simple limbal epithelial transplantation. (**a**) A 2 × 2 mm area is marked at the superior limbus of the donor eye and conjunctival flap is raised. (**b**) A sub-conjunctival dissection is carried out 1 mm into the clear cornea and limbal tissue is excised. (**c, d**) Symblephera (if any) are released, a peritomy is performed and the fibrovascular pannus is excised from the recipient ocular surface. (**e**) A human amniotic membrane graft is placed on the ocular surface and secured to it with fibrin glue. (**f, g**) The donor limbal tissue is divided into eight to ten small explants and secured to the amniotic membrane overlying cornea with fibrin glue. (**h**) A bandage contact lens is placed at the end of surgery

explants was seen on the second day and ocular surface epithelialisation was complete in all cases within 14 days [25].

On subsequent follow ups, care must be taken to note the recurrence of LSCD, clarity of the cornea, signs of rejection (in cases of allograft) as well as the health of the donor site. If the patient is on immune suppression, dosage of the same is monitored or tapered and systemic blood tests are conducted at regular intervals to detect drug induced side effects.

12.9 Complications

Intraoperatively, corneal perforation can occur during pannus dissection. A pre-operative AS-OCT can help in delineating areas of thinning. In case of intraoperative perforation, cyanoacrylate glue can be applied to the site or a tenon patch grafting can be performed. Other intraoperative complications include loss or insufficient harvesting of limbal stem cells and bleeding [26].

In the immediate post-operative complications such as loss of explants, haemorrhage under BCL or hAM, infectious keratitis, and subconjunctival haemorrhage at the donor site can be seen. Late post-operative complications include focal or total recurrence of LSCD, symblepharon formation, pyogenic granuloma and epithelial hyperplasia [27].

Risk of iatrogenic LSCD at the donor site even after multiple biopsies is low [28].

12.10 Outcomes

Primary outcome measure following LSCT is defined as achieving a stable, epithelised, avascular corneal surface at the end of follow-up period and secondary outcome measure is defined as improvement in best corrected visual acuity (Fig. 12.5).

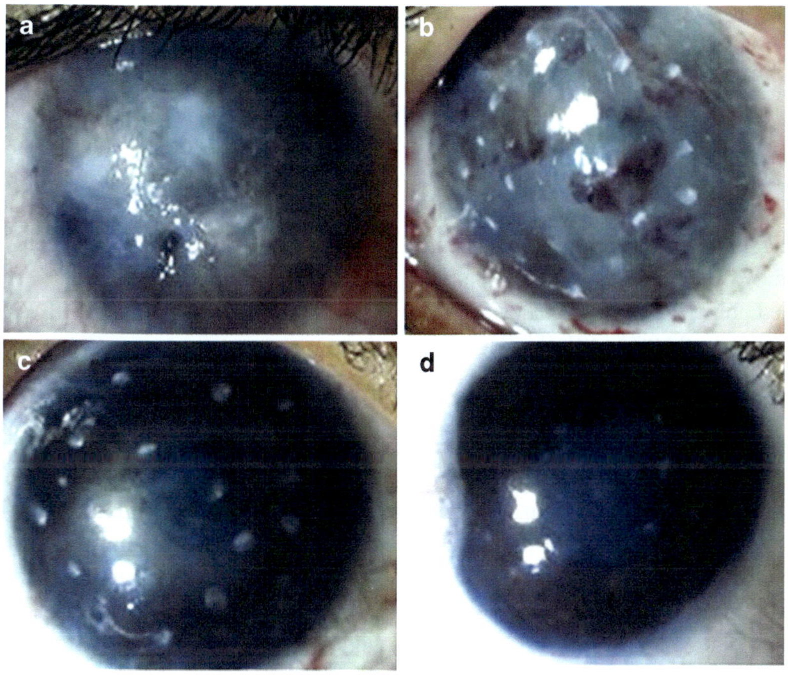

Fig. 12.5 Corneal epithelium regeneration post simple limbal epithelial transplantation (SLET). (**a**) Total limbal stem cell deficiency post lime injury in a 14 year old boy (**b**) On post-operative Day 1 after simple limbal epithelial transplantation, limbal stem cell explants can be seen well placed over amniotic membrane. (**c**) At post operative week 3, cornea is well epithelized and explants can be seen in situ. (**d**) At fifth post operative month cornea was well epithilized and there was improvement in corneal clarity with only mild central stromal haze. Patient had a BCVA 20/30 with contact lens at this time point and gradual fading of explants was noted

Outcomes of CLAu, CLET and SLET were analysed recently in a comprehensive review. In 162 eyes from 8 studies that underwent CLAu, 81% eyes were found to have a stable, fully epithelised and avascular surface while a two-line improvement in BCVA could be discerned in 74.4% eyes at a mean follow-up period of 1.56 years [29–32]. The outcomes of CLET were analysed in 581 eyes across eight studies [33–37]. At a mean follow-up period of 2.9 years, 61.4% of the eyes were successfully treated and 51.5% of the eyes had a two-line improvement in BCVA. The outcomes of SLET were analysed from 253 eyes across 4 large studies. At a mean follow-up period of 1.48 years, 78% of eyes reported success and 68.6% of eyes had a two-line improvement in BCVA. While comparing the three groups, statistically, SLET and CLAu have been reported to have significantly better outcomes compared with CLET, both in terms of anatomical and functional success. The anatomical success rates were almost identical between SLET and CLAu, while the functional success rates were marginally better with CLAu [38].

Outcomes from SLET have now been reported in various large series. Basu et al. performed autologous SLET in 125 patients (65 adults and 60 children) with unilateral LSCD due to ocular surface burns and reported that 95 of 125 eyes (76%) maintained a successful outcome [39]. A multi-centre worldwide study wherein a total of 68 patients were reviewed reported clinical success was achieved in 57 cases (83.8%) [40]. Similarly, in a study from North India with 30 eyes of 30 patients (18 adults and 12 children) 21 of 30 eyes (70%) maintained successful outcome. Visual acuity gain was seen in 71.4% of successful cases [41].

Results on outcomes of SLET in paediatric patients and in failed CLET in both adults and children are encouraging as well [28, 42]. Outcomes of Allogenic SLET reported by Iyer et al. concluded that SLET is a useful technique for LSCD wherein the mean time to epithelialisation was noted to be 22.5 ± 9.14 days and complete epithelialisation was achieved in the immediate postoperative period in 17 of the 18 eyes (94.11%) [43].

Post SLET, outcomes of DALK in the paediatrics age group have been studied with promising results. Anatomical success was seen in 72.72% of patients, and visual success was noted in 54.54% of patients [44]. Good outcomes of penetrating keratoplasty (PKP) after the ocular surface has been stabilised by SLET as an initial procedure in unilateral ocular chemical injury have been reported, with a graft survival rate of 85% at 6 months [45].

12.11 Future Directions

Therapy for limbal stem cell deficiency is an evolving science. The introduction of disease mutations into limbal stem cells by CRISPR/Cas9 genome editing has been demonstrated to create relevant cellular models of ocular disease to study novel therapeutic approaches [46].

Reprogrammed cells that secrete substances that inhibit corneal neovascularization and/or conjunctival scarring may be useful in limbal stem cell therapy in the future. Induced pluripotent stem cells derived from the corneal limbal epithelium and dermal fibroblasts have already been shown to differentiate into corneal epithelial cells [47].

Exosomes, which are nano-sized vesicles, have the ability to transfer RNAs and proteins to recipient cells and are being widely studied as a potential therapy [48].

12.12 Conclusion

Limbus is a storehouse of pluripotent stem cells. LSCD is a potentially sight threatening condition and can substantially affect quality of life. The diagnosis of LSCD is mainly clinical, and LSCT is an effective method to restore ocular surface health. The outcome of LSCT is influenced by the nature and duration of the underlying ocular pathology, the presence of ocular inflammation, as well as quantity and quality of tear film. SLET, a low cost and easily reproducible technique of LSCT provides good anatomical and functional outcomes and is a boon in managing patients with LSCD.

References

1. Sangwan VS. Limbal stem cells in health and disease. Biosci Rep. 2001;21:385.
2. Schermer A, Galvin S, Sun TT. Differentiation-related expression of a major 64K corneal keratin in vivo and in culture suggests limbal location of corneal epithelial stem cells. J Cell Biol. 1986;103:49.
3. Singh V, Shukla S, Ramachandran C, Mishra DK, Katikireddy KR, Lal I, et al. Science and art of cell-based ocular surface regeneration. Int Rev Cell Mol Biol. 2015;319:45–106.
4. Tseng SCG. Concept and application of limbal stem cells. Eye. 1989;3:141.
5. Thoft RA, Friend J. The X, Y, Z hypothesis of corneal epithelial maintenance. Investig Ophthalmol Vis Sci. 1983;24:1442–3.
6. Vazirani J, Nair D, Shanbhag S, Wurity S, Ranjan A, Sangwan V. Limbal stem cell deficiency—demography and underlying causes. Am J Ophthalmol. 2018;188:99.
7. Bobba S, Di Girolamo N, Mills R, Daniell M, Chan E, Harkin DG, et al. Nature and incidence of severe limbal stem cell deficiency in Australia and New Zealand. Clin Exp Ophthalmol. 2017;45:174.
8. Fatima A, Iftekhar G, Sangwan VS, Vemuganti GK. Ocular surface changes in limbal stem cell deficiency caused by chemical injury: a histologic study of excised pannus from recipients of cultured corneal epithelium. Eye. 2008;22:1161.
9. Baradaran-Rafii A, Javadi MA, Rezaei Kanavi M, Eslani M, Jamali H, Karimian F. Limbal stem cell deficiency in chronic and delayed-onset mustard gas keratopathy. Ophthalmology. 2010;117:246.
10. Gupta N, Singh A, Mathur U. Scleral ischemia in acute ocular chemical injury: long-term impact on rehabilitation with Limbal stem cell therapy. Cornea. 2019;38:198.
11. Dua HS, Miri A, Alomar T, Yeung AM, Said DG. The role of Limbal stem cells in corneal epithelial maintenance. Testing the dogma. Ophthalmology. 2009;116:856.
12. Dua HS, Saini JS, Azuara-Blanco A, Gupta P. Limbal stem cell deficiency: concept, aetiology, clinical presentation, diagnosis and management. Indian J Ophthalmol. 2000;48(2):83–92.
13. Sangwan VS, Tseng SC. New perspectives in ocular surface disorders. An integrated approach for diagnosis and management. Indian J Ophthalmol. 2001;49:153.
14. Deng SX, Borderie V, Chan CC, Dana R, Figueiredo FC, Gomes JAP, et al. Global consensus on definition, classification, diagnosis, and staging of limbal stem cell deficiency. Cornea. 2019;38:364.
15. Ramirez-Miranda A, Nakatsu MN, Zarei-Ghanavati S, Nguyen CV, Deng SX. Keratin 13 is a more specific marker of conjunctival epithelium than keratin 19. Mol Vis. 2011;17:1652–61.
16. Sejpal K, Bakhtiari P, Deng SX. Presentation, diagnosis and management of limbal stem cell deficiency. Middle East Afr J Ophthalmol. 2013;20(1):5–10.
17. Le Q, Xu J, Deng SX. The diagnosis of limbal stem cell deficiency. Ocul Surf. 2018;16:58.
18. Lagali N, Edén U, Utheim TP, Chen X, Riise R, Dellby A, et al. In vivo morphology of the limbal palisades of vogt correlates with progressive stem cell deficiency in aniridia-related keratopathy. Investig Ophthalmol Vis Sci. 2013;54:5333.
19. Le Q, Chauhan T, Deng SX. Diagnostic criteria for limbal stem cell deficiency before surgical intervention—a systematic literature review and analysis. Surv Ophthalmol. 2020;65:32.
20. Mehtani A, Agarwal M, Sharma S, Chaudhary S. Diagnosis of limbal stem cell deficiency based on corneal epithelial thickness measured on anterior segment optical coherence tomography. Indian J Ophthalmol. 2017;65(11):1120–6.
21. Banayan N, Georgeon C, Grieve K, Ghoubay D, Baudouin F, Borderie V. In vivo confocal microscopy and optical coherence tomography as innovative tools for the diagnosis of limbal stem cell deficiency. J Fr Ophtalmol. 2018;41:e395.
22. Siamak ZG, Reza Alizadeh RA, Deng SX. Topical interferon alpha-2b for treatment of noninvasive ocular surface squamous neoplasia with 360° limbal involvement. J Ophthalmic Vis Res. 2014;9(4):423–6.
23. Tan JCK, Tat LT, Coroneo MT. Treatment of partial limbal stem cell deficiency with topical interferon α-2b and retinoic acid. Br J Ophthalmol. 2016;100:944.
24. Sun CC, Chiu HT, Lin YF, Lee KY, Pang JHS. Y-27632, a ROCK inhibitor, promoted limbal epithelial cell proliferation and corneal wound healing. PLoS One. 2015;10:e0144571.
25. Mittal V, Jain R, Mittal R. Ocular surface epithelialization pattern after simple limbal epithelial transplantation: an in vivo observational study. Cornea. 2015;34:1227.
26. Utheim TP, Aass Utheim Ø, Salvanos P, Jackson CJ, Schrader S, Geerling G, et al. Concise review: altered versus unaltered amniotic membrane as a substrate for Limbal epithelial cells. Stem Cells Transl Med. 2018;7:415.
27. Jackson CJ, Myklebust Ernø IT, Ringstad H, Tønseth KA, Dartt DA, Utheim TP. Simple limbal epithelial transplantation: current status and future perspectives. Stem Cells Transl Med. 2020;9:316.
28. Basu S, Mohan S, Bhalekar S, Singh V, Sangwan V. Simple limbal epithelial transplantation (SLET) in failed cultivated limbal epithelial transplantation (CLET) for unilateral chronic ocular burns. Br J Ophthalmol. 2018;102:1640.
29. Keivyon KR, Tseng SCG. Limbal autograft transplantation for ocular surface disorders. Ophthalmology. 1989;96:709.
30. Rao SK, Rajagopal R, Sitalakshmi G, Padmanabhan P. Limbal autografting: comparison of results in the

acute and chronic phases of ocular surface burns. Cornea. 1999;18:164.
31. Shimazaki J, Shimmura S, Tsubota K. Donor source affects the outcome of ocular surface reconstruction in chemical or thermal burns of the cornea. Ophthalmology. 2004;111:38.
32. Özdemir Ö, Tekeli O, Örnek K, Arslanpençe A, Yalçindağ NF. Limbal autograft and allograft transplantations in patients with corneal burns. Eye. 2004;18:241.
33. Rama P, Matuska S, Paganoni G, Spinelli A, De Luca M, Pellegrini G. Limbal stem-cell therapy and long-term corneal regeneration. N Engl J Med. 2010;363:147.
34. Sangwan VS, Basu S, Vemuganti GK, Sejpal K, Subramaniam SV, Bandyopadhyay S, et al. Clinical outcomes of xeno-free autologous cultivated limbal epithelial transplantation: a 10-year study. Br J Ophthalmol. 2011;95:1525.
35. Sejpal K, Ali MH, Maddileti S, Basu S, Ramappa M, Kekunnaya R, et al. Cultivated limbal epithelial transplantation in children with ocular surface burns. JAMA Ophthalmol. 2013;131:731.
36. Ganger A, Vanathi M, Mohanty S, Tandon R. Long-term outcomes of cultivated limbal epithelial transplantation: evaluation and comparison of results in children and adults. Biomed Res Int. 2015; 2015:1.
37. Fasolo A, Pedrotti E, Passilongo M, Marchini G, Monterosso C, Zampini R, et al. Safety outcomes and long-term effectiveness of ex vivo autologous cultured limbal epithelial transplantation for limbal stem cell deficiency. Br J Ophthalmol. 2017;101:640.
38. Shanbhag SS, Nikpoor N, Rao Donthineni P, Singh V, Chodosh J, Basu S. Autologous limbal stem cell transplantation: a systematic review of clinical outcomes with different surgical techniques. Br J Ophthalmol. 2020;104:247.
39. Basu S, Sureka SP, Shanbhag SS, Kethiri AR, Singh V, Sangwan VS. Simple Limbal epithelial transplantation: long-term clinical outcomes in 125 cases of unilateral chronic ocular surface burns. Ophthalmology. 2016;123:1000.
40. Vazirani J, Ali MH, Sharma N, Gupta N, Mittal V, Atallah M, et al. Autologous simple limbal epithelial transplantation for unilateral limbal stem cell deficiency: multicentre results. Br J Ophthalmol. 2016;100:1416.
41. Gupta N, Joshi J, Farooqui JH, Mathur U. Results of simple limbal epithelial transplantation in unilateral ocular surface burn. Indian J Ophthalmol. 2018;66:45.
42. Mittal V, Jain R, Mittal R, Vashist U, Narang P. Successful management of severe unilateral chemical burns in children using simple limbal epithelial transplantation (SLET). Br J Ophthalmol. 2016;100:1102.
43. Iyer G, Srinivasan B, Agarwal S, Tarigopula A. Outcome of allo simple limbal epithelial transplantation (alloSLET) in the early stage of ocular chemical injury. Br J Ophthalmol. 2017;101:828.
44. Singh D, Vanathi M, Gupta C, Gupta N, Tandon R. Outcomes of deep anterior lamellar keratoplasty following autologous simple limbal epithelial transplant in pediatric unilateral severe chemical injury. Indian J Ophthalmol. 2017;65(3):217–22.
45. Gupta N, Farooqui JH, Patel N, Mathur U. Early results of penetrating keratoplasty in patients with unilateral chemical injury after simple limbal epithelial transplantation. Cornea. 2018;37:1249.
46. Roux LN, Petit I, Domart R, Concordet JP, Qu J, Zhou H, et al. Modeling of aniridia-related keratopathy by CRISPR/Cas9 genome editing of human limbal epithelial cells and rescue by recombinant PAX6 protein. Stem Cells. 2018;36(9):1421–9.
47. Hayashi R, Ishikawa Y, Ito M, Kageyama T, Takashiba K, Fujioka T, et al. Generation of corneal epithelial cells from induced pluripotent stem cells derived from human dermal fibroblast and corneal limbal epithelium. PLoS One. 2012;7:e45435.
48. Erbani J, Aberdam D, Larghero J, Vanneaux V. Pluripotent stem cells and other innovative strategies for the treatment of ocular surface diseases. Stem Cell Rev Rep. 2016;12:171.

13 Unsalvageable Eye: Cosmetic Rehabilitation

Kasturi Bhattacharjee, Ganesh Ch. Kuri, and Shyam Sundar Das Mohapatra

An unsalvageable eye is a blind eye, often has a structural deformity making it a cosmetic unacceptable condition for a patient. The rehabilitation of such patients is challenging, as often these patients undergo immense psychological distress arising out of this unsalvageable ocular condition.

Trauma, especially armed conflicts, are important issues that attract national and international attention. Through a variety of mechanisms, trauma results in significant ocular morbidity for victims. Ocular damage from trauma can arise either due to direct damage to the globe by projectiles or blast effects, or indirect damage via traumatic optic nerve or brain injury, which includes ruptured globe, foreign body (intraocular or orbital), orbital fracture and traumatic optic neuropathy (Fig. 13.1a). Certain injuries of the affected eye, including penetrating or perforating injuries, prolapse of ocular contents, more extensive or posterior globe lacerations and post-traumatic endophthalmitis are associated with extremely poor prognosis and ultimately lead to blindness, painful or unsightly eye [1].

When an eye is blind, painful or unsightly and unsalvageable in nature, removal of the eye may be indicated. Suitable orbital implants are used to restore orbital volume following removal of the eye with precisely fabricated ocular prosthesis fitted over it to give the best cosmetic outcome.

A number of different surgical and rehabilitation techniques are available and will be discussed here.

13.1 Surgical Techniques

Enucleation and evisceration surgeries involve permanent removal of the patient's eye.

1. **Enucleation:** Enucleation is the surgical technique of removal of the entire globe.
2. **Evisceration:** Evisceration is a surgical technique, in which the intra-ocular contents are removed entirely, leaving behind the scleral shell, extraocular muscle and optic nerve attachments intact.

13.1.1 Pre-operative Investigations

13.1.1.1 B Scan Ultrasonography

(a) To examine the ocular structure, integrity and its contents.
(b) To exclude the presence of any intraocular or orbital foreign body (FB).
(c) To measure the normal eye axial length (for calculation of the size of the orbital implant).

K. Bhattacharjee (✉)
Oculoplastics, Aesthetics and Reconstructive Surgery, Sri Sankaradeva Nethralaya, Guwahati, Assam, India

G. C. Kuri · S. S. D. Mohapatra
Sri Sankaradeva Nethralaya, Guwahati, Assam, India

S. Waikar (ed.), *Ocular Trauma in Armed Conflicts*, https://doi.org/10.1007/978-981-19-4021-7_13

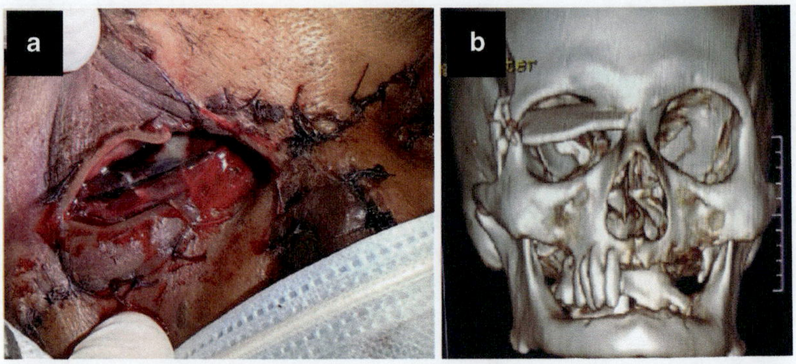

Fig. 13.1 Blast injury causing extensive direct damage to the globe, orbit and adnexal region by a projectile glass particle impacted by the right orbit (**a**) CT scan with 3D reconstruction showing a large impacted orbital FB with associated orbital wall fractures (**b**)

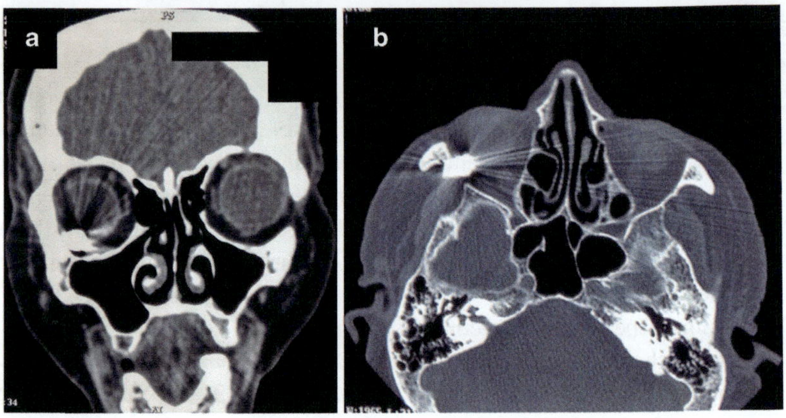

Fig. 13.2 CT scan of orbit showing a bullet in the infero-temporal part of right orbit (**a**, **b**) associated with extensive globe injury following a gunshot injury

(d) To rule out any suspected/coexisting intraocular tumor or malignancy, mandatory before evisceration surgery.

13.1.1.2 Computed Tomography (CT)/ Magnetic Resonance Imaging (MRI) Scan

(a) To assess the extent of damage to the globe, orbit and adjacent structures.
(b) In case of any intraocular or orbital foreign body (FB), for assessing exact location and extent of damage. In metallic FBs, MRI scan is absolutely contraindicated. CT scan is indicated in such cases (Figs. 13.1b and 13.2a, b).
(c) To assess the volume of the socket.
(d) In case of suspected/coexisting orbital malignancy or intraocular malignancy with orbital/extraocular spread.

13.1.2 Pre-operative Counseling

- The ophthalmologist should detail the patient about the disease condition and available management strategies before proceeding for the surgery as this causes a permanent loss of the eye.
- The patient requires reassurance and psychological support by the ophthalmologist.
- The patient needs to be explained regarding the available surgical procedures with all the pros and cons of each procedure, nature of the post-operative anophthalmic socket and about the ocular prosthesis and its fitting after a minimum period of 6 weeks after the surgery.
- The ophthalmologist should explain the indications of the surgery in detail to each patient.

13.1.3 Enucleation

Enucleation is the removal of the entire globe and optic nerve from the orbit, along with the separation of all its connections.

13.1.3.1 Indications

1. Severe trauma and risk of sympathetic ophthalmia, without any prospect of visual recovery.
2. Cosmetic deformity, blindness and unsightly eyes.
3. Other indications include painful blind eye, phthisis bulbi, intraocular tumors (where the tumor is left intact within the eye for histopathological examination) and microphthalmia with cyst.

13.1.3.2 Contraindications

1. Panophthalmitis.
2. Endophthalmitis, without any prospect of visual recovery.

13.1.3.3 Surgical Techniques

Principle

The entire globe is removed in toto by excising the extraocular muscles and transecting the optic nerve.

Method

Two surgical techniques are described here:

1. Enucleation with placement of a simple sphere implant.
2. Enucleation with placement of a donor sclera-covered porous implant for improved motility.

Enucleation with Placement of a Simple Sphere Implant

- The procedure is performed as a day care surgery under local anesthesia with a peribulbar or retrobulbar block in an adult patient. General anesthesia is required for children and apprehensive adults.
- A self-retaining lid speculum is placed to expose the entire epibulbar surface.
- A 360° conjunctival peritomy is performed (Fig. 13.3a). Tenon's fascia is bluntly dissected from the sclera in all four quadrants (Fig. 13.3b). Relaxing incisions are given at 3 and 9 o'clock positions.
- Each of the four rectus muscles are sequentially gathered on a muscle hook (Fig. 13.3c) and detached from the globe after securing them with double-armed 6-0 Vicryl sutures (Fig. 13.3d).
- The superior oblique tendon is detached directly from the globe.
- The inferior oblique muscle is secured with a 6-0 Vicryl suture and then detached. Later on, it is reattached to the inferior border of the lateral rectus muscle. This is perhaps more important as the inferior oblique muscle acts as a "hammock" for the orbital implant that provides improved motility to the anophthalmic socket.
- After detaching the extraocular muscles, the next step is to detach the optic nerve from the globe. Anterior traction across the globe helps in cutting the optic nerve. The Well's enucleation spoon with optic nerve guide is inserted laterally to identify and engage the optic nerve behind the globe.
- With the Well's enucleation spoon in place, a slender, curved pair of Metzenbaum scissors is used to transect the optic nerve, and the entire eyeball is removed (Fig. 13.3e).
- Orbital packing with direct pressure for 5-10 minutes is applied immediately to achieve adequate hemostasis.
- Polymethyl methacrylate (PMMA) orbital implant of 20 mm diameter is generally adequate for an average-sized adult orbit. The orbital implant is inserted behind the posterior Tenon's fascia through the central rent left by cutting the optic nerve.
- Multiple interrupted 6-0 Vicryl sutures are used to close the posterior Tenon's fascia that overlies the orbital implant.

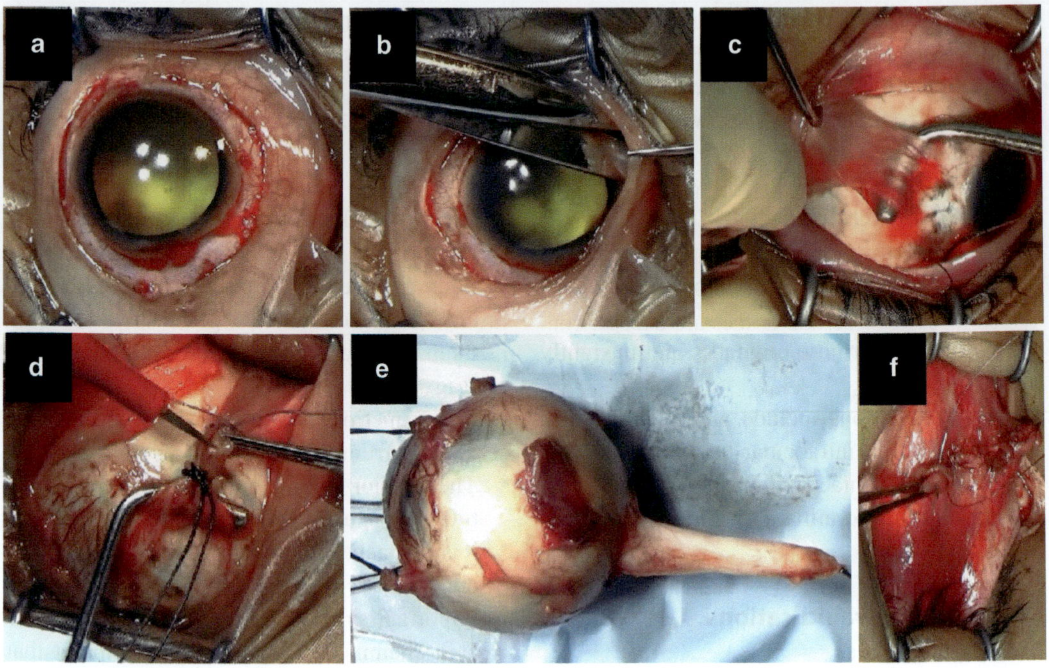

Fig. 13.3 (a–f) Surgical technique of enucleation

- Each of the four rectus muscles are sutured to the adjacent fornix through Tenon's fascia and conjunctiva using preplaced double armed 6-0 vicryl sutures (Myoconjunctival Technique). This Myoconjunctival technique will provide enhanced motility to the ocular prosthesis.
- After anterior Tenon's fascia is closed in the midline with 6-0 Vicryl sutures, the conjunctival edges are loosely approximated with a 6-0 Vicryl running suture (Fig. 13.3f).
- A broad-spectrum ophthalmic antibiotic ointment is applied to the conjunctival fornices.
- A clear, acrylic conformer of adequate size is placed and pressure bandage is applied over the socket.

Enucleation with Placement of a Donor Sclera-Covered Porous Implant

- A standard enucleation technique is performed, as already described.
- The appropriate orbital implant size may be selected by using sterile orbital implant sizers, although an 18–20 mm implant may be appropriate in most cases. Wrapping the orbital implant with sclera or fascia adds approximately 1–1.5 mm to the overall diameter of the implant.
- If a wrapping material such as sclera is used, the scleral shell should be cut to the appropriate size and shape to enclose the implant securely. Sclera is closed securely with multiple interrupted 6-0 Vicryl sutures.
- The round opening of the scleral shell from where the cornea was removed should be positioned posteriorly.
- Rectangular windows, approximately 2–4 mm, are cut through the sclera located within 8–10 mm from the anterior most apex of the implant for attachment of the extraocular muscles.
- A 20-gauge needle is used to create drill holes manually at the site of each window and at the site of the posterior round corneal window to promote further fibrovascular ingrowth into a porous hydroxyapatite implant.
- After placing the wrapped or unwrapped implant into the anophthalmic socket, the four rectus muscles are sutured to the anterior lip of the corresponding rectangular scleral windows.

- Anterior Tenon's fascia is then sutured with multiple interrupted 6-0 Vicryl sutures.
- The conjunctiva is closed with a loosely running continuous 6-0 Vicryl suture.
- A broad-spectrum ophthalmic antibiotic ointment is applied to the conjunctival fornices.
- A clear, acrylic conformer of adequate size is placed and pressure bandage is applied over the socket.

  The unique properties of porous implants allow fibrovascular ingrowth and integration of the implant with ocular prosthesis. Thus porous implants are most appropriate for patients who desire maximum prosthesis motility, for which a second-stage procedure of motility peg insertion is required. Titanium motility pegs are surgically inserted after adequate fibrovascular ingrowth has occurred into the hydroxyapatite implant.

Post-operative Care

- The pressure bandage is to be kept in place for 3–4 days postoperatively.
- After its removal, the patient can be advised for cold compression with ice.
- Systemic antibiotics and analgesics and topical antibiotic eye ointments are prescribed as appropriate.
- Ocular prosthesis is given after a period of 6 weeks once the socket is completely healed.

Complications

- Orbital implant exposure or extrusion: Meticulous closure of Tenon's fascia and proper selection of the implant material and size are important to avoid this outcome. The risk of implant extrusion is greater if there is a history of prior irradiation to the eye and orbit, severe traumatic injuries and infections in the eye and orbit.
- Generalized volume deficiency of the anophthalmic socket.
- Lower eyelid laxity with poor prosthesis support.
- Orbital implant migration.
- Upper eyelid ptosis.
- Chronic conjunctivitis with mucoid discharge.
- Integrated orbital implants (e.g., hydroxyapatite) with motility pegs have high complication rates, including pyogenic granuloma formation around the peg and chronic anophthalmic socket secretions.

Evisceration

Evisceration is a surgical technique which involves the removal of the entire intraocular content, leaving the scleral shell, extraocular muscle and optic nerve attachments intact.

Evisceration is a simpler procedure than enucleation and offers better preservation of the orbital anatomy and natural motility of the anophthalmic socket tissues.

Indications

1. Post-traumatic panophthalmitis
2. Post-traumatic endophthalmitis, without any prospect of visual recovery (Fig. 13.4a, b)
3. Anterior Staphyloma, causing cosmetic deformity, blindness and unsightly eye
4. Total sloughed out corneal ulcer in a blind eye

Contraindications

1. Severe trauma with a potential risk of sympathetic ophthalmia
2. Severely deformed eyes with phthisis or scleral contracture
3. Documented or suspected intraocular malignant tumors

13.1.3.4 Surgical Techniques

Principle

The entire intraocular contents are removed leaving the scleral shell, extraocular muscle and optic nerve attachments intact.

Method

- The procedure is performed as a day care surgery under local anesthesia with a peribulbar or retrobulbar block in an adult patient. General anesthesia is required for children and apprehensive adults.
- The procedure begins with a 360° conjunctival peritomy (Fig. 13.5a).

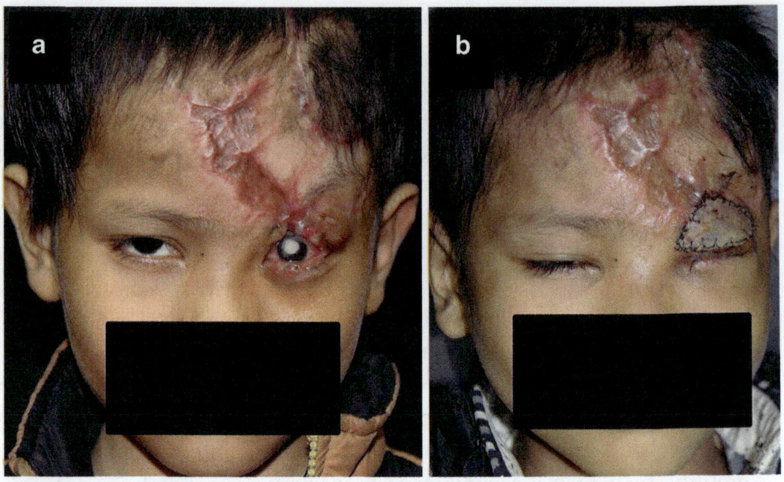

Fig. 13.4 Penetrating globe injury leading to post-traumatic endophthalmitis with no visual potential, with associated lacerations of forehead and upper eyelid (**a**), managed with evisceration of the left eye and eyelid reconstruction with skin grafting (**b**)

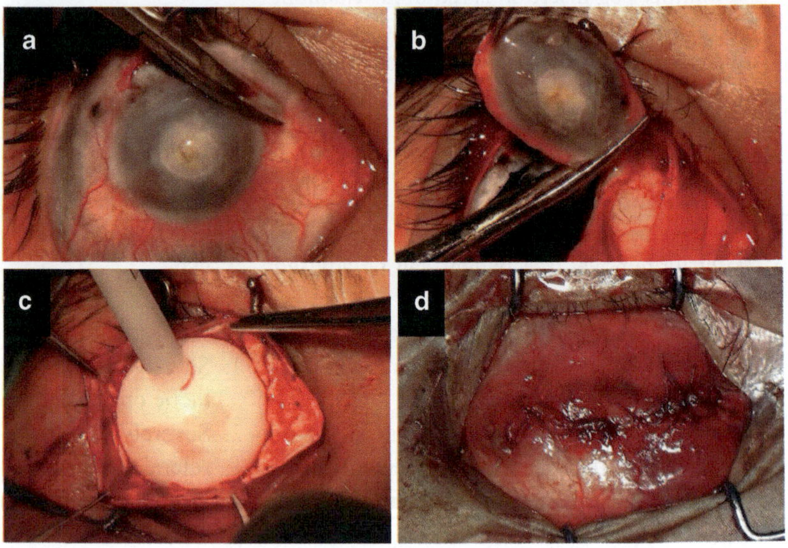

Fig. 13.5 (**a**–**d**) Surgical technique of evisceration

- Blunt dissection of Tenon's fascia from the underlying sclera is carried out in all four quadrants.
- A full-thickness incision is made around the corneal limbus with a sharp scalpel blade, followed by removal of the entire corneal button (Fig. 13.5b).
- The sclera is grasped with forceps and a cyclodialysis spatula is used to separate the iris root and ciliary body from the sclera.
- The remaining part of the uveal tissue is separated from the scleral shell back to the attachment around the optic nerve with the help of an evisceration spoon.
- The intraocular contents are removed from the scleral shell (and can be submitted for histopathological/microbiological examination if necessary).
- All remnants of uveal tissue are carefully removed from the scleral shell with an evisceration curette.
- 70% ethanol saturated in cotton-tip applicators may be used to denature any remnant of uveal tissue and to clean the interior of the scleral shell completely.
- Any oozing of blood may be controlled by application of cautery, if required.

- Orbital implant sizers are used to accurately select the orbital implant of appropriate diameter (Fig. 13.5c).
- A spherical PMMA implant is placed within the empty scleral shell. An orbital implant of 14–16 mm is usually placed when the cornea is removed.
- The scleral edges are sutured securely, with multiple interrupted 6-0 Vicryl sutures, and the medial and lateral scleral edges are cut to reduce any dog ears.
- Anterior Tenon's fascia is sutured with multiple interrupted 6-0 Vicryl sutures.
- The conjunctiva is gently closed with a running 6-0 Vicryl suture (Fig. 13.5d).
- A broad-spectrum ophthalmic antibiotic ointment is applied to the conjunctival fornices.
- A clear, acrylic conformer of adequate size is placed and pressure bandage is applied over the socket.
- If a larger implant is desired, it is necessary to perform radial relaxing sclerotomy incisions posteriorly between the rectus muscles. If a porous implant is used, such sclerotomy openings are necessary to enhance vascular ingrowth.

Sclerotomy Techniques for Evisceration

Using the conventional evisceration technique, as described previously, the largest implant that fits inside the scleral cavity without undue tension is 18 mm. If a larger implant is desired, it is necessary to perform different sclerotomy incisions.

Various sclerotomy techniques have been described, all aiming to overcome this drawback.

1. Multiple radial sclerotomy: In 1987, Stephenson reported performing multiple radial expansion sclerotomies as well as a posterior spiral sclerotomy [2].
2. Posterior sclerotomy: In 1995, Kostick and Linberg described a posterior sclerotomy [3].
3. Disinsertion of the optic nerve: In 1997, Jordan and Anderson described disinsertion of the optic nerve and small radial sclerotomies. [4]
4. Scleral quadrisection: By Huang D et al., the technique left the optic nerve intact [5]
5. Intraconal implant placement: By Long et al., placing the implant behind the sclera within the muscle cone [6].
6. Oblique splitting of the scleral cavity: In 2001, Massry and Holds described obliquely splitting the scleral cavity in two parts and releasing the flaps from their optic nerve attachments [7].
7. Four petal techniques: In 2007, Sales-Sanz and Sanz-Lopez described a technique wherein they performed four complete sclerotomies from the limbus to the optic nerve and disinsertion of the optic nerve (Fig. 13.6) [8].
8. Wedge excision of sclera: Georgescu et al. described a technique for phthisis bulbi and microphthalmos, where a 5 mm wedge of sclera was excised both nasally and temporally and a 360° equatorial scleral incision was made, dividing the sclera into anterior and posterior halves [9].

The advantage of intraconal placement of orbital implant is that it allows a larger implant placement and gives an extra barrier to the posterior sclera.

Sclerotomy openings are necessary to enhance vascular ingrowth within the orbital implant if a porous implant is used.

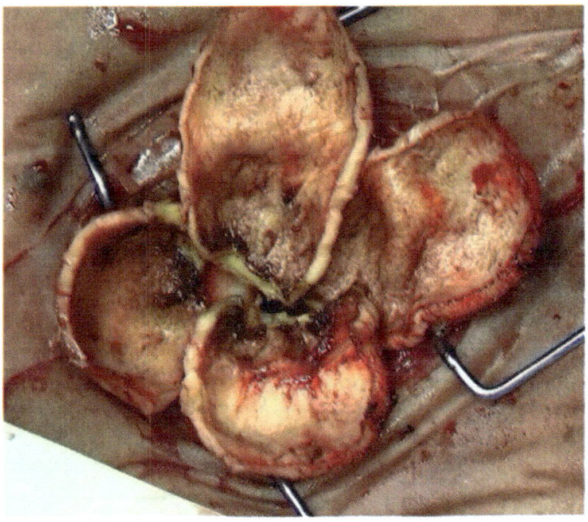

Fig. 13.6 Four petal sclerotomy techniques for evisceration

Post-operative Care

- The pressure bandage is to be kept in place for 3–4 days postoperatively.
- After its removal, the patient can be advised for cold compression with ice.
- Systemic antibiotics and analgesics and topical antibiotic eye ointments are prescribed as appropriate.
- Ocular prosthesis is given after a period of 6 weeks once the socket is completely healed.

Complications

- Postoperative infection, especially when performed in the setting of panophthalmitis or endophthalmitis. The use of broad-spectrum systemic antibiotics usually minimizes its risk and the surgeon can defer the use of a primary orbital implant.
- Postoperative extrusion of the orbital implant.
- Postoperative scleral shell shrinkage.
- Poor wound healing of the scleral edges.
- Postoperative pain is more common in cases where the cornea is retained.

13.2 Orbital Implants

Orbital implants are medical prosthesis used to replace orbital volume and allow some amount of realistic movement of the prosthetic eye following enucleation or evisceration (Fig. 13.7).

Removal or loss of an eye is immense psychological distress for any patient. Providing an appropriate implant with a well fitted prosthetic eye can go a long way to alleviate this pain.

In 1884 implants were first described by Mules [10], and ever since then different implant materials, designs and shapes have been tried [11]:

Type	Definition	Example
Non-integrated	Implant has no direct or indirect integration with orbital structures or prosthesis	PMMA, acrylic, silicone implants etc
Semi-integrated	Implant has indirect (mechanical) integration with the orbital structures, but not with the prosthesis	Allen implant
Integrated	Implant has indirect (mechanical) integration with the orbital structures and with the prosthesis	Cutler's implant
Bio-integrated	Implant has direct (biological) integration with the orbital structures, but may or may not be integrated with the prosthesis	Hydroxyapatite, Porus polyethylene, Aluminium oxide etc
Biogenic	An autograft or allograft of a natural human tissue, which has direct (biological) integration with the orbital structures, but not with the prosthesis	Dermis-fat graft (Fig. 13.8), temporalis muscle-fascia graft, cancellous bone graft, cartilage graft etc

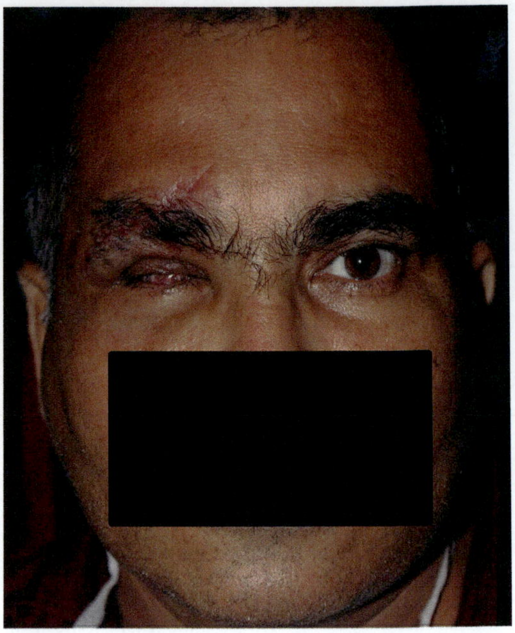

Fig. 13.7 Traumatic eyelid and globe injury with no visual potential, managed by evisceration with orbital implant

The shapes of the implants are usually spherical and the diameter ranges from 12–24 mm.

Implants can be wrapped using different materials before implantation. Wrapping of an implant and choice of wrapping materials have various advantages and disadvantages, and are still a matter of debate among the surgeons. Different wrapping materials have been tried [12, 13]:

Type	Example	Advantage	Disadvantage
Organic (autologous and heterologous)	1 Autologous materials like temporalis fascia, rectus abdominis sheath, fascia lata 2 Heterologous materials like human donor sclera (Fig. 13.9), human donor pericardium, fascia lata, sclera, bovine pericardium, and acellular dermis	1 Better integration of the implant with orbital structures 2 Reduces the chance of implant-related complications like exposure, extrusion and migration 3 Give better amount of realistic movement to the prosthetic eye 4 Increases the success rate of the surgery	1 Potential risk of disease transmission 2 Need of second surgical site for autologous materials 3 Prolongation of the surgical time 4 Increased morbidity of the patient 5 Increase the cost of the surgery. 6 Heterologous materials may not be readily available
Alloplastic	Undyed Polyglactin 910 mesh	1 Better integration of the implant with orbital structures. 2 Reduces the chance of implant-related complications like exposure, extrusion and migration. 3 Give better amount of realistic movement to the prosthetic eye 4 Increases the success rate of the surgery 5 No risk of disease transmission 6 No need for a second surgical site for autologous materials 7 No increase in morbidity of the patient	1 Prolongation of the surgical time 2 Increase the cost of the surgery

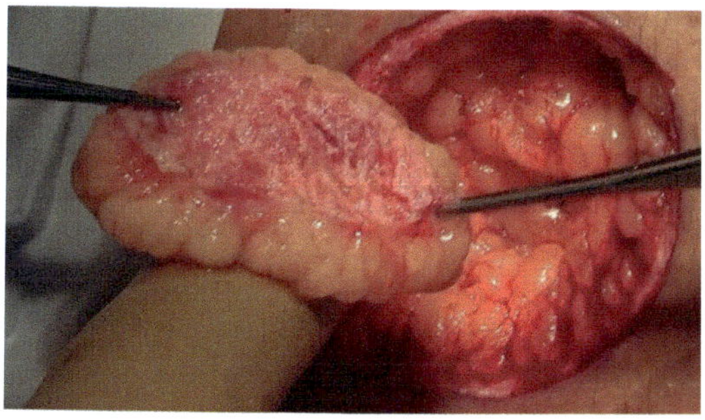

Fig. 13.8 Dermis fat graft

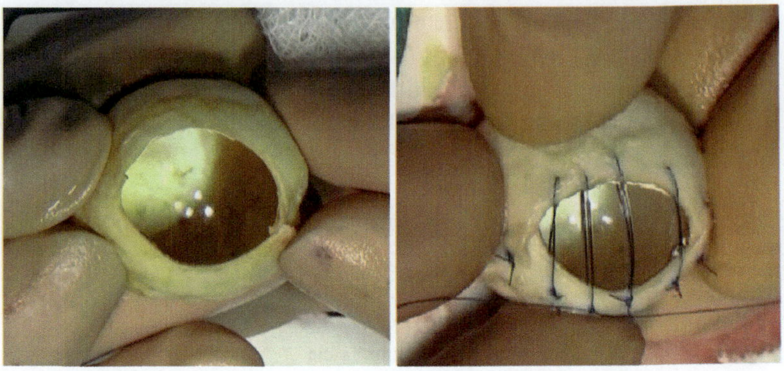

Fig. 13.9 Acrylic orbital implant wrapped with human donor sclera

13.2.1 Complications [14]

1. Implant exposure and extrusion
2. Implant migration
3. Primary or secondary infection
4. Insufficient orbital volume
5. Permanent pain
6. Thinning/erosion of conjunctive
7. Conjunctival cyst formation
8. Foreign body reaction
9. Deficiency of conjunctival fornices
10. Ptosis
11. Erosion of the implant

13.3 Ocular Prosthesis

An ocular prosthesis is an artificial substitute for the bulb of an enucleated eye ball. An optimal ocular prosthesis not only gives a good cosmetic outcome, but also improves the psychological state and confidence level of the patient [15].

13.3.1 Indications of Ocular Prosthesis

1. Status post enucleation/evisceration
2. Phthisical eye
3. Atrophic bulbi
4. Corneal Scar, causing cosmetic deformity in a blind eye
5. Congenital anophthalmia/microphthalmia

13.3.2 Types of Ocular Prosthesis

1. Conformer/Clear Shell
2. Scleral Shell
3. Full thickness prosthesis
   (a) Stock prosthesis
   (b) Custom-made prosthesis

13.3.3 Conformer or Clear Shell

After enucleation or evisceration, a clear acrylic plastic shell (Conformer) is fitted temporarily to maintain the shape of the conjunctival fornices and also allows the eye lids to blink over the shell without rubbing on the suture line. The conformer remains in situ for at least 6 weeks until the socket heals completely (Fig. 13.10).

13.3.4 Scleral Shell

Scleral shell is made of thin transparent hard plastic material with a central dark painted area resembling the cornea. This can be fitted over a minimally shrunken eyeball with total corneal opacity. The central dark painted disc shaped area hides the opacified cornea.

13.3.5 Full Thickness Prosthesis

A full thickness ocular prosthesis can be ready-made (stock prosthesis) (Fig. 13.11a) or custom-made prosthesis (Fig. 13.11b).

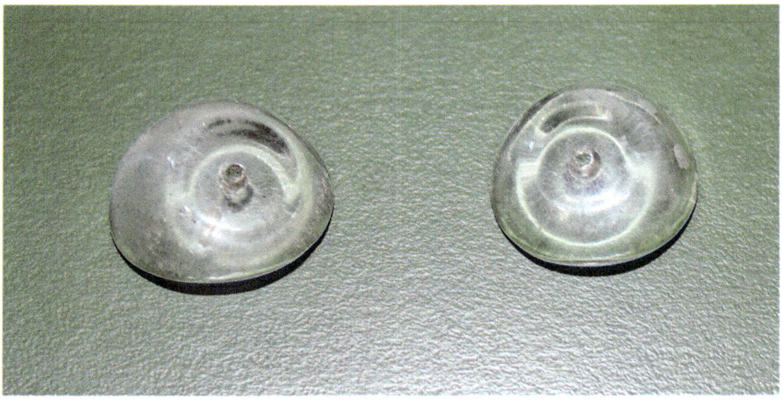

Fig. 13.10 Clear acrylic plastic shell (Conformer)

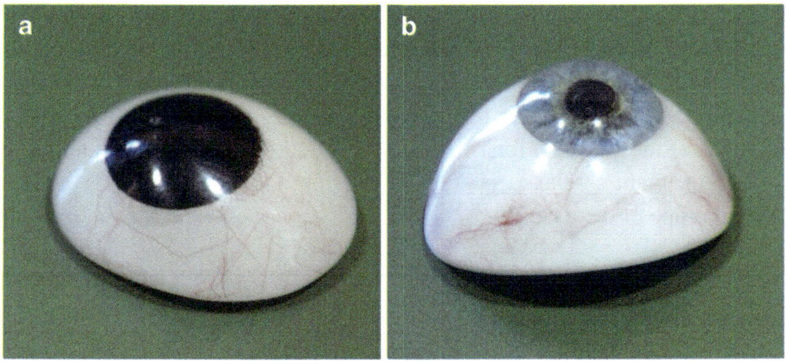

Fig. 13.11 Full thickness prosthesis. Readymade (stock prosthesis) (**a**) and custom-made prosthesis (**b**)

13.3.6 Stock Prosthesis

These are readymade prosthesis made up of acrylic material and are available in standard sizes and shapes. These are fitted to a patient when time limitation exists and the cost factor is taken into consideration.

13.3.6.1 Advantages

1. Readily available in the market
2. Available in standard sizes and shapes
3. Can be given to a patient when time limitations exist
4. Less expensive compared to custom-made prosthesis

13.3.6.2 Disadvantages

1. Made of low grade materials
2. Fitting may be improper
3. Poor symmetry with a fellow eye
4. Improper shade matching the fellow eye
5. Lesser movement of the prosthesis
6. No modification is possible

13.3.7 Custom-Made Prosthesis

These are made of high grade acrylic material and are customized for superior fitting in the anophthalmic socket. These are painted manually for accurate color matching with the fellow eye. This type of prosthesis is fabricated as per the patient's specifications to provide optimum cosmesis, excellent symmetry and color match.

13.3.7.1 Advantages

1. Prepared according to the actual measurements of the anophthalmic socket of the patient.
2. Made of high grade materials.
3. Fitting is excellent.
4. Excellent adaptiveness of the patient to the prosthesis.
5. Excellent symmetry with a fellow eye.
6. Proper shade matching the fellow eye.
7. Better movement of the prosthesis.

8. Modifications are possible to address issues like ptosis, socket expansion without surgery etc.

13.3.7.2 Disadvantages

1. Not readily available in the market
2. Can't be given to a patient when time limitations exist
3. More expensive compared to stock prosthesis

13.3.8 Method of fabrication [16]

13.3.8.1 Impression Tray Selection

Stock acrylic ocular impression trays (Fig. 13.12) or conformer is selected that fits perfectly into the confines of the socket (Fig. 13.13a). The patient should maintain a relaxed posture to provide a natural drape of the tissues.

13.3.8.2 Impression

The patient should look straight ahead, keeping all the facial muscles relaxed. Algination of a very runny consistency is filled into a syringe and then injected into the impression tray through the inlet. It is slowly filling into the socket to prevent overfilling. Adequate filling of the socket is indicated by flowing out of little amount of material through the inner canthus.

After solidification, the impression is removed by pulling the lower lid downwards and laterally and taking the impression out from the upper eyelid gently in an arc-like path. Washing and disinfection of the impression is performed then. The impression allows matching of the volume and lid contours as of the fellow eye (Fig. 13.13b).

13.3.8.3 Making a Wax Pattern

The silicone putty index is made of the impression. Once it sets, it is cut open and liquid wax is injected into it. Once the wax pattern is hardened, it is gently retrieved, cooled in cold water and smoothened. The wax pattern is then tried in the patient's socket for fitting, comfort, bulkiness of the pattern, movements of the pattern and of the eyelids over it (Fig. 13.13c). Adjustments are made as necessary. Corneal prominence is checked by standing behind the patient, retracting the eyelids and asking the patient to look downward.

13.3.8.4 Iris Painting

Paintings are done manually with acrylic pigments on a flat acrylic disc. The ocularist performs this step with the patient sitting in front so as to accurately match its color with the fellow eye. Natural daylight is preferred for coloring of the prosthesis. The base color is applied first, followed by the applicationof the other highlights in layers with fine strokes, resembling the spokes in a wheel. The pupil is represented by applying a small black dot in the center of the

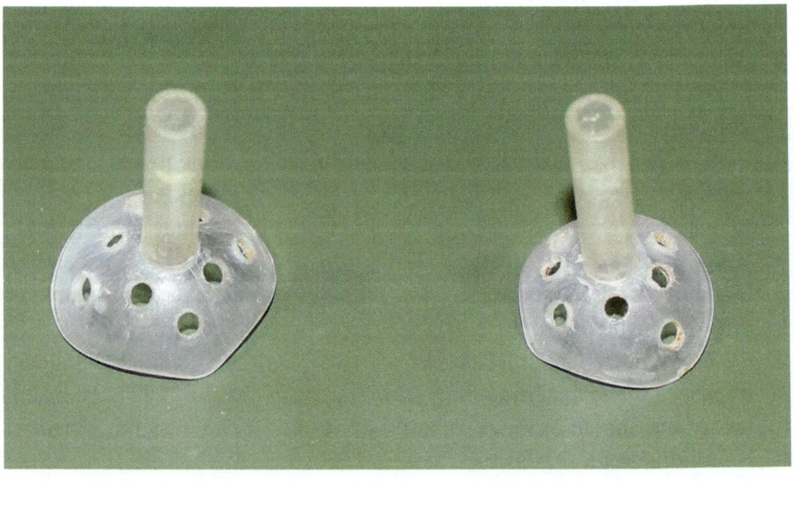

Fig. 13.12 Stock acrylic ocular impression tray

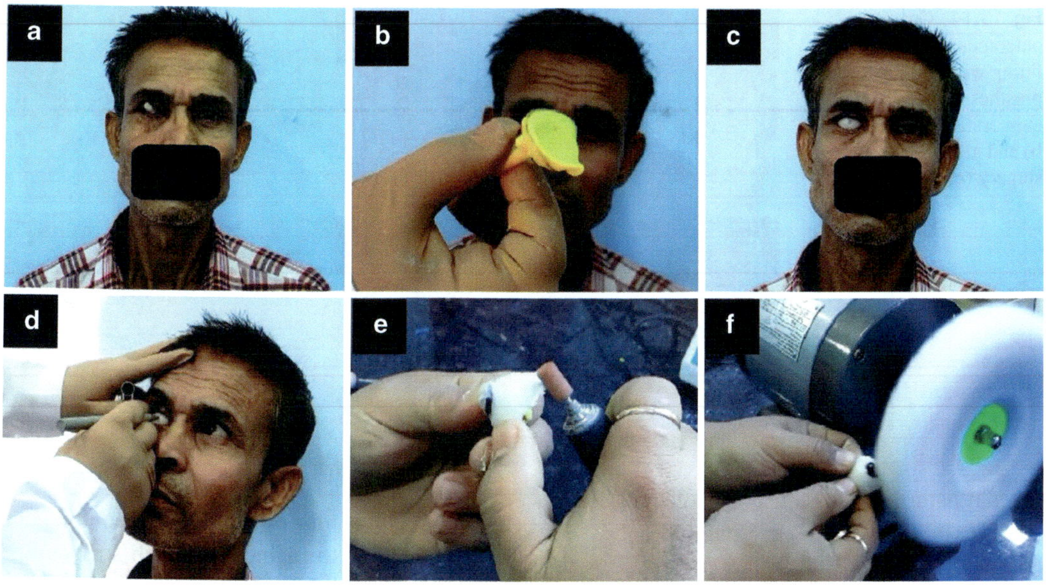

Fig. 13.13 (a–f) Fabrication of custom-made prosthesis

iris. Careful attention is given to create a realistic and accurate match with the fellow eye of the patient.

13.3.8.5 Acrylic Capping of the Iris

After the iris painting is completed, a clear acrylic dome is added over the painted surface, similar to a cornea. This dome helps in bringing up the depth and magnifies the details of the iris. The acrylic cap is precisely cut into a series of angles to blend perfectly with the scleral portion of the prosthesis.

13.3.8.6 Fabrication of Base Sclera Shell

The wax pattern is then flasked in a two-part flask using dental plaster. Once it sets, the wax pattern is removed and the flask is packed with acrylic material for fabrication of the base scleral shell. The acrylic prosthesis is then retrieved and the excess part of the acrylic surface is trimmed down. The iris portion of the acrylic prosthesis is made almost flat in correspondence to the level of the iris plane of the natural eye. Rounding off the margins and smoothening of the surface of the acrylic prosthesis are then carried out.

13.3.8.7 Positioning of the Iris

The position and the plane of the iris are marked while the patient is wearing the wax pattern (Fig. 13.13d). This step ensures that the iris position on the completed prosthesis will match perfectly with the fellow eye.

13.3.8.8 Attachment of the Iris

The iris is then attached to the base scleral shell using acrylic glue in the exact plane and position as measured previously. It is important to give the overall excellent cosmetic outcome of the final ocular prosthesis.

13.3.8.9 Coloring of the Sclera Shell and Veining

The color of the sclera is matched to the adjacent eye and veining is done to give it a natural look by replicating the blood vessels.

13.3.8.10 Clear Resin Coating and Finishing

A layer of clear resin is added onto the painted prosthesis. The clear resin coating brings up the depth and natural appearance of the prosthesis. Trimming of the rough edges of the prosthesis is performed (Fig. 13.13e). Finally, the prosthesis is

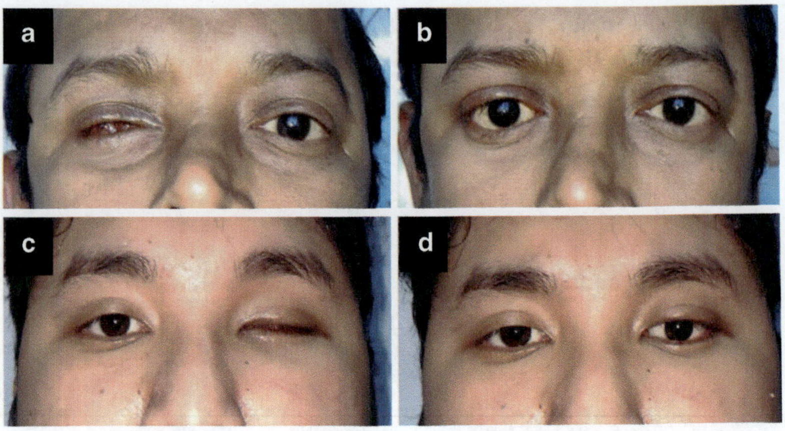

Fig. 13.14 Cosmetic outcomes following fitting with full thickness prosthesis after evisceration surgery (**a**, **b**) and after enucleation surgery (**c**, **d**)

given a natural glossy finish by polishing it with the help of polishing burs, pumice and a buff (Fig. 13.13f).

13.3.9 Patient Education Regarding Prosthesis Care

The patient is taught how to place and remove the prosthesis. Initially, patients may experience minimal discomfort, to which they get adjusted within a short span of time. Instructions regarding care and hygiene are explained in detail to the patient.

1. Handling of the prosthesis should be very minimal.
2. The prosthesis can be removed once a day for washing properly with soap and water, followed by drying and fitting again by the patients themselves.
3. Patient should be instructed to sleep with the prosthesis in place always.
4. Lubricating eye drops can be applied over the prosthesis. It ensures smooth eyelid movements over the prosthesis and also washes off the debris deposited on the surface of the prosthesis.
5. Frequent removal of the prosthesis should be avoided as this may lead to watering, discharge, eyelid laxity, eyelid eversion and inadequacy of space for fitting of the prosthesis.
6. Polishing of the prosthesis is recommended once a year to maintain smooth surface and regular rounded edges of the prosthesis, which prevents any undue friction between the eyelids and the prosthesis, thus preventing any inflammatory reaction of the socket such as a granuloma formation and giant papillary reaction in the eyelids.
7. Ideally, the prosthesis should be changed once every 5 years depending upon the morphological changes that occur in the socket.
8. Patients should use a full-framed protective polycarbonate glass to protect their fellow eyes from any kind of injury. This will also camouflage any differences between the prosthetic eye and the normal fellow eye (Fig. 13.14).

Acknowledgement Mr. Jico Gogoi, Ocularist, Sri Sankaradeva Nethralaya, Guwahati.

References

1. Morley MG, Nguyen JK, Heier JS, Shingleton BJ, Pasternak JF, Bower KS. Blast eye injuries: a review for first responders. Disaster Med Public Health Prep. 2010;4(2):154–60.
2. Stephenson CM. Evisceration of the eye with expansion sclerotomies. Ophthalmic Plast Reconstr Surg. 1987;3(4):249–51.
3. Kostick DA, Linberg JV. Evisceration with hydroxyapatite implant. Surgical technique and review of 31 case reports. Ophthalmology. 1995;102(10):1542–8, discussion 1548–9.

4. Jordan DR, Anderson RL. The universal implant for evisceration surgery. Ophthalmic Plast Reconstr Surg. 1997;13(1):1–7.
5. Huang D, Yu Y, Lu R, Yang H, Cai J. A modified evisceration technique with scleral quadrisection and porous polyethylene implantation. Am J Ophthalmol. 2009;147(5):924–8, 928.e1–3.
6. Long JA, Tann TM 3rd, Girkin CA. Evisceration: a new technique of trans-scleral implant placement. Ophthalmic Plast Reconstr Surg. 2000;16(5):322–5.
7. Massry GG, Holds JB. Evisceration with scleral modification. Ophthalmic Plast Reconstr Surg. 2001;17(1):42–7.
8. Sales-Sanz M, Sanz-Lopez A. Four-petal evisceration: a new technique. Ophthalmic Plast Reconstr Surg. 2007;23(5):389–92.
9. Georgescu D, Vagefi MR, Yang CC, McCann J, Anderson RL. Evisceration with equatorial sclerotomy for phthisis bulbi and microphthalmos. Ophthalmic Plast Reconstr Surg. 2010;26(3):165–7.
10. Mules PH. Evisceration of the globe, with artificial vitreous. Trans Ophthalmol Soc. 1885;5:200–6.
11. Bhattacharjee K, Barman MJ, Ghosh S. Orbital implants. Surgical ophthalmic oncology. Cham: Springer; 2019. p. 141–3.
12. Jordan DR, Klapper SR. Wrapping hydroxyapatite implants. Ophthalmic Surg Lasers. 1999;30(5):403–7.
13. Klapper SR, Jordan DR, Punja K, Brownstein S, Gilberg SM, Mawn LA, Grahovac SZ. Hydroxyapatite implant wrapping materials: analysis of fibrovascular ingrowth in an animal model. Ophthalmic Plast Reconstr Surg. 2000;16(4):278–85.
14. Piškinienė R, Banevičius M. Complications of orbital endoimplantation in the eye clinic of the Lithuanian University of health sciences. Acta Med Litu. 2017;24(2):101–6.
15. Raizada K, Rani D. Ocular prosthesis. Cont Lens Anterior Eye. 2007;30(3):152–62.
16. Sethi T, Kheur M, Haylock C, Harianawala H. Fabrication of a custom ocular prosthesis. Middle East Afr J Ophthalmol. 2014;21(3):271–4.

14 Orbital and Maxillofacial Injuries

N. Girish Kumar and Sabari Girish Nair

14.1 Introduction

According to the World Health Organization, injury was the cause of 5.8 million deaths worldwide in the year 2000 [1]. Injury is the main cause of death in the age group 5–44 years. in the United States. However, the effect of injury on society cannot be assessed by taking the mortality rate alone. Years of Productive Life Lost (YPLL) and Disability Adjusted Life Years (DALY) should also be considered to understand the implications of injury to society. For every death related to injury, there are an estimated 30 patients seriously injured and another 300 treated for less serious injuries. Nonfatal injuries account for a fifth of diseases being treated. In addition, a large number of injuries are not reported [2].

In 2012, an estimated 1,64,000 people died related to war and conflict, corresponding with about 0.3% of global deaths, and increasing to over 2,00,000 conflict deaths in 2014. These estimates do not include deaths due to the indirect effects of war and conflict on the spread of diseases, poor nutrition and the collapse of health services [3]. Armed violence resulting in injury has become a global health problem. Across the world, approximately 3,00,000 people die annually due to firearms in armed conflict situations, while another 2,00,000 people die every year in non-conflict situations due to firearm injury [4]. They represent a quarter of 2.3 million deaths due to violence, of which 42% are due to suicides, 38% homicide and only 26% war related [5]. At the same time, on the battlefield, 90% of the casualties are due to splinter injuries and only 15–20% due to Gun Shot Wounds (GSW) [6, 7].

The incidence and severity of conflicts are increasing throughout the world today. There is no area, region or country that is immune to terrorist attacks. These may be individual or group events; the degree may vary from a stabbing spree to a bomb blast depending on the situation. In such a scenario, it becomes imperative for every health care professional to know how to diagnose injuries afflicted by such events, the immediate emergency measures required to limit morbidity and mortality and the final definitive management and rehabilitation.

The face is an important part of our body responsible for self-recognition, vision, olfaction, hearing, mastication, breathing, verbal and non-verbal communication. It is the most prone to injuries in assaults and accidents. The psychological impact of facial disfigurement is devastating (Fig. 14.1).

N. G. Kumar (✉) · S. G. Nair (Deceased)
ECHS, Medical College, Trivandrum, India

S. Waikar (ed.), *Ocular Trauma in Armed Conflicts*, https://doi.org/10.1007/978-981-19-4021-7_14

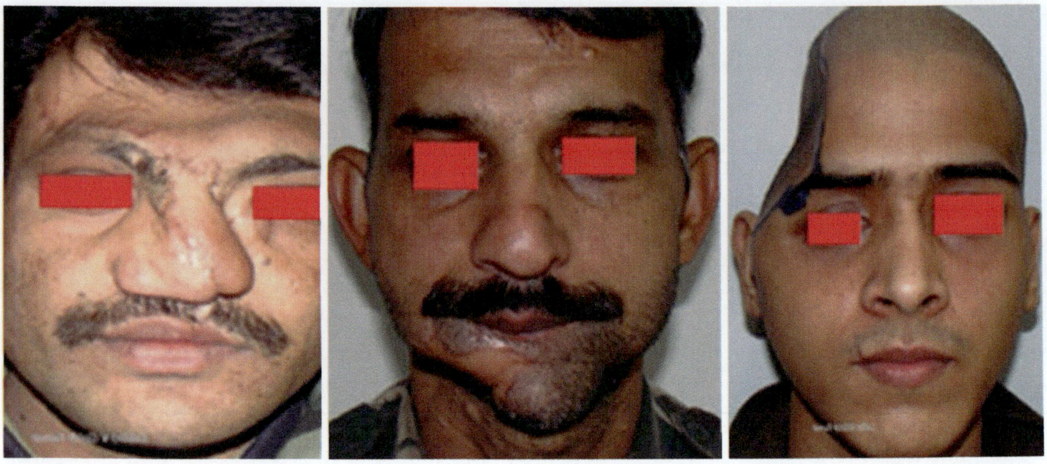

Fig. 14.1 Post-traumatic Facial defects

The brain and the cranial nerves have a close association with the face. The development and use of body armor in conflict situations has led to an increase in injuries to the extremity, head and face. In a study by Shapiro et al., 10.5% of all trauma admissions in a Level I trauma center had a facial fracture [8]. The overall mortality of patients with facial fracture was 8.7%. Even though, face accounts for only 0.035% of the total body surface area, it is commonly involved in traumatic injuries especially in conflict zones as it is left exposed and prominent. Bullet-proof vests and helmets cover most of the areas leaving the face and extremities exposed. In a study by Rai et al., 38% of patients in a conflict situation had multiple injuries leading to polytrauma. Of these, 14.2% had head and neck injuries, 13.3% chest wounds, 13.5% abdominal injury and 59% extremity wounds [9] (Fig. 14.2).

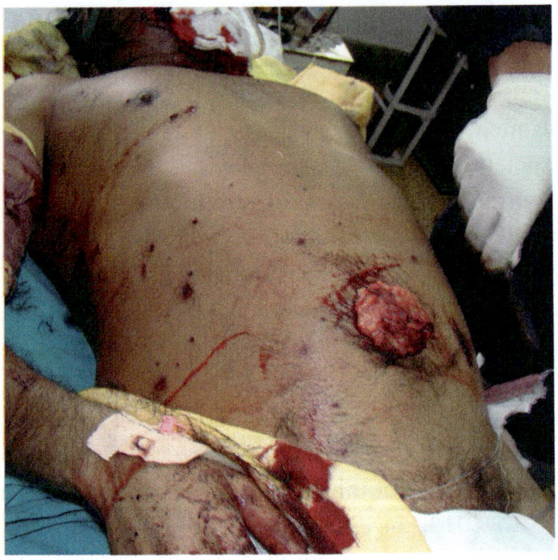

Fig. 14.2 Associated Injuries

Triage of mass casualties with multiple system injuries will have to be done by both military and civilian medical personnel as such situations will overwhelm the existing facilities. For this, all medical personnel should be prepared to provide optimum care that will save lives and morbidity. An understanding of the nature of weapons and the physiological consequences of these weapons of war and terror is essential for prompt and optimal management. The first time is the best time to achieve good results. Any secondary correction will always be suboptimal. To achieve optimal aesthetics and function with minimal morbidity, a multispecialty interdisciplinary team approach is a must.

14.2 Modes of Trauma

The main modes of trauma are blunt trauma and penetrating trauma. Blunt trauma is caused by physical assault with a blunt weapon, road traffic accidents or falls. The forces that lead to blunt trauma are due to sudden deceleration or acceleration where either the victim is in motion and strikes another object or the object is in motion and strikes the victim. Due to this, the victim may suffer a soft tissue injury, a bony injury or a combination of both. Soft tissue injuries may vary from mild abrasion to degloving injury with loss of tissue. It may lead to damage to certain vital structures or organ systems. Bony injuries may vary from an undisplaced fracture to a comminuted displaced fracture with loss of bone.

Penetrating trauma can be grouped into low velocity, medium velocity and high velocity. Examples of low velocity trauma are those due to knife attacks, impalement and low velocity bullets. In these cases, the damage is limited to the track created by the wounding object. In the case of medium velocity trauma, the projectile (high velocity bullets and shrapnel) (Fig. 14.3) enters the tissue to create a permanent cavity and a temporary cavity.

The permanent cavity is the localized area of necrosis along the tract of the bullet. The temporary cavity is a transient lateral displacement of the tissues which is caused by the shock waves generated by the bullet. The damage caused by this depends on the elasticity of the tissues. The entrance wound of a gunshot can be seen as an oval or circular wound with a punched-out clean appearance of the margins (Fig. 14.4). A contusion ring may also be present. Entrance wound

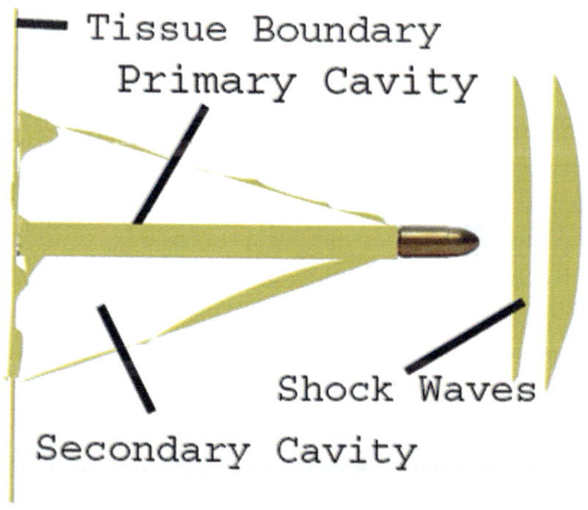

Fig. 14.3 Sketch depicting the primary and secondary cavitation caused by projectiles in the body

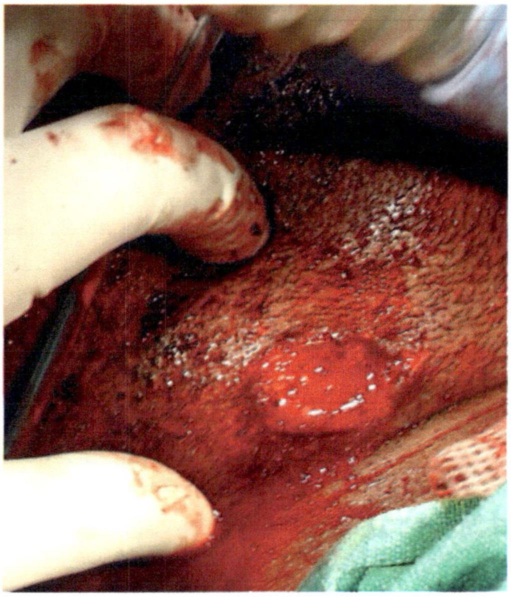

Fig. 14.4 Entrance wound of a bullet

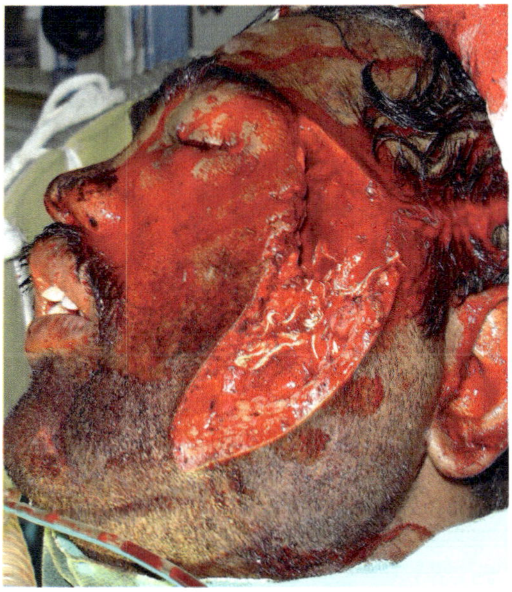

Fig. 14.5 Exit wound of the same bullet

through soft tissue overlying bone is usually stellar in appearance. Exit wounds are usually larger and more irregular. There will be eversion of the margins with irregular skin tags (Fig. 14.5). Shock waves are transmitted to the mandible when a bullet hits it, causing a fracture of the teeth at the cervical margin.

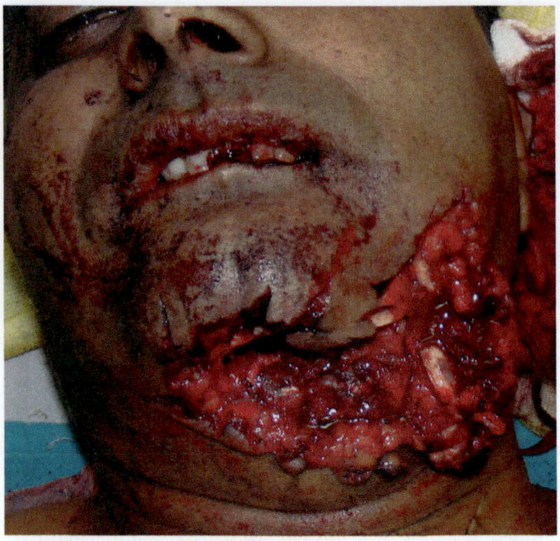

Fig. 14.6 Blast Injury of the face showing the ragged tissue margins, comminution of bone and loss of soft and hard tissue

Blast injuries are caused by bombs and Improvised Explosive Devices (IEDs). These results in the rapid release of enormous amounts of energy, leading to the generation of tremendous amounts of heat and a blast wave that travels outward at supersonic speeds. This blast wave interacts with the body tissues to create stress waves and shear waves. Stress waves create high local forces that are reinforced and reflected at tissue interfaces, thus enhancing the injury potential. Organs containing air or liquids like the lungs, auditory system and intestines are the most affected by these stress waves. Shear waves cause asynchronous movement of tissues resulting in tearing of tissue and possible destruction of attachments (Fig. 14.6). Another set of injuries in the blast trauma were caused by shrapnel released by the explosion. The material may vary from steel particles contained in the IED, automobile parts in a car bomb or fragments of wood, steel or glass from the environment. They typically cause penetrating injuries. They also carry a lot of dirt and contaminants along with them. The fourth type of injury seen is thermal injuries from the heat generated. It depends on the distance of the victim from the blast site.

14.3 Presentation

The presentation of maxillofacial injuries varies depending on the type of force applied, the angle of incidence and the site of occurrence. Generally, maxillofacial injuries appear macabre due to the high vascular supply of the tissues. However, it is not life threatening in most cases. The type of presentation depends upon the nature of force, site of application of the force and the type of tissue acted upon. The type of force may be penetrating or blunt. In penetrating injuries caused by sharp objects, the injury is usually localized and clear cut (Fig. 14.7). The extent of the injuries is clearly visible. In the case of blunt trauma (Fig. 14.8), the extent of injury is not obvious. One has to look for tissue damage in a systematic manner to avoid mistakes and misdiagnosis. In the case shown in Fig. 14.8, even though there are no lacerated wounds, there are panfacial injuries involving the frontal bone, midface and the mandible, as is evident in the three dimensional CT reformatted image (3D-CT).

14.3.1 Clinical Divisions of Face

The face is divided into upper, middle and lower thirds from a clinical point of view (Fig. 14.9). The three regions have their own peculiar features which influence the type of injury seen. The upper third arises from the hairline to the eyebrow and is formed by the frontal bone. Injuries to the upper third are characterized by the involvement of frontal sinuses and orbital roof which dictate the type of treatment required. The middle third extending from the eyebrow to the upper lip is comprised of very thin bones which crumple on impact and thus absorbs a lot of force protecting the eye and the brain except for the vertical and horizontal buttresses. These injuries can cause disturbances in vision, CSF leaks and difficulty in respiration, mastication and speech. The lower third, which extends from the lower lip to chin is the only mobile part and generally fractures at the weakest points, namely angle, the

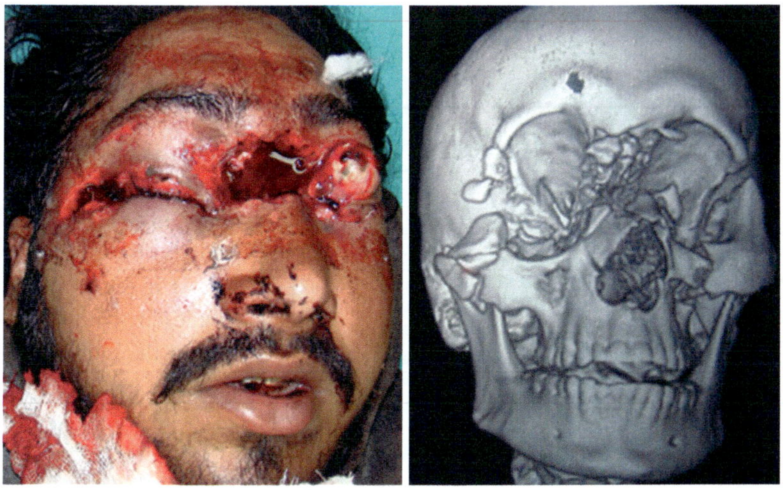

Fig. 14.7 Penetrating Injury – Clinical and Radiological picture

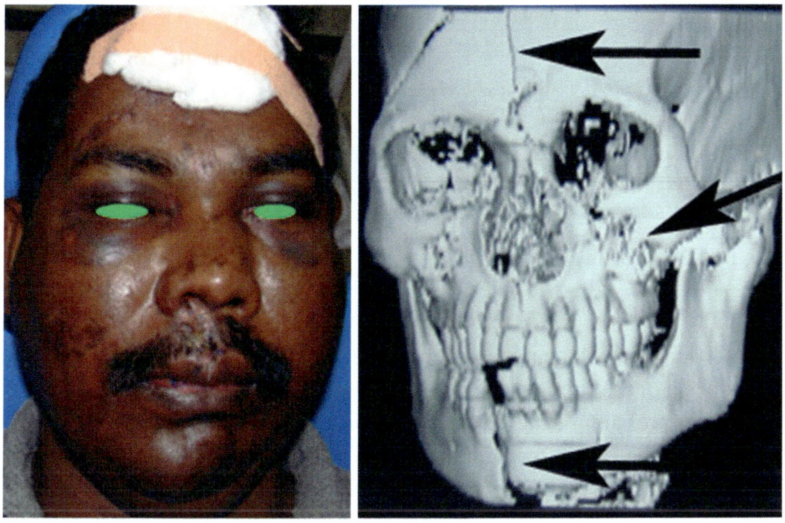

Fig. 14.8 Blunt Injury – Clinical and Radiological picture. 3D-CT shows fractured frontal bone, fractured maxilla and fractured mandible

parasymphysis region and the subcondylar region. Injuries to this region can also interfere with respiration, mastication and speech.

14.3.2 Upper Third Injuries

The upper third is mainly constituted by the frontal bone which forms the anterior cranial base and is very strong. Any fracture of the upper third is likely to have an associated head injury as the force required to fracture the frontal bone is 200 g (force of gravity) [10]. In addition, the patient may have cervical injury in up to 20% of cases and another life-threatening injury elsewhere in 30% of such cases [11]. Garg et al. suggested a novel classification of frontal bone fractures which had correlation with the severity of the head injury based on CT scan findings [12]. They found that vertical fractures with the frontal sinus and orbital extension, and fractures that penetrated the middle or posterior cranial fossa had the strongest association with intracranial injuries, optic neuropathy, disability, and death ($p < 0.05$). The presentation includes depression of contour, step deformity of the

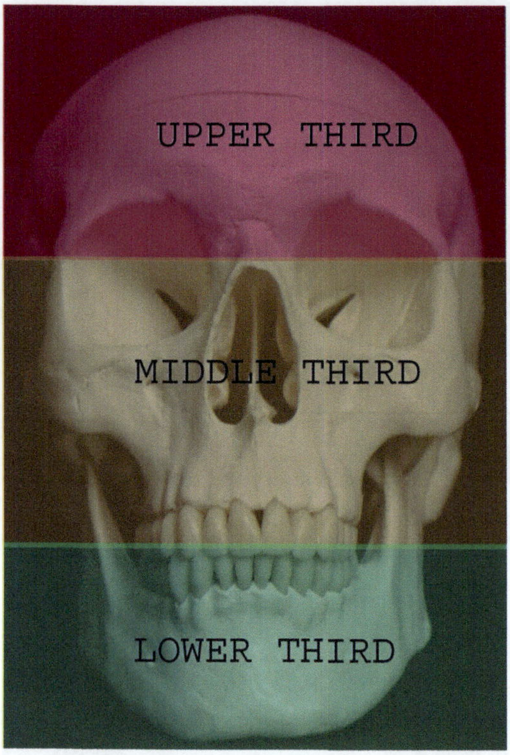

Fig. 14.9 Clinical divisions of the face

supraorbital rims, subcutaneous emphysema and paresthesia of the supraorbital and supratrochlear nerves. Depression of the forehead can be easily missed in the acute presentation due to the accompanying soft tissue oedema. In conscious patients, facial pain is a common symptom. Laceration, contusion, or hematoma to the forehead should make the surgeon suspect frontal sinus injury. In few cases, brain may be seen through lacerations. Cerebrospinal fluid (CSF), rhinorrhea or CSF in the wound can present in as many as one third of patients with frontal sinus fractures. From a surgical point of view, the frontal bone may be classified into medial fractures, lateral fractures and the combination. The medial fractures usually do not involve the cranial cavity and affect the frontal sinus (Fig. 14.10). In severe cases of trauma, both the inner table and the outer table are damaged leading to cranial involvement. For lateral fractures, the orbital roof may be involved and need special consideration (Fig. 14.11). These types of injuries are seen when the patient's head hits an object from the side. Lacrymal gland, which is also located in the region, may be affected. In combination, the trauma is so severe that the whole forehead is involved bilaterally and needs neurosurgical intervention (Fig. 14.12). In cases of gunshot wounds, the brain is usually seen through the wound if the frontal lobe is involved. Gunshot wounds in other areas of the brain may not be seen as they rarely survive. The clinical features are given in Table 14.1.

14.3.3 Middle Third Injuries

The middle third of the face is composed of a complex of bones consisting of the paired maxilla, palatine, zygomatic, lacrimal, inferior conchae and the unpaired vomer and the ethmoid bones. This region is composed of very thin bones supported by vertical and horizontal buttresses (Fig. 14.13). Most of the fractures in this region are termed complex as they involve more than one bone. The most important structure in the middle third are the eyes. They are protected by the orbital rims which are composed of dense cortical bone. The orbital walls on the other hand are usually thin except for the lateral orbital wall composed of the orbital surface of the zygoma and the greater wing of the sphenoid bone. The orbital walls are further weakened by superior and inferior orbital fissures. The floor and medial walls are the ones most frequently fractured sometimes, even without a rim fracture, leading to a blowout fracture. The weakest part of the orbital wall is the region on the floor just medial to the infraorbital groove and is the most common site of blowout fracture. The maxillary sinus and ethmoidal air cells act as airbags to protect the eye. Even though there are a wide variety of classifications of the middle third fractures, from a practical and clinical view point, middle third fractures can be grouped into naso-orbital, maxillary, zygomatic and orbital. Many a time, there may be a combination of the above.

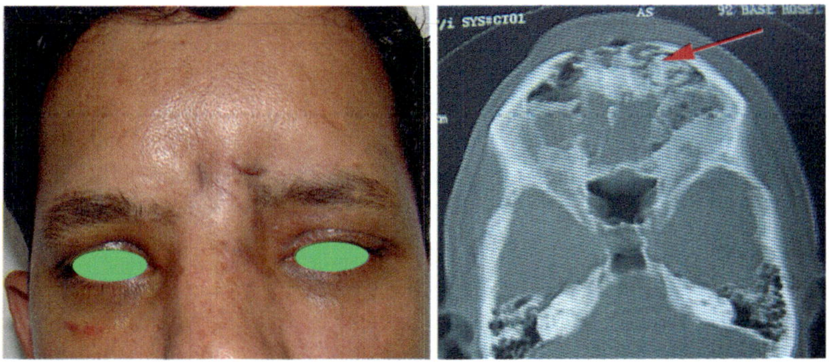

Fig. 14.10 Frontal Bone Medial fractures- clinical and CT picture

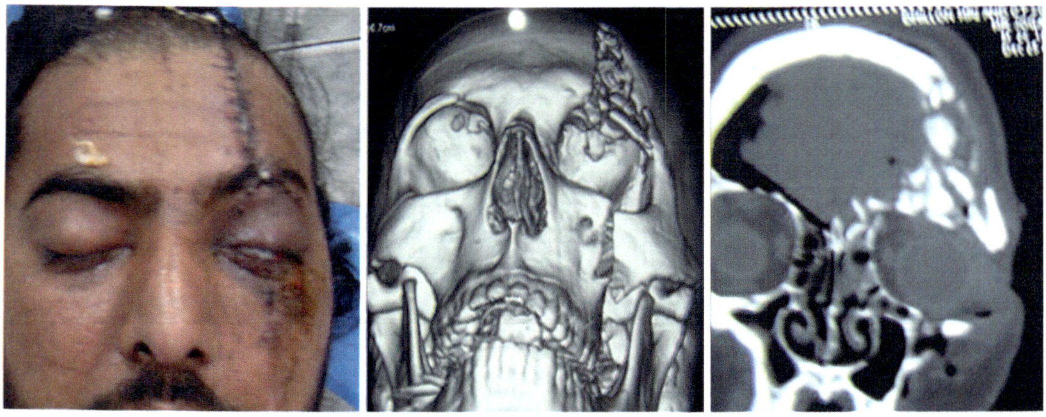

Fig. 14.11 Frontal bone lateral fracture - clinical and radiological picture

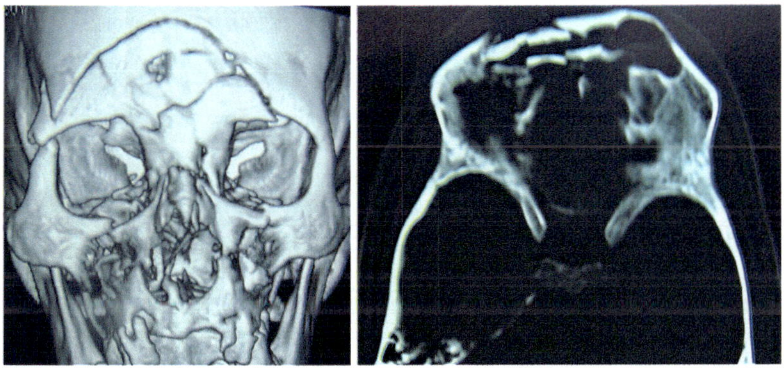

Fig. 14.12 Frontal Bone fracture- combination involving the medial and the lateral

14.3.4 Nasoorbital Fractures

Naso-orbital fractures may vary from a simple nasal bone fracture, which is the most common, to a complex fracture involving the nasal bone, frontal process of maxilla, lacrimal bone and ethmoid. This type of fracture involves the medial orbital wall and leads to disruption of the medial canthal ligament, lacrimal apparatus, fracture of the cribriform plate leading to CSF rhinorrhea and severe epistaxis from the anterior and posterior ethmoidal arteries (Fig. 14.14). The main clinical features associated with this fracture include depression of the nasal bridge, epistaxis,

Table 14.1 Clinical signs and symptoms of facial trauma

Symptoms/ signs	Upper third injuries	Middle third injuries	Lower third injuries
Symptoms	Pain, numbness, fainting, cut, swelling, bleeding, deformity	Pain, numbness, cut, swelling, bleeding, deformity, difficulty in opening eye, loss or diminished sight, double vision, difficulty in closing mouth	Pain, numbness, cut, swelling, bleeding, deformity, difficulty in opening mouth, difficulty in closing mouth, dev
Signs	Laceration, contusion, deformity, oedema, hemorrhage, loss of consciousness, hematoma / ecchymosis, sensory/motor deficit, crepitus, tenderness, step deformity,	Laceration, contusion, periorbital ecchymosis, subconjunctival ecchymosis, hemorrhage, Telecanthus, orbital dystopia, periorbital oedema, difficulty in opening eyes, restriction of eye movement, ocular injuries, enopthalmos/ exophthalmos, epiphora diminished vision, diplopia, epistaxis, subcutaneous emphysema, dystopia, CSF rhinorrhea/ otorrhea, crepitus, tenderness, step deformity, motor/sensory nerve deficit, difficulty in opening mouth/closing mouth, mobility of fractured fragments, elongation of face, dish face deformity, raccoon eyes, palatal hematoma (Guerin's sign), split palate, occlusal derangement	Pain, laceration, contusion, sensory deficit, oedema, hemorrhage, deformity, restriction in mouth opening, deviation of jaw on opening, tenderness/step deformity, deranged occlusion, open bite

Fig. 14.13 Midface Buttresses (Red arrows) and sites of stabilization

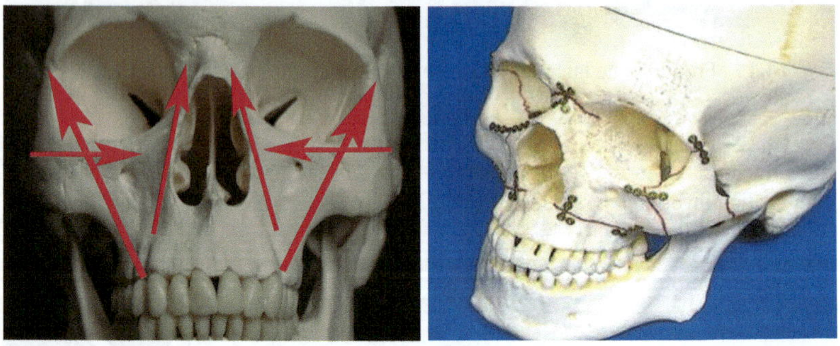

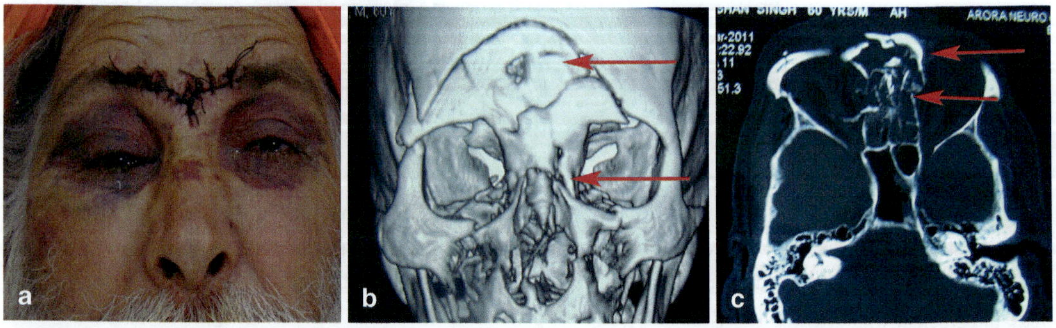

Fig. 14.14 Naso-orbital fracture – clinical and radiologic pictures. (**a**) Showing bilateral circum-orbital ecchymosis. (**b**) 3D-CT showing the nasal bone fracture. (**c**) Axial CT scan showing nasal bone fracture (White Arrow) and ethmoid fracture (Black arrow)

CSF rhinorrhea, telecanthus, shortening of the palpebral fissure, subconjunctival ecchymosis and epiphora.

14.3.5 Maxillary Fractures

The Le Fort series of fractures are those involving the maxilla above the palate and alveolus and extend through the lateral nasal wall and the pterygoid plates and are grouped into I –III depending on the extent of involvement. Le Fort- I involve only the alveolar part of maxilla and the palatine bone and so is a low-level fracture which extends from the pyriform rim backwards and outwards along the buttress and crosses the pterygomaxillary junction to fracture the lower third of the pterygoid plates (Fig. 14.15). In this type of fracture, maxilla is generally mobile and so called the floating maxilla. Sometimes there is a split of the horizontal palatine process leading to an oronasal fistula. Hematoma in the greater palatine foramen region is pathognomonic of Le Fort- I fracture. Le Fort- II fracture is a pyramidal fracture starting from the nasal bone extending laterally to involve the medial wall of the orbit, infraorbital margin around the infraorbital foramen and then down along the zygomaticomaxillary suture to end in the middle third of the pterygoid plates (Fig. 14.16). This produces the

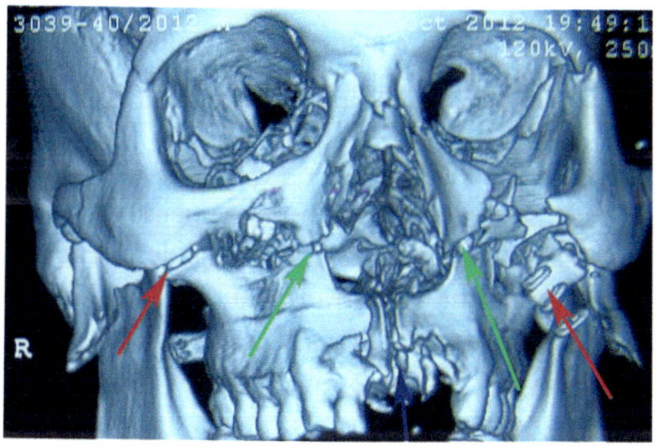

Fig. 14.15 3D-CT showing the line of fracture in Le Fort I. The red arrows show the fracture at the zygomatic buttress, the green arrows at the frontomaxillary buttress and the blue arrow at the midline split of palate

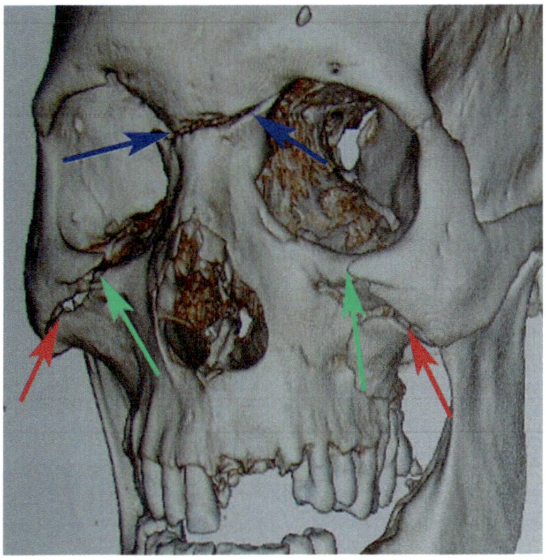

Fig. 14.16 3D- CT showing Le Fort II fracture. Red arrows at the zygomatic buttress, green arrows at the infraorbital margin and blue arrows at the nasal bone fracture

characteristic dish face deformity. In this type of fracture, maxilla is generally displaced downwards and backwards and is most commonly impacted. Hence, there may not be mobility of the fragment and at times it takes considerable force to disimpact the maxilla during reduction. The Le Fort- III fracture is actually a craniofacial dysjunction characterized by the separation of the entire face from the cranium. The fracture starts from the frontonasal suture that extends laterally to involve the frontomaxillary suture, extends posteriorly through the ethmoid bone below the optic foramen through the pterygopalatine fossa and fractures the upper third of the pterygoid plates (Fig. 14.17). The whole face is mobile, leading to lengthening of the face. Although the fractures of the maxilla have been classically grouped into these three types, Patil et al. found that only 24% of the maxillary fractures follow this pattern [13]. In a collective review of maxillary fractures, Phillips and Turco found that Le Fort I, II and III occurred in 16%, 19% and 30% of facial trauma cases. They also found that the majority of these trauma cases were due to motor vehicle accidents [14].

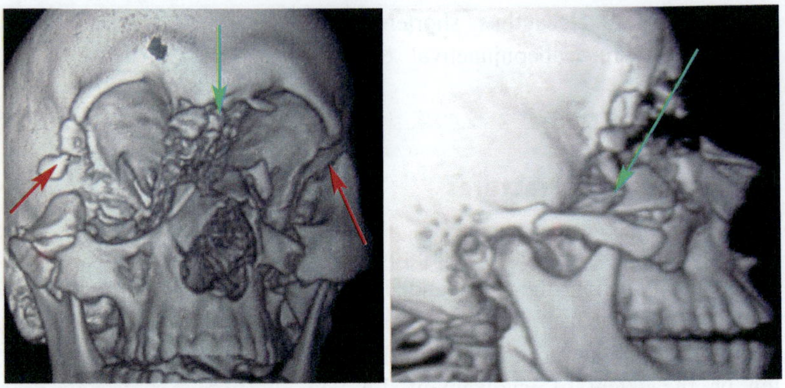

Fig. 14.17 3D CT showing the Le Fort III level fracture frontal and lateral view. The red arrows at the frontozygomatic suture, the blue arrow at the frontomaxillary suture. The green arrow in the picture on the right shows the downward and backward movement of the facial skeleton along the cranial base

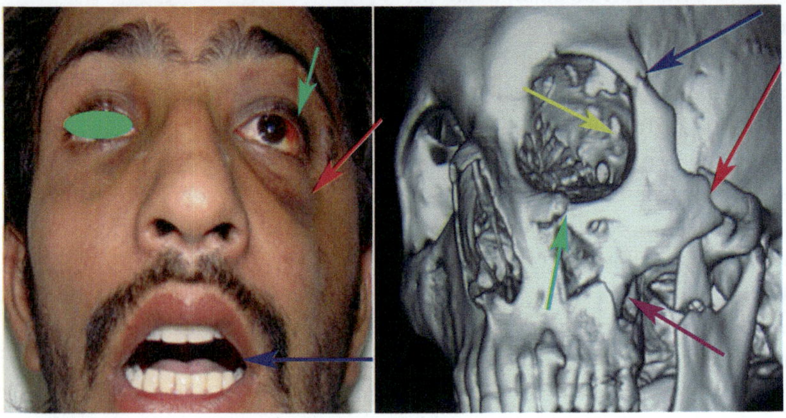

Fig. 14.18 Clinical and radiologic pictures of zygomatic complex fractures. The green arrow on the left picture shows the presence of subconjunctival ecchymoses, the red arrow depicts the malar depression and the blue arrow shows the restriction of mouth opening. The blue, red, purple, green and yellow arrows on the right show the fracture at FZ suture, zygomatic arch, zygomatic buttress, infraorbital margin and spheno-zygomatic suture respectively

14.3.6 Zygomatic Complex Fractures

The lateral group includes fractures of the zygomatic complex, again the term used because of the usual involvement of more than one bone in such fractures. This can vary from a simple fracture of the zygomatic arch to a comminuted fracture of the zygomatic complex. Sometimes the zygoma is pushed inwards and so the fracture line may not be visible in the CT. This is seen when the force is applied from the lateral aspect of the body of the zygoma. If force is applied from the front, in many cases this leads to lateral, outward and downward displacement of the zygoma leading to lowering of the eye level and enopthalmos. Fig. 14.18 depicts the typical clinical and radiological features of fractured zygoma. Any subconjunctival hemorrhage without a visible posterior limit is diagnostic of zygomatic complex fractures. Other key clinical features include restriction in mouth opening, malar depression and tenderness / step deformity in zygomatic buttress, infraorbital and frontozygomatic (FZ) suture regions. If the zygoma is significantly displaced outwards and downwards, lowering of the globe is also seen.

14.3.7 Orbital Blowout Fractures

The orbital fractures usually have some overlap with the above-mentioned middle third fractures

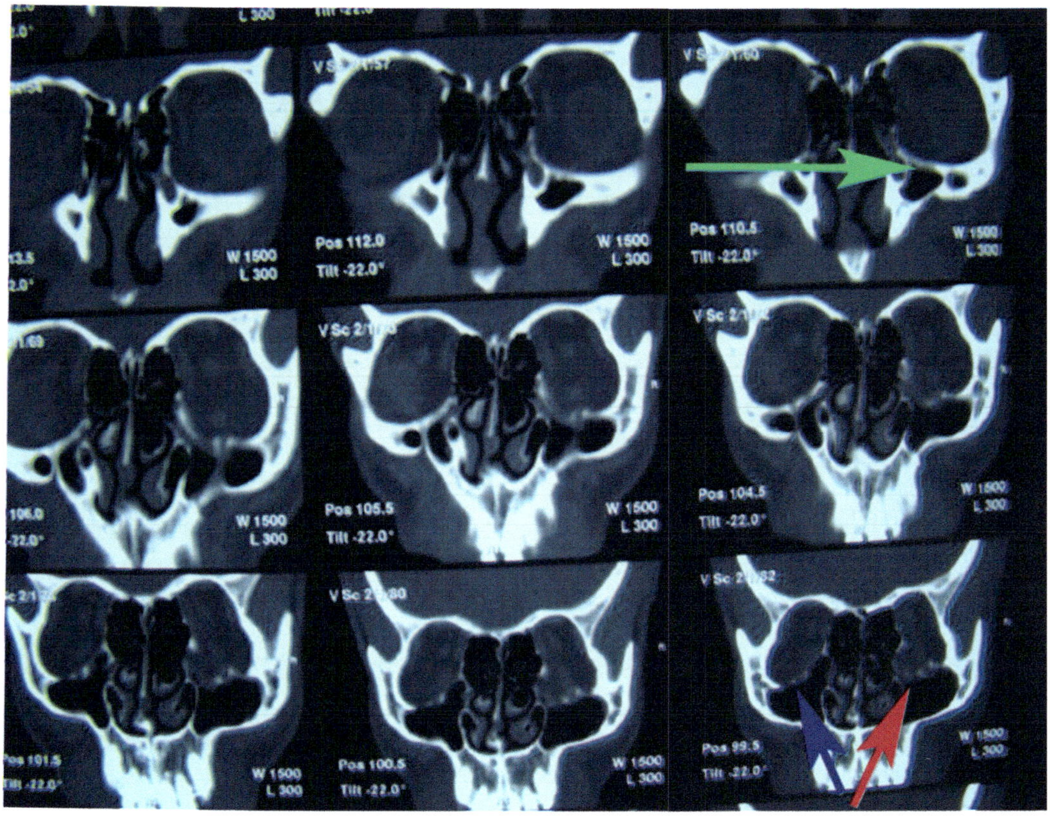

Fig. 14.19 Coronal CT scan showing a 'Blowout' fracture of the orbit. The green arrow shows the intact orbital margin, the red arrow the extrusion of orbital contents into the maxillary sinus through the floor fracture and the blue arrow shows the normal shape of the floor of the orbit at that cross section on the opposite side

as the orbital walls are formed by the zygoma, greater wing of sphenoid, maxilla, ethmoid, lacrimal and the frontal bones. However, there is a unique type of fracture in orbit called the "Blow Out Fracture". A pure blow-out fracture is one in which the orbital wall is fractured without involving orbital margins (Fig. 14.19). Usually this involves the thin upward sloping floor of the orbit leading to entrapment of orbital contents into the maxillary sinus. This may involve orbital fat or extraocular muscle. Clinically this manifests as infraorbital nerve paresthesia/anesthesia and restriction of eye movement. It is important to educate the patient to avoid blowing their nose, as air from the sinonasal tract can be forced into orbit. This can result in an orbital compartment syndrome that can cause blindness [15]. CT scans show the actual extent of the fracture. This type of fracture happens when an object having a diameter larger than the orbit hits the orbit, the eyeball is pushed inwards exerting pressure on the orbital wall which gives way. In fact, there is no clear demarcation between the floor and the medial wall. The floor ascends medially gradually to become part of the medial wall. The medial wall is also formed by thin bone (Fig. 14.19). If the extraocular muscles get entrapped in this fracture, it may lead to restriction in eye movement. This is confirmed by looking for restrictions in eye movement, usually in the upward gaze. To rule out restrictions due to nerve injuries, a forced duction test was also carried out. In some cases, even if there is no muscle entrapment, atrophy of orbital fat due to trauma can cause enopthalmos which will become evident later on. In some patients, diplopia develops and the patient walks with the head turned towards one side or with one eye closed. Even

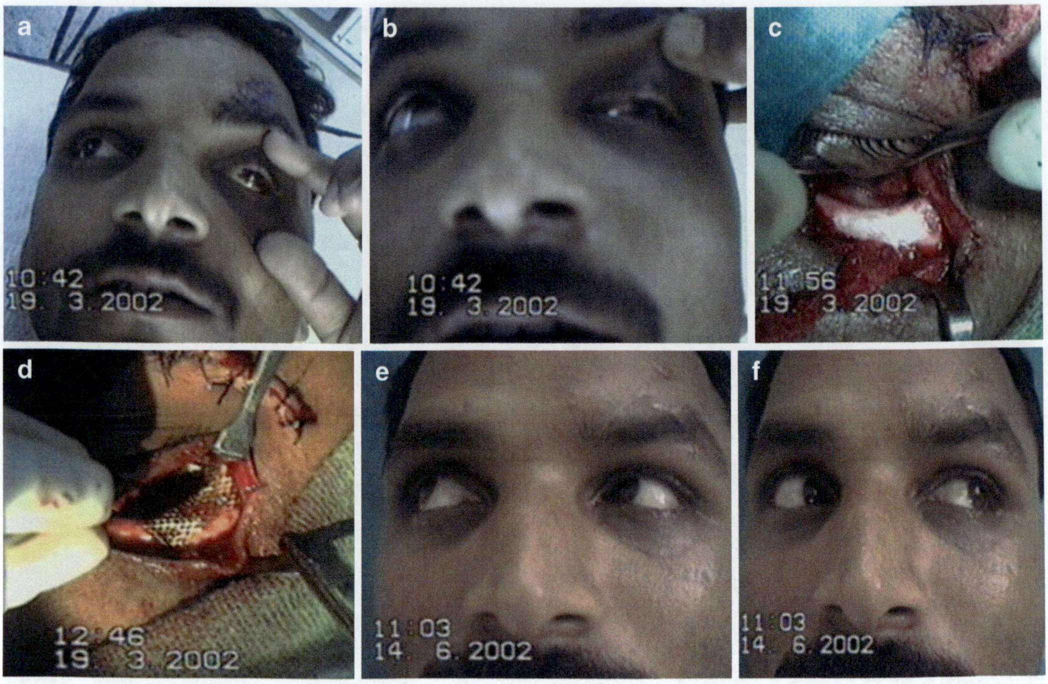

Fig. 14.20 Rare cases of blow out fractures of the lateral orbital wall. (**a, b**) showing the restriction of movement of Lt eye, (**c**) The blowout fracture of the lateral orbital wall without involving the rim, (**d**) The reconstruction of the defect with titanium mesh, (**e, f**) the restoration of full eye movement

though it involves the floor mostly, in certain cases it can involve the medial wall and rarely the lateral wall (Fig. 14.20). Occasionally, a "Blow In" fracture may occur. These is due to the fracture of the roof of the orbit in frontal bone fractures. The roof of the orbit is made of very thin bones which are easily fractured in frontal bone injury. Pure blow-out fractures are seen in 4–16% of all facial fractures while those involving the orbital rims comprise 30–55% of all facial fractures [16].

The globe is held in place in the horizontal axis by the Lockwood's suspensory ligament which is attached medially to the posterior aspect of the lacrimal bone and laterally to the medial aspect of the frontal process of the zygomatic bone at the Whitnall's tubercle located 1 cm below the frontozygomatic suture and 3–4 mm posterior to the lateral orbital margin. The shape and location of the palpebral fissure is determined by the attachment of the canthal tendons. The medial canthal tendon is attached to the anterior and posterior lacrimal crests. The lateral canthal tendon is also attached to the Whitnall's tubercle. Any disturbance in this arrangement can lead to telecanthus and dystopia. If the medial canthal attachment is detached, it will lead to telecanthus (Fig. 14.21). If the zygomatic complex is displaced downward and outward, it will lead to lowering of the globe on that side (Fig. 14.21).

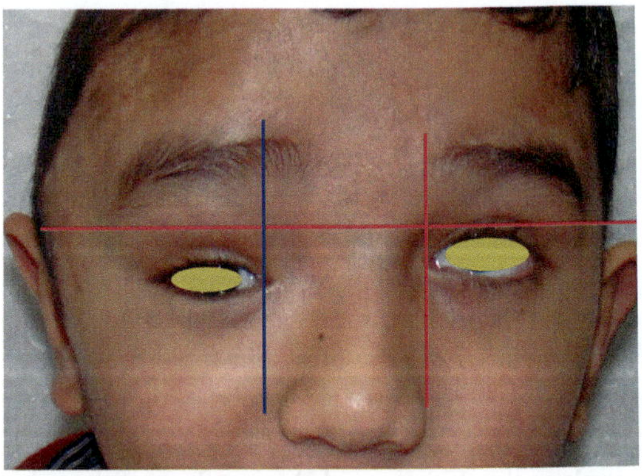

Fig. 14.21 Orbital dystopia showing the lowering of Rt Globe and telecanthus

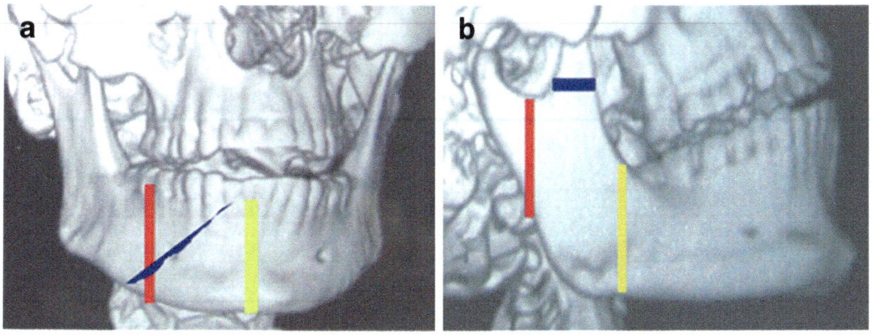

Fig. 14.22 Common sites of fracture mandible. (**a**) 3D-CT showing body fracture (red), parasymphysis fracture (blue) and symphysis (yellow). (**b**) 3D-CT lateral view showing subcondylar fracture (red), coronoid fracture (blue) and angle (yellow)

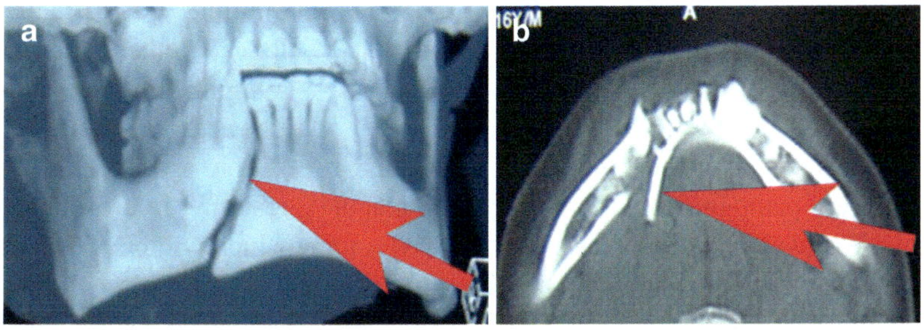

Fig. 14.23 (**a**, **b**) Fracture mandible Rt parasymphysis

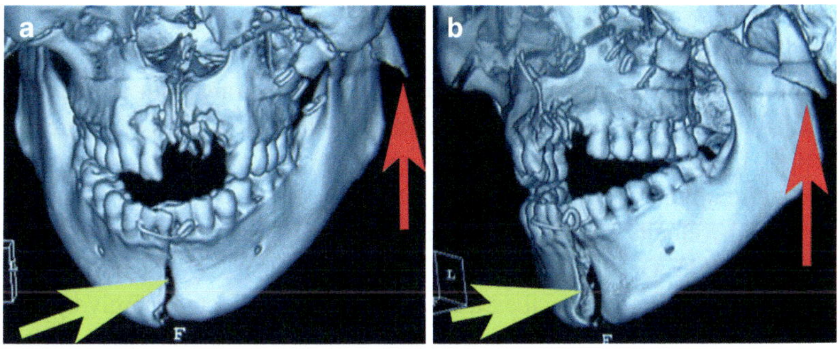

Fig. 14.24 3D-CT showing fractured mandible symphysis and subcondylar. (**a**) frontal view and (**b**) lateral view. Red arrows show the laterally displaced subcondylar fracture and the yellow arrows the torsional displacement of the symphyseal fracture

The clinical features of the middle third fractures are given in Table 14.1.

14.3.8 Lower Third Injuries

Mandible is the only movable bone in the outer facial skeleton and being very prominent in most individuals is commonly involved in maxillofacial trauma. Due to the U shape, multiple fractures are seen in more than 50% of cases. The most common fractured area depends on the type of trauma. The common sites of fracture are parasymphysis, angle, subcondylar and body (Fig. 14.22). Mild to moderate impact often causes fractures of mandible parasymphysis (Fig. 14.23). In automobile accidents and falls, subcondylar and parasymphysis fractures are commonly seen (Fig. 14.24). Assaults more often cause angle fractures (Fig. 14.25). The most common associated injuries include head injuries (39%), head and neck laceration (30%), midface fractures (28%), ocular injuries (16%), nasal fractures (12%), and cervical spine fractures (11%) [17]. Common clinical features include pain, swelling, hemorrhage, step deformity, tenderness, and difficulty in opening/closing the mouth, deviation on opening jaw, occlusal

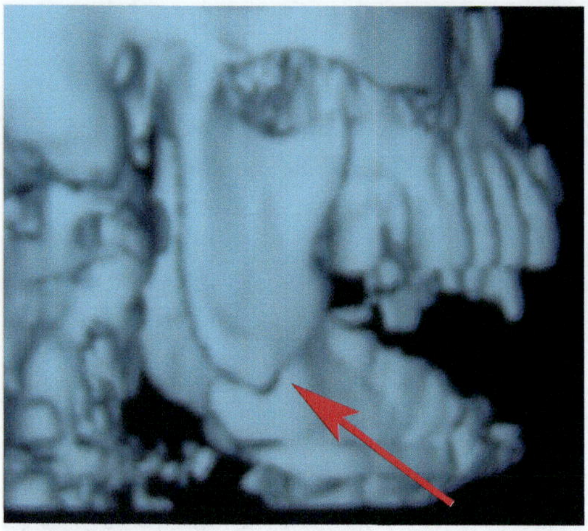

Fig. 14.25 3D-CT showing fractured angle of mandible

derangement and nerve deficit. Lingual hematoma is a pathognomonic sign of fracture mandible. Tongue blade bite test is also a useful test for detecting fracture mandible. The clinical features are given in Table 14.1.

Of 929 isolated facial fractures, the most common fracture type was a nasal bone fracture (164), followed by orbital floor (150), ZMC (76), maxillary sinus (75), mandibular ramus (48), and nasoethmoid orbital (46) [18]. In patients with orbital fractures, associated ocular injuries are present in up to 29% of the patients [19].

In high velocity injuries due to motor vehicle accidents (MVA), all three regions of the face may be involved and thus they are called panfacial trauma. It is mostly due to blunt trauma (Fig. 14.8). There may or may not be a laceration or visible injury. There are fractures in the upper third, middle third and lower third.

Similarly, Gun Shot Wounds (GSW) produce its own peculiar feature. The exact clinical picture is unpredictable. If it is due to a low velocity bullet, the bullet may enter the body and after hitting a bone may be deflected and lie without causing significant damage. Sometimes it may get deflected by bone or teeth and then take an unpredictable course inside the body. For example, in one case the bullet had entered the cheek on the right side from the front, hit the mandible and was found lying under the skin in the posterior triangle of the neck on the right side without causing any significant injury on the right side. The bullet was removed without any difficulty from the right side. Even though it had crossed over to the right side through the neck, it did not cause any major vascular injury. Arteries generally get deflected due to the resilience of the wall. For high velocity gunshot wounds, there is usually a small entry wound and a large exit wound (Fig. 14.4 and 14.5). There is extensive destruction of both hard and soft tissues along the route, causing the comminution of the bone and many a time, loss of soft tissue. However, blast injuries typically show a massive entrance wound with multiple bony fragments and foreign bodies lodged in the tissues (Fig. 14.6). There is usually a significant loss of tissue- both hard and soft. The actual extent of tissue trauma is much beyond visible as it leads to considerable micro trauma resulting in avascular necrosis of adjacent tissue which will be presented later on.

14.4 Management

Maxillofacial injuries can occur in isolation or along with injuries elsewhere. It produces local as well as systemic effects. Local effects include an inflammatory response leading to pain, tenderness, swelling and decreased function. Systemic effects include biological and psychological stress reactions. The biological reaction is affected mainly by the release of the endogenous catechol amines while the psychological reaction is of denial, shock, fear and an increased sense of vulnerability. These factors should be taken into consideration before attending to the patient.

The care received in the "golden hour" of trauma determines the final outcome. In cases of airway compromise, this take even minutes, while in patients with unstable hemorrhage, like pelvic fractures, it can take several hours. Approximately 60% of the all trauma related hospital deaths occur during this important hour. Avoidable deaths due to inadequate assessment and resuscitation contribute to the 35% of these deaths [20]. A 2016 National Academy of Science report estimated a civilian trauma Preventable Death Rate (PDR) of 20% or about 30,000 deaths per year [21]. In order to promote greater implementation of effective, affordable, and sustainable trauma systems globally, the World Health Organization (WHO) and the International Association for Trauma Surgery and Intensive Care (IATSIC) have worked collaboratively in the past to produce Guidelines for essential trauma care, which defined the core essential trauma care services that every injured person in the world should realistically be able to receive, even in the lowest income setting. In order to ensure the availability of these services, the publication went on to propose the minimum human resources, physical resources, and administrative mechanisms that should be in place in the range of health care facilities globally. The publication and the related prehospital trauma care systems have considerably catalyzed improvements in trauma systems in many countries since their release several years ago [22].

Uncontrolled hemorrhage is the most common cause of mortality in the first 48 h. With the advances in prehospital care and efficient transport, more severely injured patients are now capable of reaching hospital. The development of trauma centres has led to an increase in survival of such patients who will require reconstruction of devastating facial injuries. The craniofacial team should ideally include the anesthetist who is the first responder, neurosurgeon, ophthalmologist, maxillofacial surgeon, otorhinolaryngologist and the radiologist. A reconstructive surgeon and a pediatric surgeon can be included if required. Advances in managing severely injured patients are permitted early and definitive primary fracture treatment. The management of such cases can be considered under three heads – primary survey and resuscitation, secondary survey and definitive management.

14.4.1 Primary Management and Resuscitation

Primary management of severe maxillofacial injuries should follow the protocol advised by Advance Trauma Life Support (ATLS) to prevent loss of life and morbidity. The goals of primary management are to identify and treat threats to life, limb and eye sight, to prevent exacerbation of existing injury and to restore function to normal levels. Time is of the greatest significance. The role of a well-trained multispecialty interdisciplinary team in achieving this goal is very significant. In conflict situations, these patients have multiple penetrating injuries with severe tissue destruction. They also have profound acidosis, hypothermia and coagulopathy. In such patients, time consuming procedures for repair of all identified injuries has led to death in many cases. Today for such patients, "damage control surgery" is an option. This involves abbreviating laparotomy with rapid and precise control of hemorrhage and contamination with temporary packing if necessary, followed by physiologic resuscitation. Once the patient is stabilized, the patient can be taken up for definitive repair of all injuries, including abdominal closure.

An important point to be kept in mind is that maxillofacial trauma rarely causes hemorrhagic shock even though it appears to be very severe. In such cases, one should look for any occult hemorrhage in the thorax or abdomen or even a closed injury of the extremity. The risk of death due to maxillofacial injury is only because of airway obstruction. In many cases with severe injuries even in GSW or blast injuries, the patient is conscious and prefers to sit up in a forward position rather than lie down to maintain the airway. If such patients are made to lie down, they cannot maintain the patency of the airway. Awake fiber optic intubation is the ideal method of intubation in such patients. However, it may not be possible because of the heavy hemorrhage associated with facial injuries.

The facial soft tissue is highly vascular and bleeds from both sides. In addition, certain arteries like anterior ethmoid arteries, posterior ethmoid arteries and the internal maxillary arteries are not easily accessible for control. In such cases, packing the nose and pharynx can control the hemorrhage. There are many methods of packing. Initially, anterior and posterior packing with gauze was the only option which was difficult and time consuming. A wide variety of materials are available now. The most widely used and

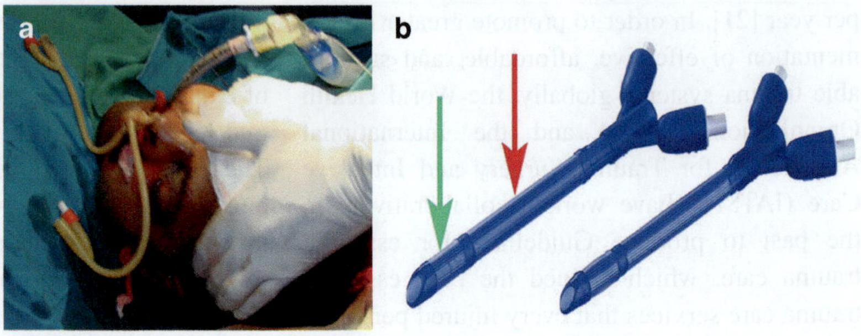

Fig. 14.26 Management of hemorrhage by packing. (**a**) Use of Foley's Catheter as a nasal pack. (**b**) Epi-Max Catheter with anterior cuff (Red Arrow) and posterior cuff (Green Arrow)

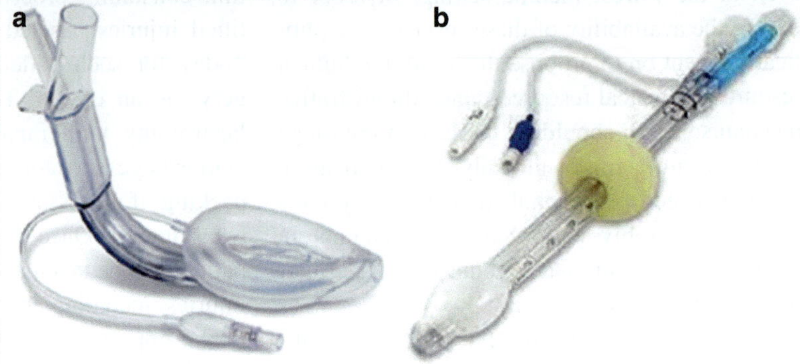

Fig. 14.27 Airway for difficult intubation in trauma. (**a**) Laryngeal mask, (**b**) Combitube

the easiest to use is the epistaxis catheter to achieve anterior and posterior nasal pack (Fig. 14.26). The lubricated epistaxis catheter is inserted through the nostril after cleaning the nasal cavity of foreign bodies and blood clot in such a way that the posterior balloon extends into the nasopharynx. The posterior cuff is inflated with 4–8 mL of air. The catheter is then pulled out gently until it engages the posterior choanae to form the posterior seal. Then the anterior cuff is inflated with 10–25 mi of air and the catheter taped to the nose. An oral tube is then passed as early as possible. Once the patient's condition stabilizes, the oral tube can be changed to a nasal tube so that occlusion can be obtained by intermaxillary fixation. In mandibular fractures, hemorrhage from the fractured fragment can be controlled by temporarily stabilizing the fracture.

The American Society of Anesthesiologists (ASA) has come out with a Practice guideline for management of difficult airway [23]. In case of difficulty in vision due to excessive hemorrhage, oral intubation under direct laryngoscopy should be attempted. Once the patient's condition is stabilized, it can be converted to nasal intubation or submental intubation. Other options for control of the airway in the emergency setting are the use of laryngeal mask airway and Combitube (Fig. 14.27). The use of intervention radiology to arrest such deep hemorrhage by embolization is also being studied. Planned tracheostomy can be carried out once patient's condition stabilizes where the need for prolonged intubation is expected postoperatively. In a study by Beogo et al., it was found that tracheostomy was required in 22.4% of all Le Fort fractures and 43.5% of all Le Fort -III fractures [24].

Once the patient's condition is stabilized, the secondary survey is carried out. A head to toe examination is done to note all injuries obvious and otherwise. The potential for missing an injury or failing to appreciate the significance of an injury is great, especially in an unresponsive or unstable patient. A detailed ophthalmic examination should be carried out at the earliest as it may not be possible later on due to lid edema. Examination of the face should start from the upper third, then middle third and then the lower third in a systematic manner. Soft tissues are examined to detect any asymmetry, swelling, hemorrhage, contusion, laceration and avulsion. Any bleeding from the ear and nose should be noted. Hearing and acuity of vision should be checked. Jaw movements are checked for restriction/ deviation. Restrictions can be due to an angle fracture, subcondylar fracture or a Le Fort-II fracture. Deviation of the jaw to the same side occurs in unilateral subcondylar fracture. An open bite or inability to close mouth fully can be seen in bilateral subcondylar fractures as well as Le Fort-II fractures of the maxilla (Fig. 14.28 and 14.29). All bony margins are palpated to look for tenderness, step deformity and crepitus. The presence of crepitus in the soft tissues suggests the involvement of the paranasal sinus. Both sensory and motor nerves are checked for deficit at this stage and recorded clearly as changes may occur in their status after surgical treatment. The intraoral examination should reveal the presence of step deformity, occlusal derangement, unilateral or bilateral open bite, soft tissue laceration/ hematoma and the fracture of teeth (Fig. 14.28, 14.29 and 14.30). Missing teeth to be noted. Any mobile anterior teeth in the maxilla may be dislodged accidentally during intubation. Intrafragmentary movements, if any, should be noted. Mobility of the maxilla is assessed by placing the head securely against a headrest, grasping the upper teeth and alveolus and moving it gently but purposefully in all directions. In the case of a mandible the mandible is pushed down while the mouth is open. Any fracture of the mandible if present, will cause pain. In the case of symphyseal fractures, the fracture fragments will be distracted upon opening the jaw. It can also be checked by gently pushing both angles inwards when patient will experience pain in the symphysis. Split palate can lead to an oronasal fistula.

14.4.2 Imaging

The primary imaging modality of maxillofacial trauma today is CT scan. Previously, the PNS view of the skull was a basic radiograph of the middle and upper third fractures. Due to the multiple bones involved and their overlap, a two-dimensional radiograph in middle third and upper third fractures led to many fractures being missed. In addition, the severity of the fracture and the degree of involvement of the cranial and orbital cavities cannot be assessed with a conventional two-dimensional radiograph. Today, the coronal section of the facial bone gives the surgeon enough idea about the actual extent of the middle

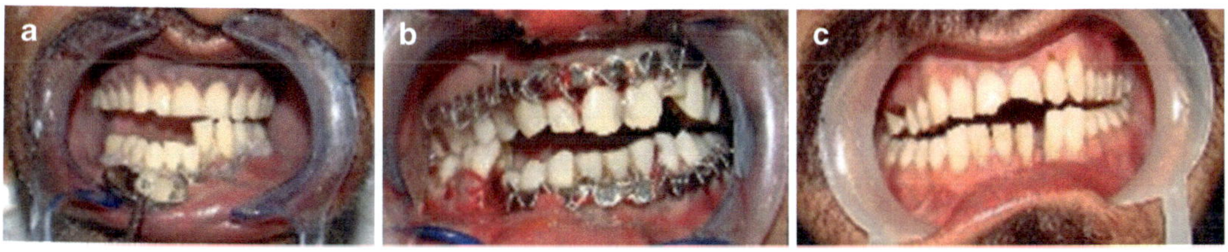

Fig. 14.28 Clinical presentation of fracture mandible. (**a**) step deformity seen in fractures of parasymphysis and angle of the mandible. (**b**) step deformity seen in the fractured body of the Mandible Rt. (**c**) Anterior open bite seen in bilateral subcondylar fracture

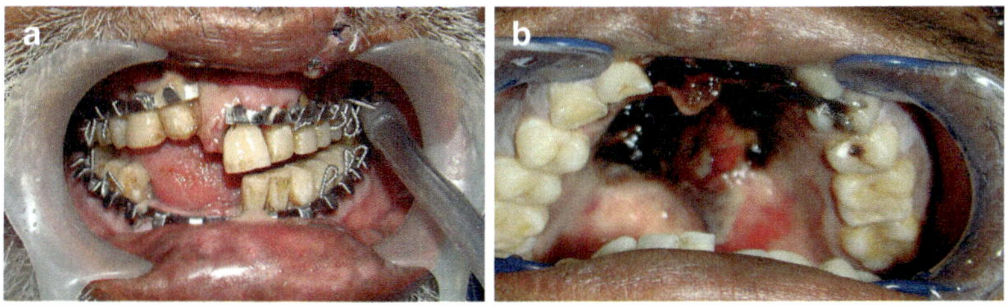

Fig. 14.29 Clinical presentation of fractured maxilla Le Fort I. (**a**) step deformity due to vertical displacement of maxillary fragments. (**b**) Horizontal displacement due to split palate

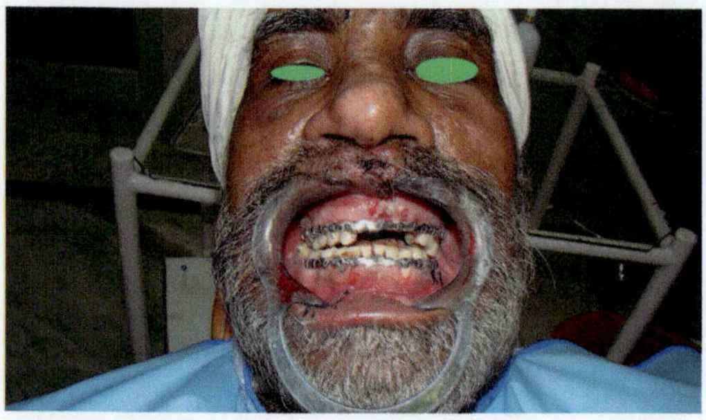

Fig. 14.30 Fracture maxilla Le Fort II clinical picture showing elongation of face, anterior open bite and downward and backward displacement of maxilla

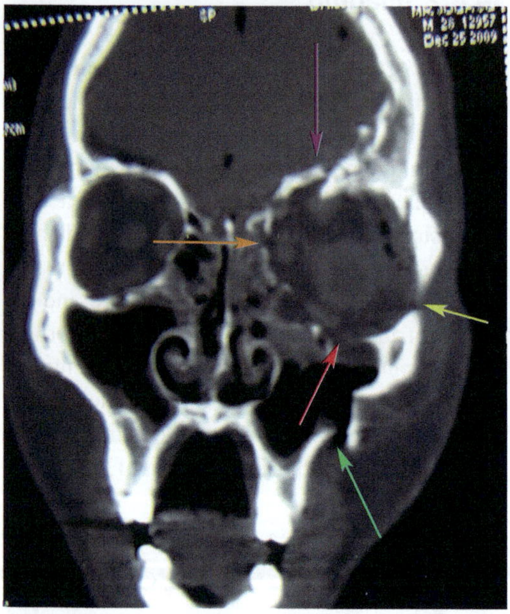

Fig. 14.31 Coronal section CT showing the involvement of all four walls in the orbit

third fractures (Fig. 14.19). For frontal bone fractures, it is important to know the anteroposterior involvement of the fracture. An axial section of the region will clearly show the involvement of the anterior as well as the posterior table of the frontal sinus which is an important information required for planning the type of surgery required (Fig. 14.10 and 14.12). A good coronal section of the same region will give a clear idea of the involvement of the orbital roof (Fig. 14.31). A CT scan is equally important for fractures involving orbit to assess the degree of reconstruction required. In fact, the requirement of reconstruction of the orbital floor can be easily predicted after visualizing a coronal section which gives a clear idea about the anteroposterior and the transverse width of the floor defect. This will clearly show the entrapment of the soft tissue in the orbital floor fracture. In maxillary fractures also, coronal sections give a clear idea of the type of fracture and the involvement of the maxillary sinus and the orbital floor which is important to plan surgical management. The axial sections give a clear idea of the involvement of the pterygoid plates in the fracture as well as the type of fracture of the horizontal palate. Even though Orthopantomograph gives a good picture of pure mandibular fractures, in fractures involving the condylar region, a CT scan is an essential diagnostic modality. The CT scan will clearly show the type of fracture which is important in deciding the approach to the fracture as well as the difficulty in management. Today with the availability of 3D modeling and manufacture of patient specific implants, CT scans have a greater role to play [25, 26]. This is also true with the increasing use of interventional radiology in controlling hemorrhage from deep seated tissues like internal maxillary artery. An MRI may be required in select cases to explore the possibility of nerve injury as well as ocular injuries.

14.4.3 Definitive Management

The face has several important functions like nutrition, respiration, vision, taste and communication. The importance of these functions can be understood by the fact that 11 of the 12 cranial nerves supply the face. Its proximity to the vital structures of the head and neck is also of great significance. It is responsible to a great extent for the personality of the individual and any disfigurement will lead to considerable psycho-social problems. The earlier definitive treatment is started, the better the result will be. This is due to rounding of bony ends with time leading to difficulty in approximation later on. It is especially important in the middle third fractures as the bone fragments are too thin in most of the regions and it is difficult to realign the structure if these bones are lost. Three dimensionally restoring the middle third when there is multiple fragmentation as seen in severe trauma is a big challenge. Soft tissue contracts with time and it becomes difficult to approximate the tissues leading to dehiscence postoperatively. The best time to achieve good results is the first attempt. Any compromise in the quality of primary repair will lead to secondary deformity which is very difficult to correct at a later stage.

The goal of definitive management is to establish form and function through:

- Anatomic reduction of fracture fragments after achieving occlusion followed by stabilization.
- Preservation of width, projection and height of the face.
- Preservation of vital structures of the face like facial nerves, parotid ducts, lacrimal ducts, eyeballs, cranial nerves.
- Early return to function.

14.4.4 Soft Tissue Repair

Soft tissue wounds may be cleaned, contused or punctured wounds, or any combination of these three. The first step in wound management is wound debridement. This is done by exploring the wounds by placing incisions where necessary, followed by thorough debridement with diluted chlorhexidine and a brush to remove all dirt and foreign bodies to prevent tattooing. After this the wound is irrigated copiously with saline followed by antibiotics. It should be remembered that glass particles may not be easily visible and have to be looked for. Then necrotic tissues are excised conservatively. With face being very vascular, excision is limited to tags of loose, dead skin or mucous membrane at the edge of the wound. No area should be allowed to dry. Placement of wet gauze in between procedures will prevent the desiccation of the soft tissue flaps. Wherever possible, primary closure must be done. This is true even for gunshot wounds and blast injuries, unlike other areas of the body where it is best to leave it open due to excessive contamination and contusion. Where there is extreme loss of tissue and facilities for harvest of flaps to cover the defect is not available, skin can be sutured to mucosa to limit the contraction of the wound. Care should be taken to preserve vital structures like parotid duct and the facial nerve during debridement, especially in injuries involving the cheek. Once the soft tissues are debrided properly, the hard tissues must be restored to its original form before closing primarily. In facial regions, generally drain placement is not necessary. However, if the wound is extensive and tissues appear traumatized, a suction drain can be placed. Primary closures can generally be obtained by giving adequate release incisions. The cleansed wound is first loosely assembled, in order for an assessment of any tissue loss to be made. In the face, approximately 5 cm advancement can be obtained by releasing incisions. Where advancement will lead to excessive tension, local or regional flaps may be used to achieve closure. No bones should ideally be left exposed. Lingual mucosa is notorious for giving away in the postoperative period. To prevent that, some reduction of bone level can be attempted to reduce tension. For severe injuries, it is best to start with landmarks easily identifiable like corner of mouth, eyebrow, eyelid, vermillion border and angle of the eye to achieve reasonable esthetics (Fig. 14.32). Tetanus toxoid should be administered if indicated.

14.4.5 Hard Tissue

The principles of hard tissue management are wide exposure of all the fractures, mobilization, reduction and stabilization. Management of hard tissue injuries involves the mobilization, reduction and stabilization of fracture fragments. In tooth bearing areas, occlusion must be ensured before stabilization of the fractures.

14.4.6 Approaches to the Facial Skeleton

There are numerous methods for exposure of the facial skeleton [27]. As far as possible, incisions

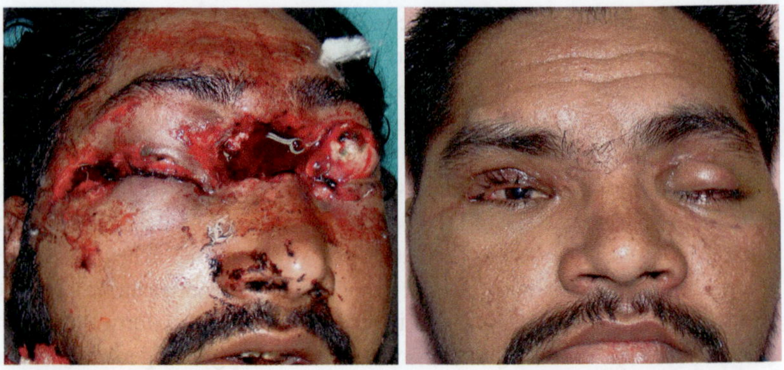

Fig. 14.32 Preoperative and postoperative photos showing restoration of form with direct primary closure

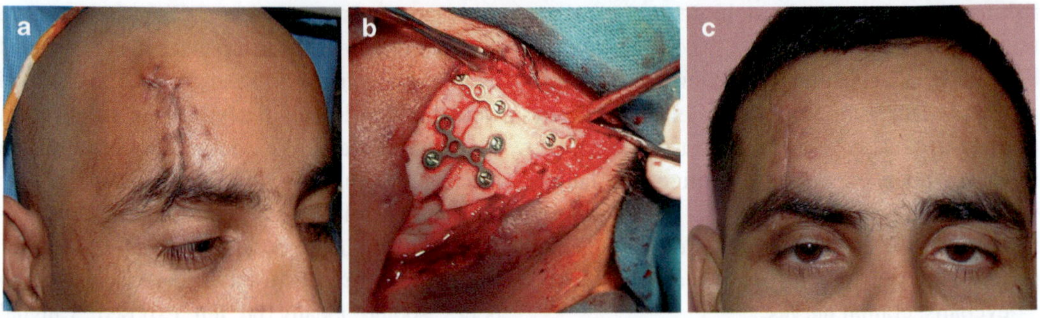

Fig. 14.33 Approach through existing lacerations. (**a**) Existing laceration. (**b**) Intra-operative exposure. (**c**) Postoperative appearance

should not be placed in the face to avoid disfiguration as well as injury to the facial nerve branches. The exception to this rule is when there are existing lacerations (Fig. 14.33) and it is possible to get adequate exposure of the fracture either through the laceration or by very little extension to it. However, in the naso-orbital region, even in the presence of a laceration, it would be better to approach through a coronal incision to get enough advancement of the tissue for closure without tension and to avoid an ugly scar in the most prominent part of the face. The selection of the method depends to a large extent on the part to be exposed, the type of fracture (degree of fragmentation and stability) and the training, skill and comfort level of the operating surgeon. Intra-oral incisions are used wherever possible.

The best approach to upper third fractures is the coronal or hemicoronal incision which gives adequate exposure, does not leave visible scars, minimizes the risk of facial nerve injury and helps the management of complex fractures (Fig. 14.34). Among the middle third fractures, the fractures of the nasoorbital complex and Le Forte III fractures of the maxilla are again approached from the coronal incision which gives the best results. For the maxillary, Le Forte II fractures intra oral incision along with an incision in the

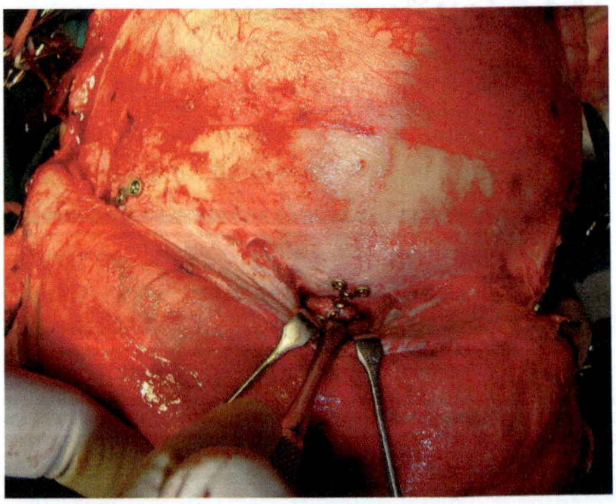

Fig. 14.34 Coronal approach for upper third and middle third fractures

infraorbital region will give optimum results. The incision in the infraorbital region can be transconjunctival, subciliary, midpalpebral or infraorbital. Each has its own advantages and disadvantages. In the hands of a good surgeon all these incisions give good results. For fractures of the zygomatic complex and Le Forte I fracture of maxilla, an intra-oral vestibular incision gives wide exposure for mobilization, reduction and stabilization of the fractures. In the case of zygomatic complex fractures additional incision in the lateral brow, infraorbital region or a hemicoronal incision may be required depending on the extent of fragmentation and the resultant stability of the reduced fractures. Accordingly, one point, two point, three point and four point fixation is planned. For mandibular fractures involving the angle, body and parasymphysis, intraoral vestibular incision is good enough. For subcondylar fractures, Hind's retromandibular incision gives the best access.

14.4.7 Upper Third Fractures

Once all fracture fragments are exposed through a suitable incision, the next step is the mobilization of all fractures. In the upper third fractures, the fragments are very difficult to mobilize. Burholes may be required to mobilize fracture fragments in frontal bone fractures. In some cases where the posterior table is not involved, it may be wise to do camouflage surgery by applying a titanium plate over the depressed fracture without mobilizing the anterior table for reduction. The main consideration in frontal bone fractures involving the frontal sinus is the management of the frontal sinus to prevent infection. The frontal sinus is ideally obliterated to prevent infection of the nasal cavity. If the bone pieces are too small and are not attached, it may be better to remove them and replace them with a titanium mesh/plate.

14.4.8 Middle Third Fractures

The middle third is composed of multiple very thin bones and few strong vertical and horizontal buttresses. The horizontal buttresses include the supraorbital margin, the zygomatic arch, the infraorbital margin and the piriform rim. The vertical buttresses are the zygomatico-fronto-maxillary and the fronto-maxillary buttresses. So, during reduction, these areas are best to reassemble as well as stabilize.

The fracture at the frontozygomatic suture is usually a dysjunction and not a true fracture. However, in some cases of direct hit, fragmentation of this region is also encountered. Similarly, in naso-orbital fractures, usually the medial canthal tendon is detached along with a piece of bone which can be refixed. In zygomatic complex fractures, if there is no dysjunction at the fronto-zygomatic suture, one-point fixation at the zygomatic buttress will provide stability. If there is dysjunction at the fronto-zygomatic suture, a two-point fixation at the buttress and the fronto-zygomatic suture is good enough (Fig. 14.35). However, when there is severe fragmentation, it may be advisable to stabilize the fractures at the buttress, frontozygomatic suture and infraorbital margin (Fig. 14.36). If the zygomatic arch is also comminuted, a four-point fixation through a hemicoronal approach may be required (Fig. 14.37). In rare instances, direct hits at the lateral orbital rim cause an isolated fracture of the lateral orbital wall, which is difficult to manage as there is usually a collapse in the orbit at that point (Fig. 14.38). Reducing it requires considerable force, which if not controlled will lead to avulsion of the fragment.

The management of orbital blow-out fractures is controversial; some advocate late intervention if symptoms do not improve [28] while others advocate early (less than 2 weeks) intervention, the rationale being that late intervention leads to a compromised result [29]. Indications for immediate surgical intervention are diplopia present with CT evidence of an entrapped muscle or periorbital tissue associated with a nonresolving oculocardiac reflex (bradycardia, heart block, nausea, vomiting, or syncope), "White-eyed blow-out fracture", Young patients (< 18 years)with history of periocular trauma, little ecchymosis or edema (white eye), marked extraocular motility vertical restriction, and CT

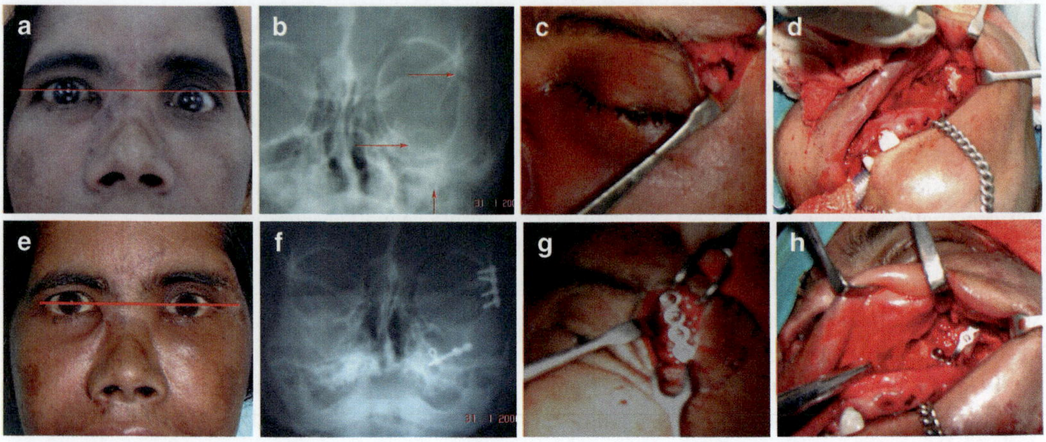

Fig. 14.35 Two point fixation of Zygomatic complex fractures. (**a**) Preoperative photo showing the lowering of the left eyeball due to downward and outward displacement of Lt Zygomatic complex. (**b**) Preoperative PNS View Xray showing the frontozygomatic dysjunction and downward displacement at zygomatic buttress and infraorbital margin. (**c**) Intraop photo showing the frontozygomatic dysjunction. (**d**) Intraop photo showing the downward displacement at zygomatic buttress. (**e**) Postoperative photo showing the restoration of eye level. (**f**) Postoperative X ray PNS view skull showing the two point fixation. (**g**) Intraop photo showing the reduction and stabilization at FZ suture. (**h**) Intraop photo showing reduction and stabilization of the buttress

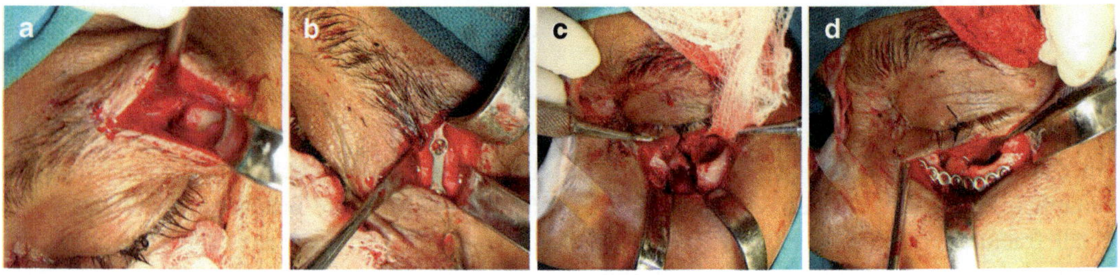

Fig. 14.36 Three point fixation of zygomatic complex fracture. (**a**) Fracture displacement at FZ suture. (**b**) Reduction and stabilization. (**c**) Fracture displacement infraorbital margin. (**d**) Reduction and stabilization

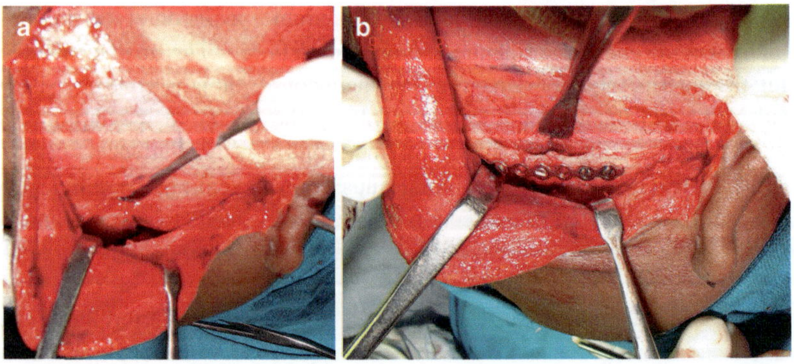

Fig. 14.37 Four point fixation. (**a**) a depressed fracture of the zygomatic arch. (**b**) reduced and stabilized

examination revealing an orbital floor fracture with entrapped muscle or perimuscular soft tissue and early enopthalmos/hypoglobus causing facial asymmetry [30].

Brucoli et al. found that the incidence of diplopia, enopthalmos, and infraorbital nerve dysfunction is decreased by immediate intervention and early surgical repair of the orbital blow-out fractures. Patients who had surgery within 2 weeks of trauma have a lower risk to develop postoperative complications; this study supports an early surgical treatment of orbital blow-out fractures, when it is indicated [31]. Early surgery minimizes progressive fibrosis and contractures of the prolapsed tissues and fat atrophy and gives the best results. Other authors report the same data [32, 33]. The most common surgical approach reported was a preseptal transconjunctival approach (32.0%), followed by the subciliary (27.9%) and postseptal transconjunctival (26.2%) approaches. The most commonly reported implants for orbital reconstruction was titanium (65.4%), followed by Medpor (43.7%) and composite Medpor and titanium (26.4%) [34] (Fig. 14.39).

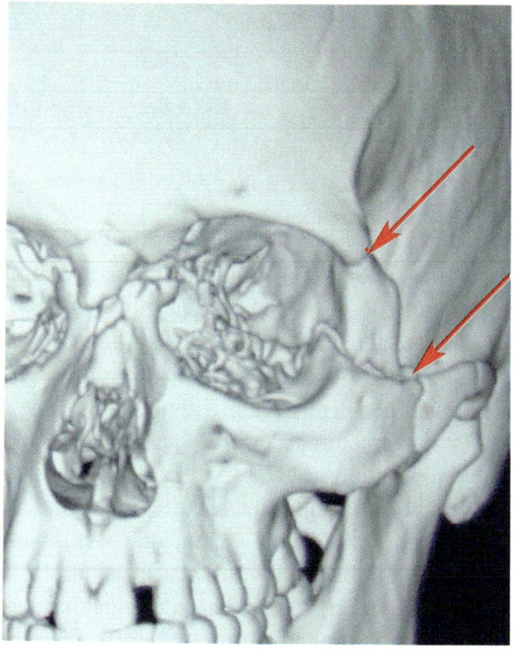

Fig. 14.38 Isolated fracture of the lateral wall of the orbit

Regarding orbital floor fractures, reconstruction of orbital floor defects of more than 2 cm requires the use of an autogenous graft or alloplasts. The commonly used autogenous grafts are the calvarial graft, mandibular symphysis grafts (Fig. 14.40) and iliac bone graft. The alloplastic materials that have been successfully used are the titanium mesh and porous polyethylene sheets. Currently, patient specific implants are available manufactured as per the patient's specification using CAD/CAM based on CT scans. This gives better results as the orbital floor anatomy is com-

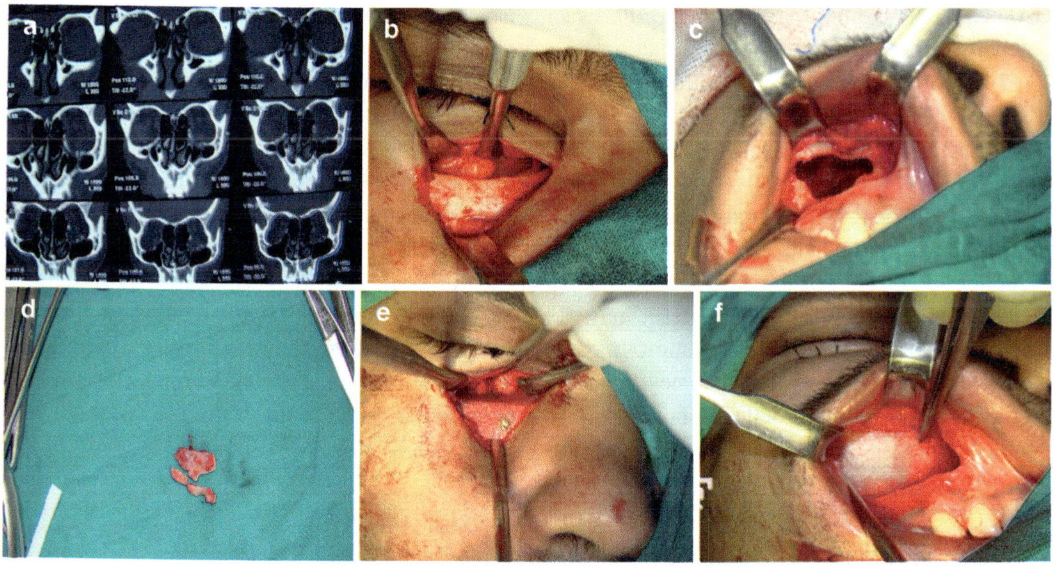

Fig. 14.39 Blowout fracture of orbit. (**a**) Coronal section CT shows blowout fracture of Rt Orbit. (**b**) Intraop photo showing entrapment of orbital tissues in the fracture. (**c**) Tissues cannot be disengaged from the fracture site without further traumatizing. Caldwell Luc approach was used to remove interfering bony spicules. (**d**) Bony fragments interfering with reduction removed. (**e**) Orbital floor reconstructed with Medpore Sheet. (**f**) Caldwell approach closed with Medpore sheet

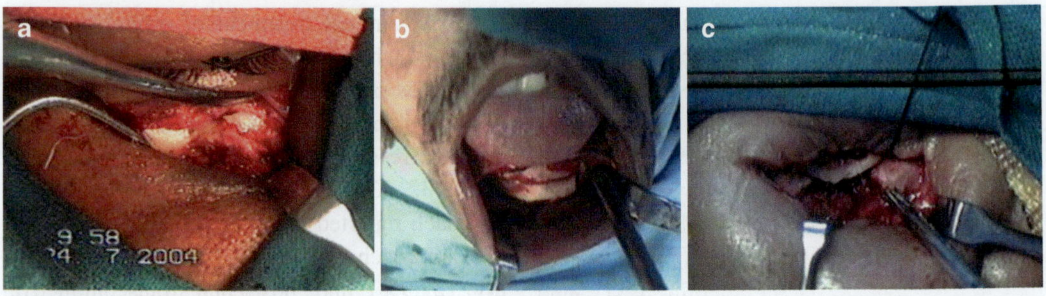

Fig. 14.40 Orbital floor reconstruction with Mandibular Symphysis graft. (**a**) Orbital floor defect. (**b**) Mandibular symphysis graft harvested. (**c**) Reconstruction of orbital floor with graft

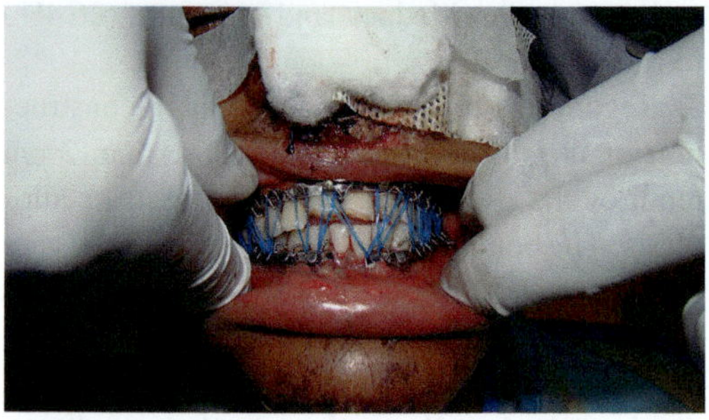

Fig. 14.41 Intermaxillary Fixation using arch bars to achieve occlusion

plicated with depression followed by an upward slope which is difficult to recreate manually. In CAD/CAM, it is possible to recreate the exact defect by mirror imaging [25, 26].

In Le Fort fractures, after mobilization of the fractures, occlusion is achieved before reducing the other fractures. This was achieved by approximation of the upper and lower jaw using wires and elastics (Fig. 14.41). Another point in complex fractures to be noted is that the fracture reduction should start from the inner to the outer. Without mobilizing all the fractures, it may not be possible to achieve correct reduction. In cases with gross comminution, small bone fragments with attachment loss are better removed to prevent their necrosis and infection in the postoperative period. Either bone grafts or titanium plates can be used to bridge the gaps. Once the bone fragments are reduced, they are stabilized with miniplates and screws. In the infraorbital margin, even micro plates and screws can be used. In a few cases, especially with associated fracture mandibles, it may be advisable to perform open reduction and fixation of the palate also to ensure restoration of the width of the alveolar arch. Otherwise, the mandible will also be restored with greater width leading to deformity as well as functional problems. Phillips found that 60% of the Le Fort fractures required open reduction and internal fixation (ORIF), while 30% required conservative management and 10% no treatment. The majority of Le Fort – I fractures were managed using an intraoral vestibular incision, while Le Fort –II and III required an additional infraorbital (transconjunctival/sub ciliary) incision along with lateral brow/coronal incisions (Fig. 14.42). Minimally invasive techniques have recently been introduced for the management of isolated zygomatic complex fractures and orbital fractures. However, they are not of use in severe maxillofacial injuries. Le Fort I, II, and III fractures had mortality rates of 0%, 4.5%, and 8.7%, respectively [33]. Le Fort fractures are associated with significant morbidity, including the development of visual problems (47%), diplopia (21%), epiphora (37%), difficulty with breathing (31%), and difficulty with mastication (40%) [35]. Satisfactory outcomes with regards to function and aesthetics were achieved in 89.1% of patients, while long term infection, temporary temporomandibular joint stiffness, or facial deformity were seen in 10.9% of patients [36].

14.4.9 Lower Third Fractures

Compared to upper third and middle third fractures, lower third fractures are complicated by severe muscle pull displacing the fracture frag-

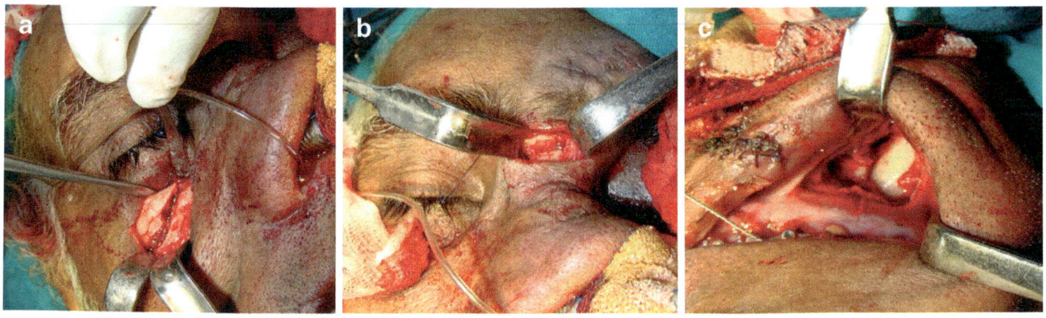

Fig. 14.42 Fracture maxilla – approaches. (**a**) Infraorbital incision. (**b**)'W' incision. (**c**) Vestibular incision

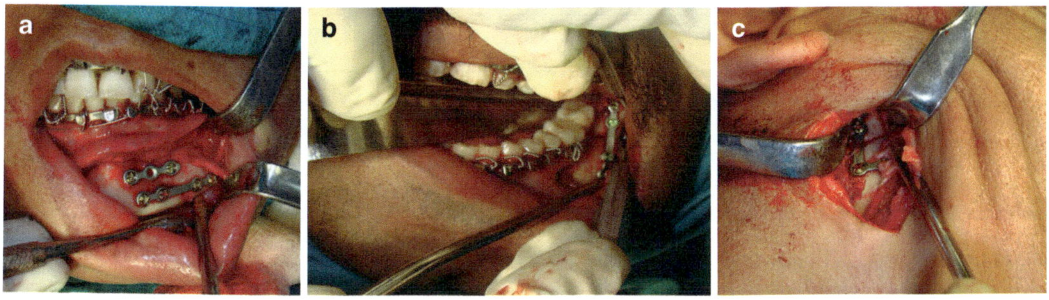

Fig. 14.43 Approaches to Mandible. (**a**) Vestibular incision for parasymphysis fractures. (**b**) Vestibular incision for angle fractures. (**c**) Hind's approach for subcondylar fractures

ments. The most common fractures of the mandible are parasymphysis, body, angle and subcondylar. In most cases there is more than one type of fracture depending on the nature of the force acted upon. These multiple fractures may be unilateral or bilateral. Commonly associated with multiple fractures are parasymphysis and angle/subcondylar, bilateral subcondylar and bilateral body. Once the fracture fragments are mobilized, occlusion is achieved by intermaxillary fixation. Then the fragments are reduced and stabilized starting from the dentate portion (Fig. 14.43). The stabilization is achieved using the miniplates and screws as described by Champy et al. [37]. In cases of severe loss of bone, a reconstruction plate is used.

14.4.10 Panfacial Fractures

In Panfacial fractures, management becomes more difficult as there is no stable base. The situation is similar to solving a jigsaw puzzle. Look for the easiest part to align first. It is impossible to reduce such fractures anatomically without mobilizing all fracture fragments. Different approaches have been advocated – inside out or outside in. in a clinical situation, all fractures are exposed and mobilized first. If mandible and maxilla are fragmented, mandible is fixed first anatomically. Then the maxilla is fixed based on mandible. If frontal bone is intact or stable, zygoma is aligned to the frontal bone and stabilized. Then the rest is arranged as if you are doing a jigsaw puzzle.

14.4.11 Blast Injuries and GSW

The management of gunshot and blast injuries requires more experience and skill. In GSW, the tract of the bullet should be carefully explored to get a complete picture of the injury. The entry wound and the exit wound may not be in a straight line. Usually, GSW is easier to manage to achieve a reasonable restoration of form and function (Fig. 14.44). Important vessels tend to escape

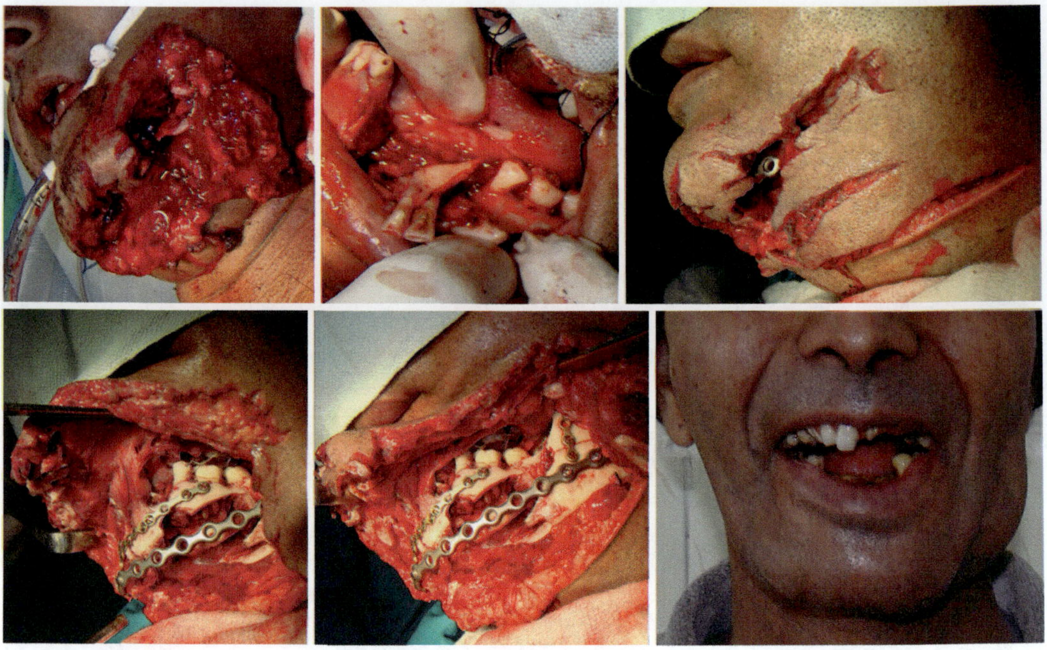

Fig. 14.44 Blast injury of mandible

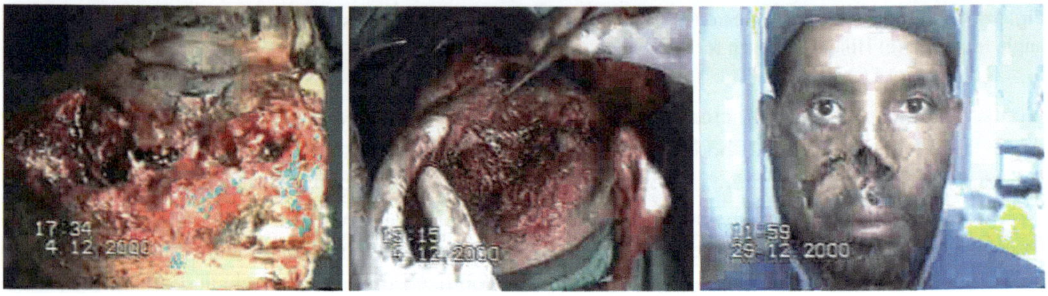

Fig. 14.45 Blast injury of maxilla

injury in most cases. Blast injuries have a different set of problems. They include loss of hard and soft tissues, contamination of the wound by multiple types of foreign bodies and lastly the contusion effect. The contamination may be soil, wood and metal splinters or even glass particles. The viability of the adjacent tissues cannot be ascertained immediately. They suffer contusion due to the shock waves and the vitality of these tissues will become evident only after a week or so. In blast injuries with severe loss of hard and soft tissues in US and UK, an external Jackson's crib is used to prevent infection at the fracture site [38, 39]. In India, direct fixation with bone plates and screws have been used to get good results [40] (Fig. 14.44 and 14.45).

14.5 Rehabilitation

Rehabilitation of patients with maxillofacial injuries with secondary deformities is very challenging. Optimum primary management is the best way to avoid such deformities. This is due to the fact that there is significant soft tissue contraction during healing which will increase the defect as well as make the tissue fibrotic leading to difficulty in advancing the flaps for closure of the defect. In

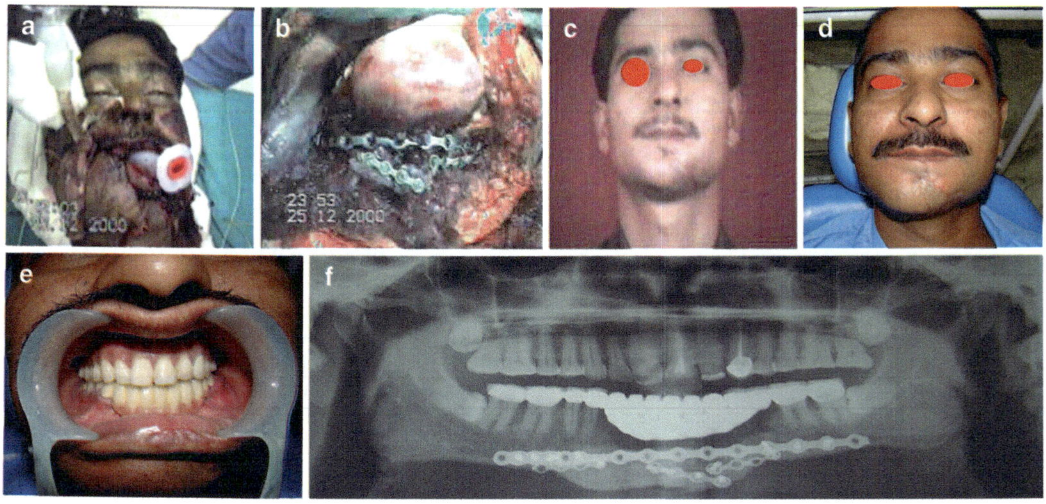

Fig. 14.46 Rehabilitation of GSW. (**a**) Preop. (**b**) Intraop showing the fixation of multiple bone fragments with titanium plates and screws. (**c**) Postop photo 3 months. (**d**) Postop photo 16 years. (**e**) Provision of Fixed Prosthesis immediately after surgery helped hold mandible in place avoiding the collapse of the arch in comminuted symphysis fractures due to the strong muscle pull. (**f**) OPG 16 years. postop showing the multiple bone fragments held in place with titanium miniplates and good bony healing

addition, due to scarring, vascularity of the soft tissue is compromised leading to increased incidence of dehiscence postoperatively. The most difficult to correct are the deformities involving the orbit. Enopthalmos take almost a month to settle down and be visible. It is almost impossible to assess the volume replacement required to achieve correction because of the 3-dimensional nature of the defect. To prevent this, it is always advisable to explore the orbital floor whenever the CT scan shows the presence of defects irrespective of the fact whether signs and symptoms are present. In severe fragmentation of bone, virtual surgical planning and fabrication of patient specific implants will give the best results. For blast injuries in the mandible where there is significant loss of bone in the symphysis region, it is ideal if a dental fixed prosthesis is placed replacing the missing teeth at the earliest (Fig. 14.46). Otherwise, due to the muscle pull, even the screws placed in the reconstruction plates can come out leading to collapse of the arch. In addition, the reconstruction plate bridging the gap is replaced with a bone graft for consolidation. This can be an iliac crest bone graft if the defect is less than 8 cm. For bony defects greater than 8 cm, a free fibula bone graft is the best option. Dental implants can be placed on this bone graft to restore mastication.

14.6 Conclusion

Maxillofacial trauma is an increasingly common phenomenon leading to significant morbidity, YPLL and DALYS. Optimal primary management by a multispecialty interdisciplinary team will minimize mortality and morbidity as well as restore function at the earliest. Any disfigurement of the region can have very serious psychosocial consequences. Correction of secondary deformities is very challenging and leads to compromised results. With the recent advances in materials, technology and techniques, it is possible to restore optimum function as well as esthetics if handled by an expert team in the first attempt.

References

1. Peden M, Mcgee J, Krug E, editors. Injury: a leading cause of the global burden of diseaes-2000. Geneva: World Health Organization; 2002.
2. Krug E, Etienne G. Injury—a leading cause of the global burden of disease. Geneva: World Health Organization; 1999.
3. WHO. Health in 2015: from MDGs to SDGs.
4. Cukier W. Firearms/small arms: finding common ground. Can Foreign Policy. 1998;6:73–87.

5. Krug EE, editor. World report on violence and health, vol. 360. Geneva: World Health Organization; 2002. p. 1083.
6. Reza A, Mercy JA, Krug EE. Epidemiology of violent deaths in the world. Inj Prev. 2001;7:104–11.
7. World Health Organization (WHO). Small arms and global health. Paper prepared for SALW talks. Geneva: WHO; 2001.
8. Shapiro A, Johnson R, Miller S, McCarthy MC. Facial fractures in a level I trauma Centre: the importance of protective devices and alcohol abuse. Injury. 2001;32:353–6.
9. Rai KM, Kale R, Mohanty SK, Chakrabarty A, Waghray MR, Kumar R, Prasad D, Lahiri AK. Treatment of casualties in a forward hospital of Indian Army: nine years experience. Med J Armed Forces India. 2004;60:20–4.
10. Pappachan B, Alexander M. Biomechanics of craniomaxillofacial trauma. J Maxillofac Oral Surg. 2012;11(2):224–30.
11. Bentley RP. Craniofacial trauma including management of frontal sinus and nasoethmoidal injuries. In: Langdon JD, Arnold H, et al., editors. Operative oral & maxillofacial surgery. London: CRC; 2017. p. 513.
12. Garg RK, Afifi AM, Gassner J, et al. A novel classification of frontal bone fractures: the prognostic significance of vertical fracture trajectory and skull base extension. J Plast Reconstr Aesthet Surg. 2015;68(5):645–53.
13. Patil RS, Kale TP, Kotrashetti SM, Baliga SD, Prabhu N, Issrani R. Assessment of changing patterns of le fort fracture lines using computed tomography scan: an observational study. Acta Odontol Scand. 2014;72(8):984–8.
14. Phillips JB, Turco LM. Le fort fractures: a collective review. Bull Emerg Trauma. 2017;5(4):221–30.
15. Boyette JR, Pemberton JD, Bonilla-Velez J. Management of orbital fractures: challenges and solutions. Clin Ophtalmol. 2015;17(9):2127–37.
16. Kim HS, Jeong EC. Orbital floor fracture. Arch Craniofac Surg. 2016;17(3):111–8.
17. Yuen HW, Hohman MH, Mazzoni T. Mandible fracture. [updated 2019 Oct 30]. In: StatPearls [internet]. Treasure Island, FL: StatPearls Publishing; 2020.
18. Erdmann D, Follmar KE, Debruijn M, et al. A retrospective analysis of facial fracture etiologies. Ann Plast Surg. 2008;60(4):398–403.
19. Kreidl KO, Kim DY, Mansour SE. Prevalence of significant intraocular sequelae in blunt orbital trauma. Am J Emerg Med. 2003;21(7):525–8.
20. Jeroukhimov I, Cockburn M, Cohn S. Facial trauma: overview of trauma care. In: Thaller SR, WS MD, editors. Facial trauma. New York: Marcel Dekker; 2004. p. 1–17.
21. National Academies of Sciences [NAS]. A national trauma care system: integrating military and civilian trauma systems to achieve zero preventable deaths after injury. 2016. http://www.nationalacademies.org/hmd/Reports/2016/A-National-TraumaCare-System-Integrating-Military-and-Civilian-Trauma-Systems.aspx.
22. WHO. Guidelines for trauma quality improvement programmes 2009.
23. Practice Guidelines for Management of Difficult Airway. An updated report by the American Society of Anesthesiologists Task Force on Management of Difficult Airway. Anesthesiology. 2013;118(2):1–20.
24. Beogo R, Bouletreau P, Konsem T, Traore I, Coulibaly AT, Ouedraogo D. Wire internal fixation: an obsolete, yet valuable method for surgical management of facial fractures. Pan Afr Med J. 2014;17:219.
25. Vignesh U, Mehrotra D, Dichen Anand A, Howlader D. Three dimensional reconstruction of late post traumatic orbital wall defects by customized implants using CAD-CAM 3D stereolithographic models. A case report. J Oral Biol Craniofac Res. 2017;7:212–8.
26. Parthasarathy J. 3D modeling, custom implants and its future perspectives in craniofacial surgery. Ann Maxillofac Surg. 2014;4(1):9–18.
27. Ellis E III, Zide MF. Surgical approaches to the facial skeleton. 3rd ed. Philadelphia: Wolters Kluwer; 2018.
28. Matteini C, Renzi G, Becelli R, et al. Surgical timing in orbital fracture treatment: experience with 108 consecutive cases. J Craniofac Surg. 2004;15:145–50.
29. Putterman AM, Stevens T, Urist MJ. Nonsurgical management of blow-out fractures of the orbital floor. Am J Ophthalmol. 1974;77:232–9.
30. Burnstine MA. Clinical recommendation for repair of isolated orbital floor fracture. Opthalmology. 2002;109:1207–13.
31. Brucoli M, Arcuri F, Cavenaghi R, Benech A. Analysis of complications after surgical repair of orbital fractures. J Cariofac Surg. 2011;22(4):1387–90.
32. Hossal BM, Beatty RL. Diplopia and enophthalmos after surgical repair of blow-out fracture. Orbit. 2002;21:27–33.
33. Jin HR, Lee HS, Yeon JY, Suh MW. Residual diplopia after repair of pure blow-out fracture: the importance of extraocular muscle injury. Am J Rhinol. 2007;21:276–80.
34. Christensen BJ, Zaid W. Inaugural survey on practice patterns of orbital floor fractures for American Oral and maxillofacial surgeons. J Oral Maxillofac Surg. 2016;74(1):105–22.
35. Girotto JA, MacKenzie E, Fowler C, Redett R, Robertson B, Manson PN. Long term physical impairment and functional outcomes after complex facial fractures. Plast Reconstr Surg. 2001;108(2):312–27.
36. Jarupoonphol V. Surgical treatment of Le Fort fractures in Ban Pong hospital: two decades of experience. J Med Assoc Thail. 2001;84(11):1541–9.
37. Champy M, Lodde JP, Schmitt R, Jaeger JH, Muster D. Mandibular osteosynthesis by miniature screwed plates via buccal approach. J Maxillofac Surg. 1978;6(1):14–21.

38. Gokel T. Improvised explosive devices and the oral and maxillofacial surgeon. Oral Maxillofac Surg Clin North Am. 2005;17:281–7.
39. Gibbons AJ, Breeze A. The face of war: the initial management of modern battlefield ballistic facial injuries. J Mili Veteran Health. 2011;19(2):15–8.
40. Girish Kumar N, Vijaya N, Jha AK. Blast injuries of mandible: a protocol. J Maxillofac Oral Surg. 2012;11(2):191–4.

Injuries of the Nasolacrimal Drainage System

15

Apjit Kaur and Ankita

15.1 Introduction

The lacrimal drainage pathway is frequently involved in blunt and penetrating trauma of the periorbital area and face. Both accidental and iatrogenic traumas are reported to cause soft tissue and bony anatomical changes resulting in tear drainage abnormalities [1, 2]. Epiphora and dacryocystitis are common presentation [1, 3]. With the advances in radiology, it is possible to localize, classify, and plan the management in such cases [4]. As facial trauma is associated in a subset of cases, the need of comprehensive management cannot be ignored.

15.2 Anatomy of the Lacrimal Drainage Pathway

Knowledge of the antomy of the medial canthal area, both soft tissues and bones encompassing lacrimal passage, is crucial for diagnosis and proper management of injuries in the area.

15.2.1 Osteology

The medial wall of orbit is formed of frontal process of maxilla, lacrimal bone, lamina papyracea of ethmoid, and body of sphenoid. The anteromedial wall of orbit harbors the lacrimal sac, which lies in the lacrimal fossa. The fossa is formed by maxillary bone anteriorly and lacrimal bone posteriorly, bounded by the anterior and posterior lacrimal crest. The anterior lacrimal crest is rounded and projects from the maxillary bone, while the posterior lacrimal crest is sharp and projects from the lacrimal bone. Maxillary-lacrimal suture lies vertically in the lacrimal fossa, corresponding to the maxillary line in the lateral wall of nose and roughly bisecting the fossa. Its position in the fossa is dependent upon the size of the individual bone [5]. The lacrimal fossa is about 12 mm long, 4–6 mm antero-posteriorly and 2–3 mm wide. The fossa is widest at the base and tapers into a depression, which leads to the bony nasolacrimal canal in the lateral wall of the nose [1].

A. Kaur (✉)
Department of Ophthalmology, Oculoplasty and Orbit Unit, King George Medical University, Lucknow, India

Ankita
Department of Ophthalmology, Sanjay Gandhi PGIMS, Lucknow, India

S. Waikar (ed.), *Ocular Trauma in Armed Conflicts*, https://doi.org/10.1007/978-981-19-4021-7_15

The nasolacrimal canal is bounded laterally by the maxillary bone and medially by the lacrimal bone and inferior turbinate. The nasolacrimal canal is directed downward, backward, and laterally into the bony canal and in the lateral wall of nose to open into the inferior nasal meatus. The bony canal measures about 12 mm. The duct diameter is about 4–6 mm at the superior end. The lower end is situated 25–30 mm posterior to lateral margin of anterior nares or 35 mm posterior to insertion of inferior turbinate head [6, 7].

15.2.2 Soft Tissue Anatomy

Lacrimal passage drains tears from conjunctival cul-de-sac into inferior meatus of nose. Lacrimal punctum lies on lacrimal papilla, an elevation at the medial end of eyelid margin. Lacrimal punctum is located at the medial end of both upper and lower eyelids, 5 and 6 mm from medial canthus, respectively [8]. The canaliculus of each eyelid travels 2 mm vertically (downwards in the lower eyelid and upwards in the upper eyelid). It then continues horizontally for 8 mm, in close proximity to the eyelid margin. The canaliculi either join to form common canaliculus, or may separately enter the lateral wall of lacrimal sac just above the vertical midpoint of the sac. The medial canthal tendon (MCT) delineates the fundus of the lacrimal sac, which lies up to 3–5 mm superior to it, the body of the sac extends approximately 10 mm beneath it. The sac continues into nasolacrimal duct inferiorly. The membranous part of the duct in the lateral wall of nose is about 5 mm long [9].

Insight of soft tissue anatomy in the medial most part of the eye is also important. The MCT provides the fibrous strength to the medial most part of the eyelids. The superficial heads of the pretarsal and preseptal orbicularis oculi augment the MCT. The superficial head of pretarsal fibres lies anterior to the canaliculi. The deep head of the pretarsal fibres (constituting Horners muscle) inserts onto the posterior lacrimal crest and the lacrimal fascia. The deep head of preseptal fibres also inserts into the deep fascia of the sac [6, 9].

15.3 Lacrimal System Injuries

15.3.1 Etiology

Lacrimal drainage pathway injuries commonly result from trauma due to high-energy impact on the upper part of the nasal bridge, resulting from physical assault or road accidents (Figs. 15.1 and 15.2). Laceration injuries due to animal bite like dog and bear are also not uncommon (Fig. 15.3) [1, 10, 11]. Dog bite is the most common cause of penetrating trauma,

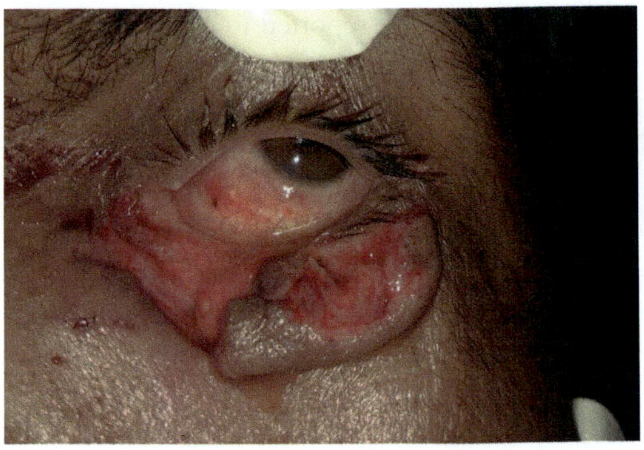

Fig. 15.1 Clinical picture illustrating left lower eyelid laceration: medial full-thickness laceration involving the lower canaliculus and horizontal partial thickness laceration below the lash line

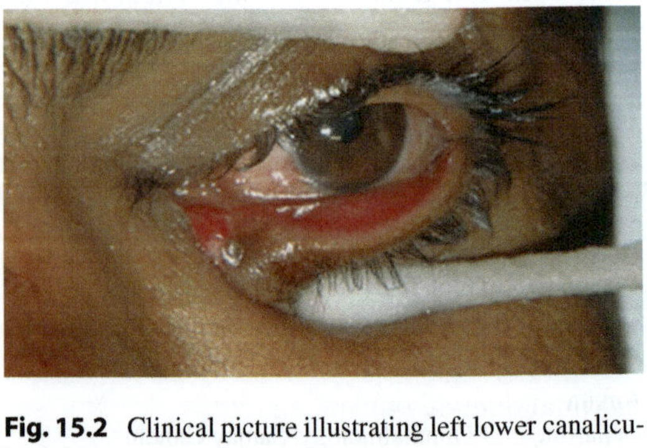

Fig. 15.2 Clinical picture illustrating left lower canalicular injury

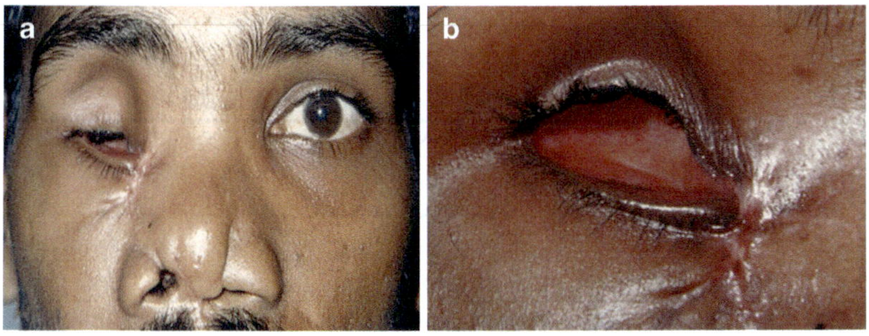

Fig. 15.3 Clinical picture illustrating (**a**) Bear paw injury with telecanthus and lower eyelid scar extending to upper cheek (right side) and ala of nose (**b**) Eviscerated right eye and right lower canalicular involvement

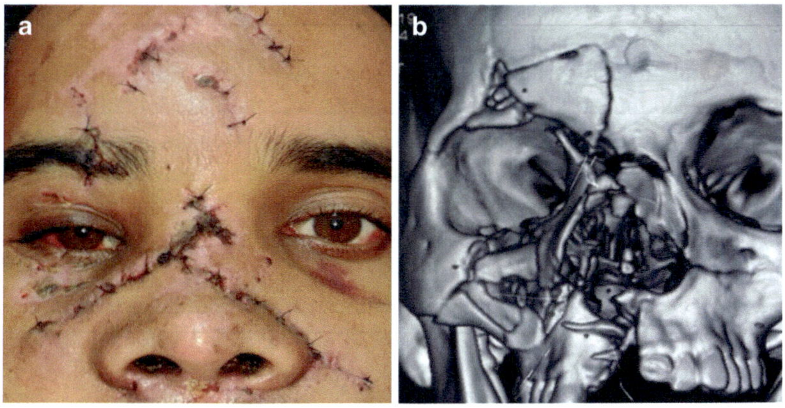

Fig. 15.4 (**a**) Clinical picture of patient with right eye dystopia, mild right upper lid ptosis, saddle nose deformity, and multiple sutured lacerations over face following road accident. (**b**) 3-D reconstruction CT image of the patient illustrating fracture roof, medial wall and floor of orbit, fracture maxilla, zygoma, and nasal bone of right side

while fist fight is for blunt trauma. It can include either a soft tissue injury or may be complicated with orbital fractures. Orbital fractures can be categorized as simple/isolated fractures and complex fractures. Complex orbital fractures are associated with orbitofacial fractures. The naso-orbital-ethmoid (NOE), Le Fort II and Le Fort III fractures are frequently associated with lacrimal drainage pathway injuries [4, 12–17] (Fig. 15.4).

Surgical procedures of the face and nose are reported to cause nasolacrimal duct injury. Mid-face procedures, which involve reflection of the medial wall of the orbit, like Le Fort III osteotomy, can injure the apparatus [10]. Functional endoscopic sinus surgery (FESS) used for treatment of chronic and acute complicated rhinosinusitis can also cause injury to the lacrimal duct due to anatomical predispositions in the area. The lacrimal bone can be thin in areas near attachment of the uncinate process. Also, pnuematization of agger nasi cells may extend up to the lacrimal or even the maxillary bone in the lacrimal fossa, rendering the bones thin and thus predisposing to surgical trauma [2, 7].

15.3.2 Mechanism of Injury

The anatomical location of the lacrimal drainage pathway predisposes it to both soft tissue and bony injuries. Lacrimal drainage obstruction can occur at any level starting from punctum to the nasolacrimal duct. A surgical classification system exists to delineate the location and extent of injury and for planning management system. Presaccal obstruction refers to injuries involving the puncta, the canaliculi, and/or common canaliculi; saccal obstruction refers to injuries localized up to the lacrimal sac; and postsaccal obstruction can be due to injuries of the nasolacrimal duct [18]. Due to lack of tarsal plate support at the medial most end of the eyelid, the canalicular part easily succumbs to injury. Penetrating trauma causes direct canalicular injury, while blunt trauma causes stretching in the area and subsequent injury. Trauma in males (both children and young adults) is more common, and lower canaliculus involvement is frequent [19, 20]. The distal part of the nasolacrimal duct is protected by bony structures, and almost never affected by trauma [1].

Several mechanisms are involved, which may be classified into soft tissue or bony trauma. Soft tissue may develop scarring and fibrosis, and bones may be displaced or obstruct other surrounding bone segments. Most of the symptoms are a result of progressive fibrosis of soft tissue and do not present immediately after trauma. In addition to lacrimal drainage pathway obstruction, several lid deformities in the form of entropion, ectropion, and punctal causes like stenosis can also result in epiphora [12].

15.4 Clinical Manifestations

The main presenting symptom of lacrimal drainage system injury is a watery eye. Presence of telecanthus and dystopia of canaliculus and punctum are suggestive of involvement of deeper tissues like the medial canthal tendon (Figs. 15.4 and 15.5). Early post traumatic phase is associated with edema, hematoma, and transient canalicular stenosis. Persistent watering, associated with development of localized sac swelling, which drains through the punctum on pressure, points toward nasolacrimal duct obstruction. A sac swelling that does not drain on pressure could be associated with canalicular block or encystment of the lacrimal sac. Malar contour abnormality with enophthalmos results from associated orbital fractures (Fig. 15.6) [1, 3, 12]. The presenting complaints depend upon the location of injury. While punctal stenosis and unrepaired canalicular trauma may present only with epiphora, trauma in lacrimal sac and nasolacrimal duct can present with symptoms of acute or chronic dacryocystitis, telecanthus, and even facial functional and cosmetic deformities if associated with Le Fort or NOE fractures [3, 21–24] (Figs. 15.7 and 15.8).

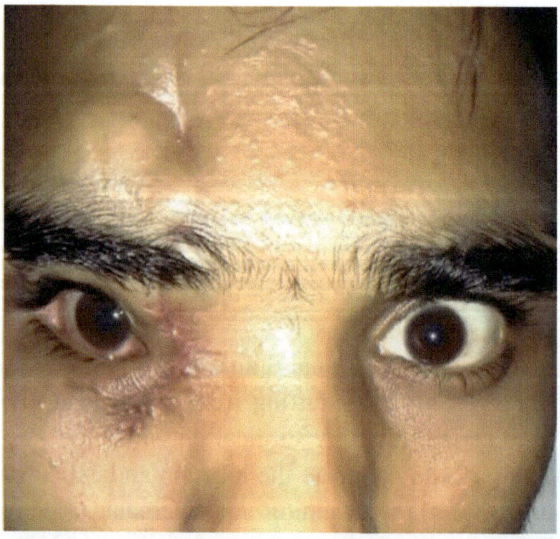

Fig. 15.5 Clinical picture illustrating posttraumatic telecanthus (right side) and scar over medial part of lower eyelid, medial to medial canthus, and upper eyelid extending to forehead, left upper eyelid retraction, and saddle nose deformity

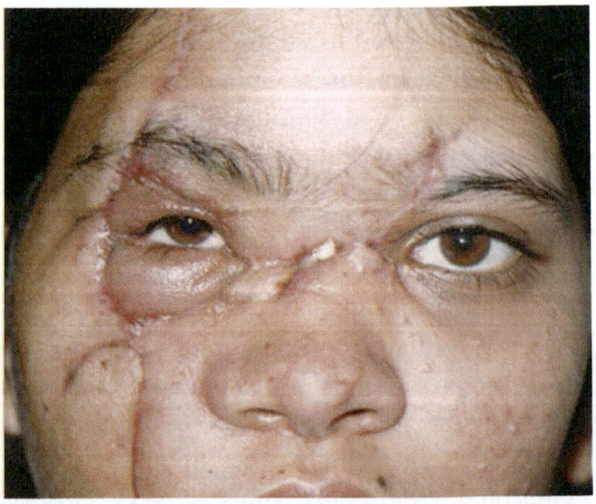

Fig. 15.6 Clinical picture illustrating post traumatic telecanthus, medial canthal deformity (Rt), malar flattening (Rt), and nasal bridge deformity

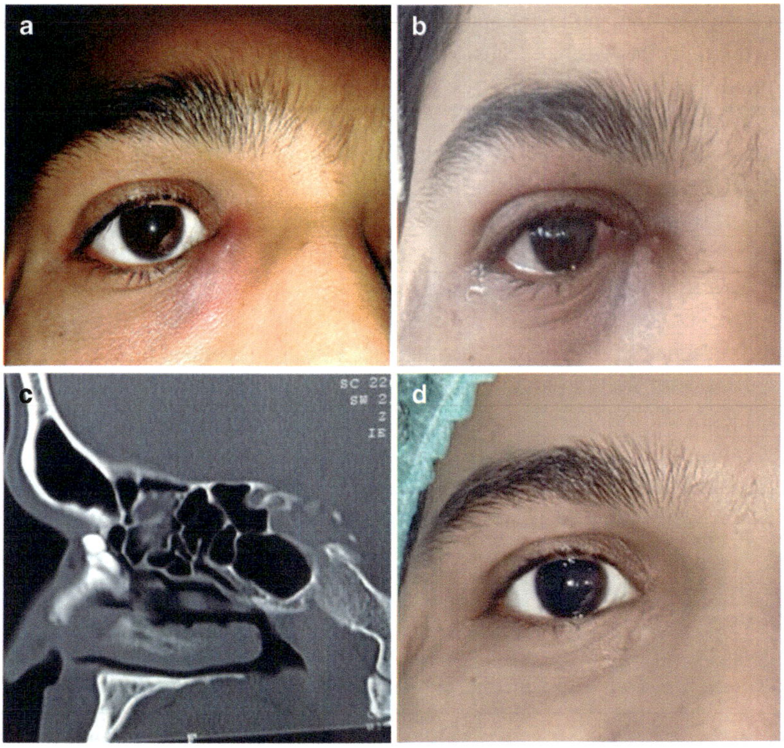

Fig. 15.7 Posttraumatic dacryocystitis with telecanthus (right side) (**a**) Clinical picture of acute stage; (**b**) Clinical picture of chronic stage; (**c**) CT-DCG sagittal section image showing obstruction distal to the lacrimal sac; (**d**) One month follow-up image with good post-op results

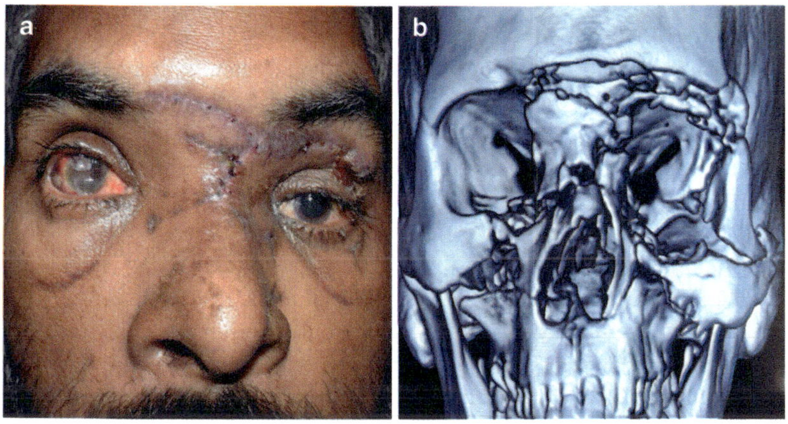

Fig. 15.8 (**a**) Clinical picture of a patient with road accident showing ocular injury and telecanthus (right side), multiple sutured lacerations over forehead, nose, and left upper eyelid with saddle nose deformity. (**b**) 3-D reconstruction CT image of the same patient illustrating multiple facial fractures (Le Fort Type II and NOE Type III with bilateral orbital roof fracture)

15.5 Diagnosis

15.5.1 Clinical Assessment

Emergency trauma management consists of ensuring airway, breathing, and circulation of the patient. Significant facial injuries are often associated with thoracic, abdominal, or neurological injury [1]. A detailed history and physical examination is required in every case of trauma, to differentiate between hypersecretion and epiphora. History should focus on enquiring about the nature, duration, mode of trauma, and any associated risk factors likely to cause the resultant conditions [4].

A thorough slit-lamp evaluation of eyeball and eyelid should be performed before rushing to the lacrimal area evaluation. In cases of recent trauma, soft tissue edema and ecchymosis may mask underlying bony trauma. Lacerations in the medial canthal area should be further examined to see the extent of injury and presence of tissue loss. Cotton tipped swab can be used for palpation and examination of tissues. The identification of proximal end becomes crucial in lacrimal canaliculus transection. The “Calameri ring” sign demonstrates the proximal edge of transected canaliculus as rolled epithelium [19].

The lacrimal sac is encased by the anterior and posterior limbs of the medial canthal tendon, endangering its integrity in canthal trauma [25]. “Traction test” is used to check medial canthal tendon disruption. It is performed by pulling the eyelid against the medial attachment, after holding upper or lower eyelid margin at lateral end. The margin should become taut in cases with intact tendon. If edema precludes the view, any asymmetry in medial canthal position should be considered indicative of MCT disruption. Palpation in cases with traumatic telecanthus may sometimes reveal crepitus, suggestive of an associated medial orbital wall fracture [1].

Protrusion of fat from cutaneous laceration points towards orbital penetration. In such cases concurrent globe injuries should also be looked for and managed [25]. Bony dislocation and displacement is suspected in cases with post traumatic facial deformity, shifting or flattening of the orbital and naso-orbital regions and associated traumatic telecanthus [12]. Saddle nose deformity after trauma suggests loss of bony support on the sac area [1]. Medial orbital wall fractures produce lacrimal passage injuries due to disruption of medial canthal tendon, emphysema due to damaged ethmoid air sinuses, and vascular compromise due to damage to ethmoidal arteries. This can also result in sight-threatening complications [25].

In cases with delayed presentation, evidences of changes due to chronic inflammation, infection, and scarring should be evaluated for. Punctal non-apposition, eyelid malposition, periocular scarring, and discharging sinuses are indicators of breach in lacrimal drainage integrity. Irrigation of lacrimal system is contraindicated in presence of acute inflammation and edema. In the setting of midface trauma, irrigation fluid may extravasate through the breach in lacrimal system and produce false results. In such scenario, therapeutic probing may yield better details about patency of the pathway. Tear meniscus height and fluorescein dye disappearance test can also yield high false-positive results. Jones dye test I and II may help evaluate site and extent of block [4].

15.5.2 Role of Imaging

Radiological evaluation has limited contributory role in evaluation of presaccal trauma. Extent and nature of saccal and postsaccal injuries are satisfactorily delineated by radiological tests like CT and MRI. NOE fractures need to be evaluated with a CT scan, with axial and coronal sections spaced 1.5 mm. High resolution imaging avoids missing subtle pathologies, which may affect the future prognosis. Structural integrity of drainage system beyond canaliculus is delineated adequately by dacryocystography (DCG), either using CT or magnetic Resonance imaging (MRI) with topical Gadolinium (Fig. 15.9). It helps ascertain the relative position in relation to displaced bony fragments and/or plates/meshes that may have been used. The latter indicates impingement of grafts/meshes on the lacrimal system [4]. 3-D reconstruction CT images offer excellent image resolution in associated facial trauma [26] (Fig. 15.4b and 15.8b). Radionucleotide scintigraphy can highlight physiological functioning of the sac but is less practical due to high cost and nonavailability [4, 7]. Nasal endoscopy provides information regarding concurrent nasal pathology. Newer continuous view endoscopes aid in complex lacrimal surgical procedures and in cases where nasal pathologies are also to be dealt

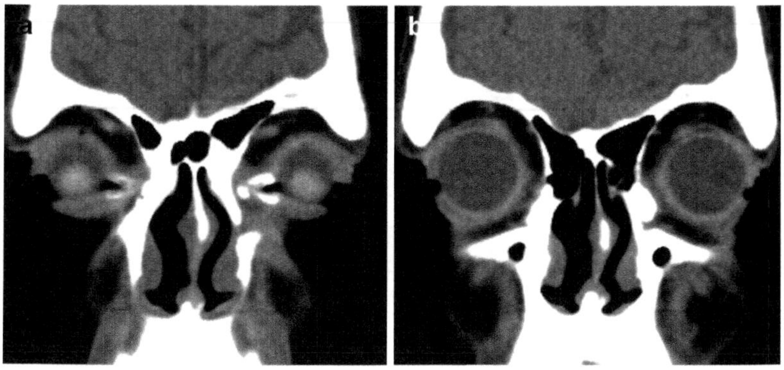

Fig. 15.9 Illustrating the CT-DCG coronal section images (**a**) With dye filling the upper and lower canaliculi and lacrimal sac of left side; (**b**) Pooling of dye in the lacrimal sac

with [27, 28]. The role of stereotactic navigation in lacrimal abnormalities, often referred to as image guided dacryolocalization, is helpful in understanding the precise lacrimal and peri-lacrimal anatomical abnormalities in posttraumatic cases [23, 29, 30].

15.6 Management

All ocular and optic nerve injuries should be addressed prior to managing lacrimal trauma as bony manipulation may worsen the preexisting damage [1]. Lacerations and bony trauma repair can be categorized into primary and secondary repair. Primary repair is regarded as early when done within 24–48 h and delayed within 2 days to 2 weeks. Repair after 2 weeks is referred to as secondary repair. Though early repair is advocated in majority of lacrimal injuries, delayed repair can be advantageous as posttraumatic edema is less [31]. Tissue ecchymosis and edema may sometimes mask underlying bony disfigurement and also pose difficulty in identification of soft tissue structures [1]. Secondary repair, planned or unplanned, has its own advantages and disadvantages [17].

Early single-staged repair with precise fracture reduction and bone grafting (if required) provides best results. Local anesthetic block is preferred, though simultaneous management of extensive injuries of face requires general anesthesia. Surgery in children and elderly patients also needs general anesthesia [1].

15.6.1 Canalicular Trauma

Single functional canaliculus is sufficient to drain basal tear secretion. Also, upper canalicular obstruction rarely produces epiphora in normal environmental conditions. It is said that lower canaliculus should be preserved for the patient and upper canaliculus for the ophthalmologist [3]. All presaccal lacerations injuries should be attempted to repair in the first place, within 24–48 h of injury [1].

Reanastomosis of cut canalicular ends is of prime importance [1]. Proximal end of lacerated canaliculus can be identified by injecting air, saline, viscoelastic substances or dye (fluorescein or trypan blue) through the ipsilateral intact canaliculus and observing its egress from the transected end. Some authors also advocate the use of topical sympathomimetic drugs to blanch surrounding tissue, lacrimal probing from opposite punctum, which pushes the proximal end laterally and 23G fibreoptic pipe illumination through uninjured canaliculus [32–34]. Alternatively, pigtail probe can also be used in a similar way. Stent is passed in order to maintain proper alignment and patency of the canalicular system. Various types of stents are available depending on the material and design. Minimonoka (monocanalicular) and Crawford (bicanalicular) are commonly used synthetic stents. Other types of stent used are Mono-Crawford, Ritleng and Goldberg bicanalicular stents, etc [24]. Monocanalicular stents are passed from the punctum and traverse only the cut canaliculus. The other end may either

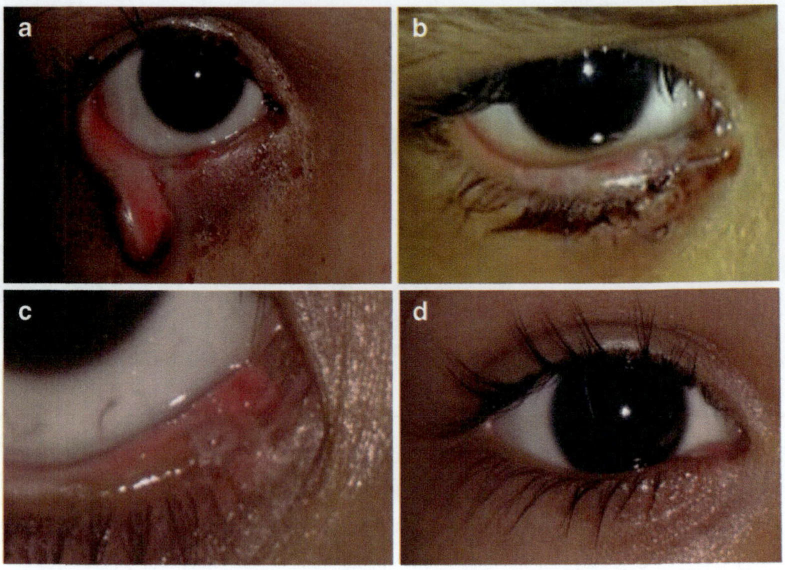

Fig. 15.10 Clinical picture of patient illustrating: (**a**) Right lower lid full-thickness laceration involving lower canaliculus. (**b**) Same patient after eyelid and canalicular repair and stenting with Minimonoka stent. (**c**) One week post-op image of the patient with stent in place. (**d**) One month follow-up image with stent in situ

rest in the sac or may extend into nose. Bicanalicular stents cannulate both canaliculi and are fixed in a similar fashion. Lid repair is done after suturing the canalicular wall. Silicon stents are removed 2–6 months after the procedure [34] (Fig. 15.10). If the transected canalicular end cannot be localized, lid laceration repair with canalicular laissez-faire is used.

Conventionally, monocanalicular stents work for lacerations of single canaliculus and bicanalicular stents for both upper and lower canaliculi. But it is reported that bicanalicular lacerations have better outcomes both functionally and cosmetically with separate monocanalicular intubation of the injured canaliculi [35]. Proximal canalicular lacerations produce epiphora more often as compared to distal lacerations. Damage to lacrimal pump, which has more action in proximal part of canaliculus, is a possible explanation for the same [19]. The vectors of the medial canthal tendon encasing the lacrimal passage need to be re-established. One commonly used technique is to pass a double-armed suture through the precanalicular pretarsal muscle fibers followed by the periosteum medially and tying a knot after exteriorizing the suture laterally through the skin [32].

In cases of delayed repair, often the proximal end can be more visible due to contrast from surrounding tissue, but the overall results are poor. Poor outcomes can be attributed due to granulation tissue surrounding canaliculus and associated eyelid and canthal deformity [1, 31, 34, 36].

Canaliculodacryocystorhinostomy is indicated in cases with obstruction at the level of common canaliculus. The patent common canaliculus and lacrimal sac are anastomosed with stent to maintain patency [20].

15.6.2 Lacrimal Sac and Duct Trauma

Post traumatic dacryocystitis results from blockage of NLD. Postinflammatory stricture of the soft tissues and misalignment of the osseous part contribute to the block. Swelling in mucosal walls of lacrimal sac in early phase contributes to luminal block [1, 12]. Traumatic chronic dacryocystitis due to nasolacrimal duct injury occurs almost about 4 weeks following trauma [36]. All cases with acute dacryocystitis should be managed with antibiotic therapy, and dacryocystorhinostomy (DCR) should be performed after 4 weeks at least [12]. Re-assessment should be performed after edema resolves, preferably 1–3 months after trauma. FDDT is suggestive of NLD block, but CT-DCG provides details about

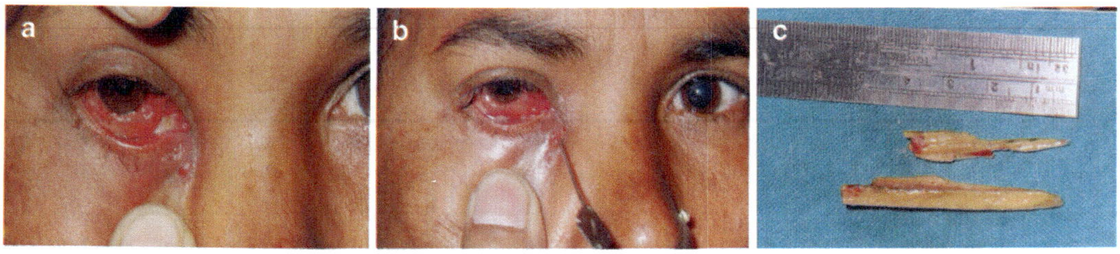

Fig. 15.11 Clinical picture of foreign body in inferior orbit masquerading as lacrimal sac abscess and cutaneous fistula. (**a**) Lower eyelid retraction reveals inferomedial subconjunctival abscess with cutaneous fistula; (**b**) Probe passed from fistula and the direction was found to be toward subconjunctival space; (**c**) Wooden foreign body retrieved from subconjunctival space

anatomical changes in the sac, surrounding bones, and nose with bony deformity if present [1, 12].

Due to the disturbed anatomical configuration, the surgery of posttraumatic dacryocystitis surgery becomes challenging. External dacryocystorhinostomy is preferred over endoscopic procedure (Fig. 15.7). A larger skin incision with minimal tissue damage should be practiced to preserve lacrimal pump function. Bone removal may be tougher due to inflammation and impaction following trauma. Larger osteotomy size (>15 mm) is advocated [37]. Delayed secondary repair, 5–6 months from primary repair and subsequent DCR, decreases sac friability [1, 12]. Application of mitomycin-C at the osteotomy site, preferably circumosteal, provides superior results [38, 39]. The role of dacryocystectomy is limited only in patients with multiple failed external DCR surgeries and extensive intranasal synechiae [21].

Dacryocystorhinostomy may not be helpful in cases with widespread scarring in the lacrimal sac or displaced lacrimal bones. Conjunctivodacryocysorhinostomy (CDCR) procedure is usually done in such cases. Jones tube or similar bypass stent is placed from the caruncle into the lateral nasal mucosal wall, directly, after making a large osteotomy [1, 27].

There are several instances when unusual presentations in the lacrimal sac have been seen following trauma. Sac pneumatocoele has been reported to occur in medial wall fractures due to anatomical proximity. Lacrimal sac trauma is not uncommon after endoscopic transnasal DCR. Iatrogenic foreign bodies in lacrimal sac and posttraumatic orbital foreign bodies mimicking as sac abscess have also been reported (Fig. 15.11) [40, 41].

15.6.3 Concurrent Facial Trauma

Saccal and postsaccal injuries are often associated with facial fractures, especially NOE fractures. The complex anatomy of the NOE region is often reported to have many anatomical variations. Radiology has helped evaluate various complexities in nasolacrimal system fractures. Fracture of lacrimal fossa, avulsion of anterior or posterior lacrimal crest, bony fragment in the lacrimal fossa, nasolacrimal canal fracture, bony fragment in canal or distraction of fractured canal, nasomaxillary buttress displacement, midface displacement, and periosteal stripping have been identified [42]. (Fig. 15.8).

Dacryocystitis due to trauma in NOE region is usually managed by external DCR if it does not resolve spontaneously after 4–6 weeks or after fracture reduction [43, 44] Early repair (within 2 weeks) and prophylactic intubation of the ipsilateral nasolacrimal system during any maxillofacial surgery (trauma, tumors, or any chronic infection of lacrimal drainage system) is advocated in several studies [42]. Although intubation in such cases may be difficult, risky, and traumatizing to the drainage pathway, late intervention cannot rule out the same [45]. The role of intraoperative navigation in orbital and orbitofacial trauma management is also emerging. It ensures

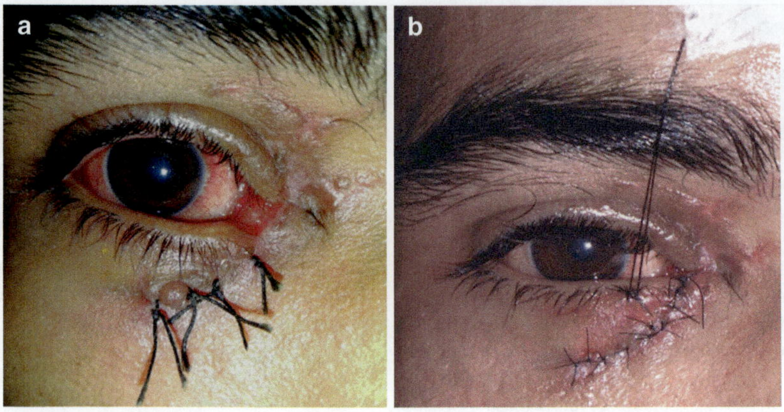

Fig. 15.12 (**a**) Illustrating sutured eyelid laceration of right lower eyelid: eyelid notching, unopposed canalicular ends, puckering of skin in lower lid, scar over medial part of upper eyelid, and medial ankyloses. (**b**) Illustrating secondary repair of lower lid laceration: well apposed eyelid margin, repaired lower canaliculus with Minimonoka stent, improved lower eyelid skin pucker. Medial ankyloses, however, couldn't be released

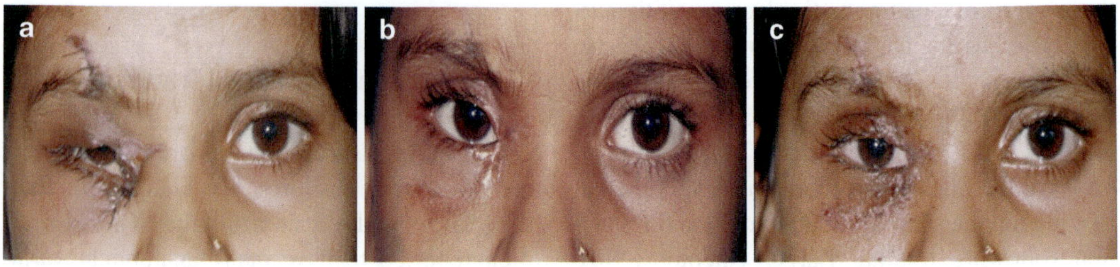

Fig. 15.13 (**a**) Illustrating sutured eyelid laceration of right forehead, upper and lower eyelid: lower eyelid notching, unrepaired canaliculi, puckering of skin in lower lid, telecanthus, mechanical ptosis, and medial ankyloses. (**b**) Illustrating secondary repair of lower lid laceration: well apposed upper and lower eyelid margin with repaired lower canaliculus and telecanthus. (**c**) The same patient after release of medial ankyloses

accuracy of reduction of fractured fragments and, thus, good postoperative outcomes [15, 39].

15.6.4 Secondary Repair

Secondary repair of lacrimal injuries is challenging owing to dense scarring and fibrosis and inability to identify normal anatomical details. Repair involves excision of all scar tissues and identification of lacrimal passage using probe and dye, if possible. All injuries with bony fracture and displacement need to be addressed first. In canalicular trauma, reanastomosis of lacerated canalicular ends with stenting is tough, but possible. Lacrimal sac and duct injuries can be managed with external dacryocystitis and bicanalicular stenosis [17]. (Figs. 15.12 and 15.13).

15.7 Complications and Sequelae

Silicon tube intubation in lacrimal apparatus is well tolerated. However, complications like cheese wiring of punctum and canaliculus are reported. Removal of stent is then indicated. Pyogenic granuloma may form near the punctum, which can be removed with cautery at base (Fig. 15.14). Intubation can cause keratoconjunctivitis due to chronic irritation of the ocular surface, warranting its urgent removal. A prolapsed and extruded tube, if can't be positioned through any approach, should be removed [1].

Presence of persistent epiphora after DCR surgery is reported as resulting from eyelid laxity or lacrimal pump failure and can be managed by eyelid-tightening procedures and lacrimal stenting, respectively [46].

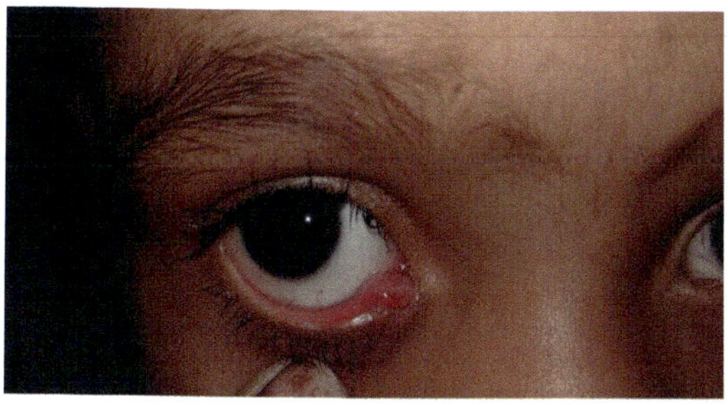

Fig. 15.14 Clinical picture of patient of right lower canalicular injury with pyogenic granuloma and Minimonoka stent in situ

References

1. Della RDA, Ahmad S, Preechawi P, Schaefer SD, Della RRC. Nasolacrimal system injuries. Berlin: Springer; 2007. p. 91–103.
2. Bolger MWE, Parsons CDS, Mair MEA, Kuhn FA. Lacrimal drainage system injury in functional endoscopic sinus surgery. Arch Otolaryngol Head Neck Surg. 1992;118:1179–84.
3. Linberg JV, Moore CA. Symptoms of canalicular obstruction. Ophthalmology. 1988;95:1077–9. https://doi.org/10.1016/S0161-6420(88)33057-5.
4. Lelli GJ. Trauma lacrimal sac and nasolacrimal duct. In: Encyclopedia of ophthalmology. Cham: Springer; 2017. p. 1–4.
5. Tripathy K, Sharma YR, Chawla R, Basu K, Vohra R. Triads in ophthalmology: a comprehensive review. Semin Ophthalmol. 2015;00(00):1–14. https://doi.org/10.3109/08820538.2015.1045150.
6. Burkat CN, Lucarelli MJ. The lacrimal system. Cham: Springer; 2015. p. 1–14.
7. Cohen NA, Antunes MB, Morgenstern KE. Prevention and management of lacrimal duct injury. Otolaryngol Clin N Am. 2010;43:781–8.
8. Machiele R, Czyz CN. Anatomy, head and neck, eye lacrimal gland. Treasure Island, FL: StatPearls; 2020. p. 1–4. http://www.ncbi.nlm.nih.gov/pubmed/30422509.
9. Paulsen F. Anatomy and physiology of the nasolacrimal ducts. Ophthalmologe. 2008;105:1–13.
10. Balaji SM. Management of nasolacrimal duct injuries in mid-facial advancement. Ann Maxillofac Surg. 2015;5(1):93–5.
11. Anthony CM. Eyelid laceration. San Francisco: American Academy of Ophthamology; 2014. p. 1–7.
12. Gruss JS, Hurwitz JJ, Nik NA, Kassel EE. The pattern and incidence of nasolacrimal injury in naso- orbital-ethmoid fractures : the role of delayed assessment and dacryocystorhinostomy. Br J Plast Surg. 1985;38:116–21.
13. Phillips BJ. Le fort fractures: a collective review. Bull Emerg Trauma. 2017;5(4):221–30.
14. Esmaeelinejad M. Maxillofacial fractures: from diagnosis to treatment. In: Trauma surgery. London: InTech; 2018. p. 53–71.
15. Udhay P, Bhattacharjee K, Ananthanarayanan P, Sundar G. Computer—assisted navigation in orbitofacial surgery principle of intraoperative navigation. Indian J Ophthalmol. 2019;67(7):995–1003.
16. Sh E, Shahnaseri S, Soltani P, Reza M, Motamedi K. Management of naso-orbito-ethmoid fractures : a 10-year review. Trauma Mon. 2017;22(3):e29230.
17. Drnovšek-Olup B, Beltram M. Trauma of the lacrimal drainage system: retrospective study of 32 patients. Croat Med J. 2004;45(3):292–4.
18. Passos E, De JF, Cristina A, Santos G. Endoscopic dacryocystorhinostomy : our experience and literature review. Rev Bras Oftalmol. 2013;724:1–7.
19. Singh M, Gautam N, Ahir N, Kaur M. Is the distance from punctum a factor in the anatomical and functional success of canalicular laceration repairs ? Indian J Ophthalmol. 2017;65(11):1114–9.
20. Burkat CN, Stewart K, Stewart K. Canalicular obstruction. San Francisco: American Academy of Opthamology; 2020. p. 1–7.
21. Varghese CM, Varghese AM, Syed KA, Paul RR. Dacryocystectomy: an uncommon indication—a case report. Int J Pediatr Otorhinolaryngol. 2014;78(1):139–41. https://doi.org/10.1016/j.ijporl.2013.10.046.
22. Mukherjee B, Dhobekar M. Traumatic nasolacrimal duct obstruction: clinical profile, management, and outcome. Eur J Ophthalmol. 2013;23(5):615–22.
23. Ali MJ, Naik MN. Image-guided Dacryolocalization (IGDL) in traumatic secondary acquired lacrimal drainage obstructions (SALDO). Ophthal Plast Reconstr Surg. 2015;31(5):406–9.
24. Mukherjee B, Dhobekar M. Management of lacrimal system trauma. In: Emergencies of the orbit and adnexa. Cham: Springer; 2017. p. 77–87.
25. Roth FS, Koshy JC, Goldberg JS, Soparkar CNS. Pearls of orbital trauma management. Semin Plast Surg. 2010;24:398–409.
26. Udhay P, Noronha OV, Mohan RE. Helical computed tomographic dacryocystography and its role in the diagnosis and management of lacrimal drainage system blocks and medial canthal masses. Indian J Ophthalmol. 2008;56(1):31–7.
27. Sweeney A, Sweeney A, Burkat CN, Yen MT, Yen MT. Secondary acquired nasolacrimal duct obstruction. San Francisco: American Academy of Ophthalmology; 2020. p. 1–11.
28. Ali MJ, Singh S, Naik MN. The usefulness of continuously variable view rigid endoscope in lacrimal surgeries: first intraoperative experience. Ophthal Plast Reconstr Surg. 2016;32(6):477–80.
29. Nair AG, Singh S, Kamal S, Ali MJ. The importance of endoscopy in lacrimal surgery. Expert Rev Ophthalmol. 2018;13(5):257–65. https://doi.org/10.1080/17469899.2018.1520635.
30. Ali MJ, Singh S, Naik MN, Kaliki S, Dave TV. Interactive navigation-guided ophthalmic plas-

tic surgery: navigation enabling of telescopes and their use in endoscopic lacrimal surgeries. Clin Ophthalmol. 2016;10:2319–24.
31. Chu Y, Wu S, Tsai Y, Liao Y, Chu H. Early versus late canalicular laceration repair outcomes. Am J Ophthalmol. 2017;182:155–9. https://doi.org/10.1016/j.ajo.2017.08.006.
32. Murchison AP, Bilyk JR. A practical approach to canalicular lacerations. Rev Ophthalmol. 2017;2017:1–7.
33. Cho SH, Hyun DW, Kang HJ, Ha MS. A simple new method for identifying the proximal cut end in lower Canalicular laceration. Korean J Ophthalmol. 2008;22(2):73–6.
34. Reifler DM. Management of canalicular laceration. Surv Ophthalmol. 1991;36(2):113–32.
35. Ejstrup R, Wiencke AK, Toft PB. Outcome after repair of concurrent upper and lower Canalicular lacerations. Orbit. 2014;33(3):169–72.
36. Bai F, Tao H, Zhang Y, Wang P, Han C, Huang Y, et al. Old canalicular laceration repair: a retrospective study of the curative effects and prognostic factors. Int J Ophthalmol. 2017;10(6):902–7.
37. Ali S, Rizvi R, Sharma SC. Management of traumatic dacryocystitis and failed dacryocystorhinostomy using silicone lacrimal intubation set. Indian J Otolaryngol Head Neck Surg. 2011;63(3):264–8.
38. Nair AG, Ali MJ. Mitomycin-C in dacryocystorhinostomy: from experimentation to implementation and the road ahead: a review. Indian J Ophthalmol. 2015;63(4):335–9.
39. Kamal S, Ali MJ, Naik MN. Circumostial injection of mitomycin C (COS-MMC) in external and endoscopic dacryocystorhinostomy: efficacy, safety profile, and outcomes. Ophthal Plast Reconstr Surg. 2014;30(2):187–90.
40. Yuksel N, Akcay E, Kilicarslan A, Ozen U, Ozturk F. A surprise in the lacrimal sac. Middle East Afr J Ophthalmol. 2016;23:268–70.
41. Zhou L, Li SY, Cui JP, Zhang ZY, Guan LN. Analysis of missed diagnosis of orbital foreign bodies. Exp Ther Med. 2017;13(4):1275–8.
42. Garg RK, Hartman MJ, Lucarelli ÞMJ, Leverson G, Afifi AM, Gentry LR, et al. Nasolacrimal system fractures a description of radiologic findings and associated outcomes. Ann Plast Surg. 2015;75(4):407–13.
43. Balaji SM, Balaji P. Epiphora drainage by DCR—long—term results. Indian J Dent Res. 2019;30(3):337–41.
44. Oppenheimer AJ, Monson LA, Buchman SR. Pediatric orbital fractures. Craniomaxillofac Trauma Reconstr. 2013;1(1):9–20.
45. Spinelli HM, Shapiro MD, Wei LL, Elahi E, Hirmand H. The role of lacrimal intubation in the management of facial trauma and tumor resection. Plast Reconstr Surg. 2005;115(7):1871–6.
46. Shams PN, Chen PG, Wormald PJ, Sa FCS, Sloan B, Wilcsek G, et al. Management of functional epiphora in patients with an anatomically patent dacryocystorhinostomy. JAMA Ophthalmol. 2014;5000(9):1127–32.

16 Neuro-ophthalmology of Head Trauma

Kumudini Sharma and Ved Prakash Maurya

16.1 Introduction

Neuro-ophthalmic symptoms and signs may be the presenting features of traumatic brain injury (TBI). TBI is caused by an impact to the head from an external force or from combat blast exposure. During blast exposure, the blast waves and acceleration forces damage brain, eye, and orbit. In children and young adults, fall, motor vehicle accident, and sports activities are the commonest causes of TBI. Sixty to Seventy percentage of cases of postconcussion syndrome may have visual symptoms [1]. Neuro-ophthalmic manifestations of TBI may be due to structural changes (subdural, epidural, or subarachnoid or parenchymal bleed) or may be due to the specific area of the brain injured during trauma.

The frequently occurring TBI is concussion resulting from rapid acceleration and deceleration of the brain inside the fixed skull, resulting in injury to cerebral cortex (Frontal & occipital lobes) or structures in the inferior surface of the brain (optic nerve, optic chiasma, cranial nerves, and brainstem). In the brain, 38% of the white matter carry the visual information; hence, in mild, moderate, and severe TBI, the visual abnormalities are common [2].

In Facio-cranial injuries by missiles, these enter into cranium and cause the defect in basal dura and result in the formation of CSF fistula. Nearly 10% of military cranial injuries damage the dural sinus and cause subdural hemorrhage. Gunshot injury to intracranial arteries may result in hemorrhage (sub arachnoid, intraventricular hemorrhage) or traumatic aneurysm. Gunshot wound is the common penetrating injury to head and brain.

The patients who sustain less severe form of TBI such as concussion can have long-lasting visual symptoms and they are the ones who present to ophthalmologists. The Neuro-ophthalmic symptoms may be blurred vision, diplopia, difficulty in reading, eye pain, and field defects. A complete Neuro-ophthalmic examination should be carried out in all symp-

K. Sharma (✉)
Department of Ophthalmology, Hind Institute of Medical Sciences, Lucknow, India

V. P. Maurya
Department of Neurosurgery, Sanjay Gandhi Postgraduate Institute of Medical Sciences, Lucknow, India

S. Waikar (ed.), *Ocular Trauma in Armed Conflicts*, https://doi.org/10.1007/978-981-19-4021-7_16

tomatic cases of TBI. These include the tests for optic nerve function, perimetry, accommodation, stereopsis and supra nuclear ocular movement assessment, ocular motor nerves examination. Supranuclear movements dysfunction is mostly seen in mild TBI, while optic nerve and ocular motor nerve palsy are seen in moderate-to-severe TBI [1].

TBI can be classified depending on CT, Glasgow coma scale score, duration of loss of consciousness, eye opening response on stimulation into mild, moderate, severe. Various types of traumatic brain injuries are as follows:

(a) Concussion
(b) Contusion (Fig. 16.1)
(c) Diffuse axonal injury
(d) Traumatic intracranial hemorrhages – subarachnoid hemorrhage (Fig. 16.2)
(e) Hematoma formation – Extradural (Fig. 16.3), Subdural (Fig. 16.4), Intracerebral

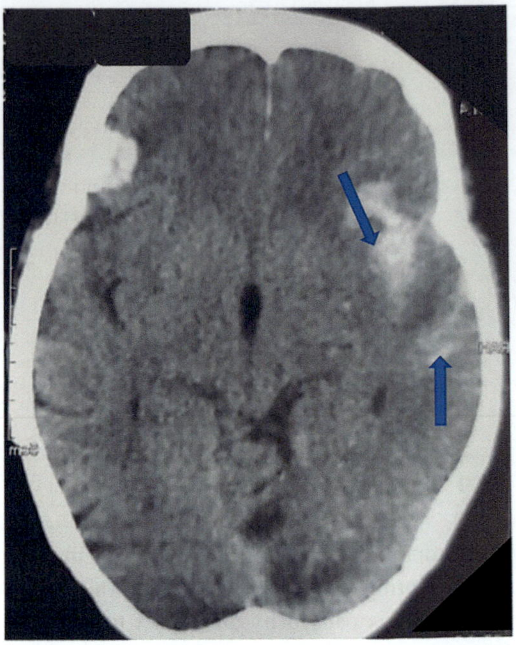

Fig. 16.2 CT scan of head showing hyperdensity in the left frontal and temporal lobe area corresponding to the sulci of the sylvian fissure. The hyperdensity follows the pattern in the subarachnoid space of the corresponding sulcus. Impression: Posttraumatic subarachnoid hemorrhage (SAH)

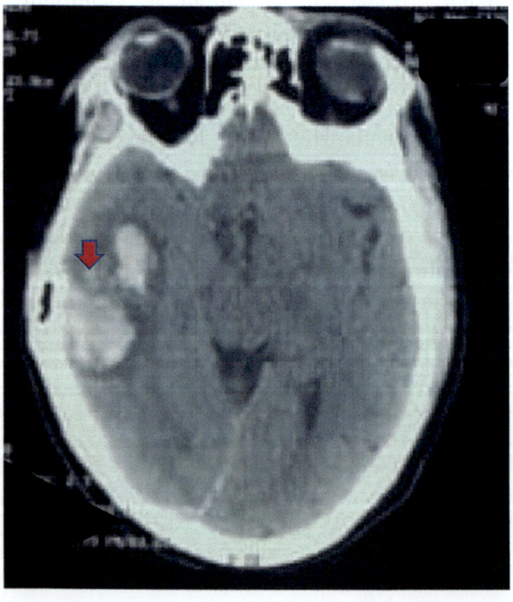

Fig. 16.1 CT scan of head showing hyper dense, intra-axial lesion in the right temporal lobe. The lesion is causing hypodensity (edema) in the surrounding area with compression over adjacent structures. Impression: Right temporal contusion

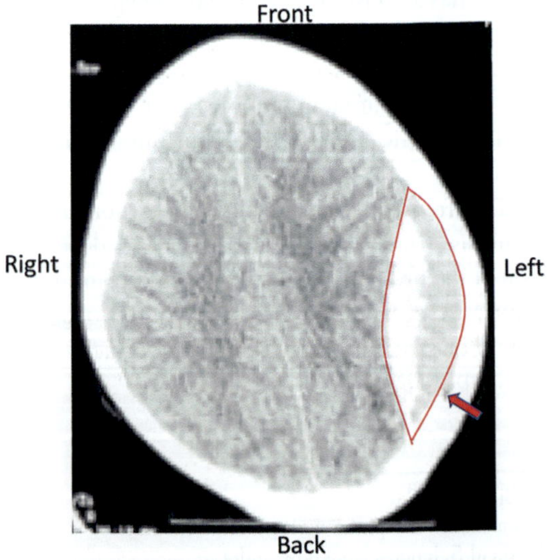

Fig. 16.3 Computerized tomography (CT) scan of head showing biconvex, extra axial, hyperdense lesion (acute hematoma) in the left parietal region (the hematoma is outlined with red color for the sake of understanding). The red arrow is indicating the fracture line in parietal bone. Impression: Left parietal extradural hematoma (EDH)

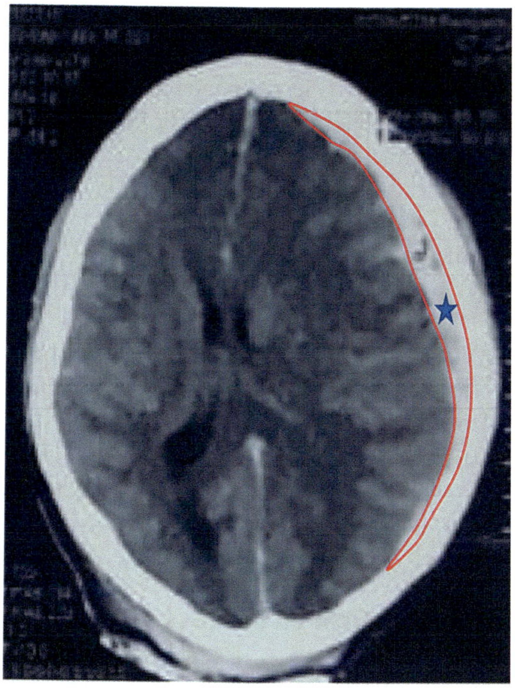

Fig. 16.4 CT scan of head showing convexo concave, hyperdense, extra-axial lesion (acute hematoma) in the left fronto parietal region (the hematoma is outlined with red color for the sake of understanding). The star indicates the location of hematoma and there is mass effect in the form of midline shift. *Impression*: Left fronto parietal acute subdural hematoma (SDH) with midline shift

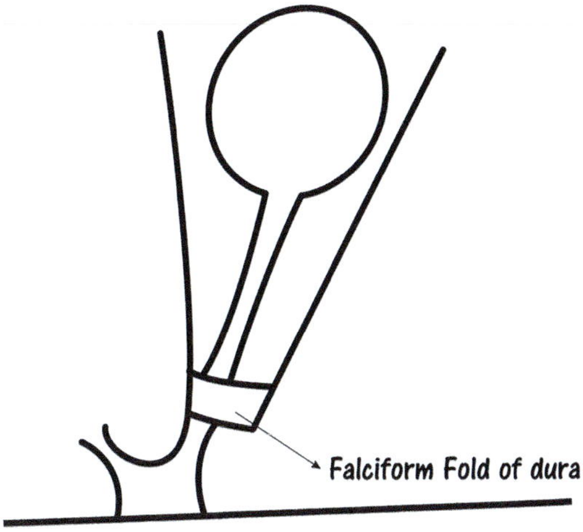

Fig. 16.5 Intracanalicular part of optic nerve, falciform fold of dura when optic nerve exits from the canal

16.2 Neuro-ophthalmic Features of Head Trauma Can Be Considered

(a) Injury to sensory visual pathway
(b) Injury to motor visual pathway

Injury to sensory visual pathway
(a) Optic nerve injury
(b) Papilledema
(c) Injury to optic chiasma
(d) Injury to optic tract and radiation
(e) Traumatic cortical visual loss

16.3 Optic Nerve Injury/Traumatic Optic Neuropathy (TON)

Traumatic Optic nerve injury (TON): The optic nerve may get damaged by direct or indirect trauma. The injury to ON may vary from simple contusion and hematoma to complete avulsion of the optic nerve. Direct injury to ON occurs by penetrating object, while indirect injury occurs by the transmitted waves from an external force. Indirect ON injury has been reported in 0.5–0.8% of cases of head injury. Any part of ON can be involved, but most commonly, injury occurs to intracanalicular part of the optic nerve. Second common site of injury to ON is its intracranial part as there is a falciform fold of dura at the cranial end of the optic canal. Indirect injury to the optic nerve causes compression of ON against this falciform fold of dura (Fig. 16.5).

TON is seen mainly in young men by motor vehicle or bike accident, or gunshot. In war injury, missiles can enter the intracranial compartment through the eye balls and damage the eyeball irreversibly. They may injure the optic nerve, cavernous sinus, and internal carotid artery. Diagnosis is made by testing acuity, color vision, pupillary reaction, field, and visual evoked potential. Fundus is normal initially, but optic atrophy appears 3–6 weeks after trauma. CT scan of orbit is performed to rule out hematoma or bony fragment compressing the Optic nerve. The presence of aforementioned finding on CT scan requires surgical intervention.

Treatment of TON is controversial; high-dose corticosteroids sometimes given but are not of proven benefit. Experimental and clinical studies did not find high dose of steroids to be beneficial in TON [3, 4]. The international ON Trauma study included 133 patients and divided them into three groups: patients with no treatment, patients on steroids, patients subjected to surgery with or without steroids. The authors did not find steroids or surgery beneficial to them [5]. Review of all studies carried out on traumatic optic neuropathy did not show statistically significant results to suggest that surgery, steroids, or combination of both are more effective than no treatment [6]. Surgery is indicated in cases where there is hematoma of ON or a bony fragment impinging on the optic nerve on neuroimaging [7].

16.4 Papilledema

Occurs when there is thrombosis of Superior sagittal sinus (SSS)/Transverse sinus or there is chronic subdural hematoma. The intracranial venous sinus thrombosis affects CSF (cerebrospinal fluid) absorption and causes increase in intracranial pressure (ICP). The patient presents with headache and sixth nerve palsy. Neuroimaging (CT/MRI along with venography) is needed to make the diagnosis. Treatment of venous sinus thrombosis includes anticoagulant, ICP-lowering drugs.

Sometimes, the thrombus after resolution causes narrowing of the sinus, which, several months later, may present with headache and papilledema and is diagnosed as benign intracranial hypertension. Magnetic resonance venography (MRV) will help in making the diagnosis of venous sinus narrowing and measurement of venous sinus pressure proximal and distal to narrowing should be performed. If gradient in pressure is more than 10 mmHg, then angioplasty with or without stenting is indicated. If pressure gradient is less than 10 mmHg, then medical treatments with ICP-lowering drugs such as Diamox, glycerol, etc. should be given.

16.5 Optic Chiasmal Injury

Chiasmal injury is less common than ON injury, seen in blunt injury to mid brow or face with basilar skull fracture.

Clinically there will be:

- Bitemporal hemianopia.
- CSF rhinorrhea.
- Diabetes Insipidus.
- Visual loss is irreversible, while diabetes insipidus and CSF rhinorrhea requires treatment.

Traumatic damage of optic tract, radiation, and occipital lobe may also occur.

16.6 Cortical Visual Loss

Cortical visual loss was reported in 0.4–0.6% following trauma to the head. There is bilateral visual loss with normal fundus and pupillary reaction. Mild close head injury may cause temporary visual loss in both eyes which is associated with irritability and confusion [8]. In occipital lobe trauma, when bullet passes from superior part of occipital lobes from one side to other, it causes inferior altitudinal defects in both eyes (Fig. 16.6).

If the bullet passes through the inferior part of both occipital lobes and misses the dural sinus confluence, then patient will have superior altitudinal defects in both eyes, which is very uncommon as the penetrating bullet commonly hits the torcular of dural sinuses. Then the patient dies due to massive intracranial hemorrhage (Fig. 16.7). Optokinetic nystagmus, mirror test, visual-evoked response, and neuroimaging help in making the diagnosis of cortical visual loss.

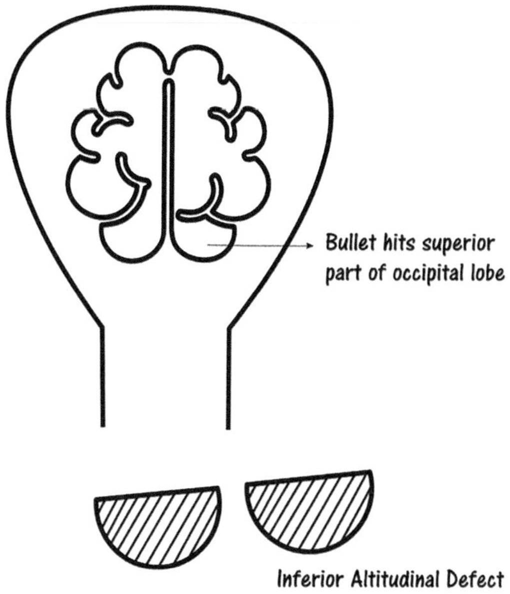

Fig. 16.6 Inferior altitudinal defect

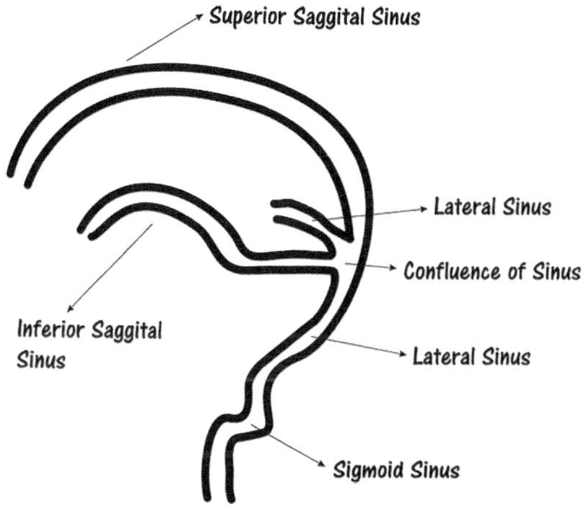

Fig. 16.7 Torcular of Dural sinuses

16.7 Motor Visual Pathway Injury Includes

(a) Injury to 3, 4, 6 cranial nerves
(b) Injury to brainstem
- Internuclear ophthalmoplegia
- Dorsal mid brain syndrome
- Skew deviation

(c) Supranuclear movement disorders

16.8 Ocular Motor Nerve Palsy

Seen mostly in moderate-to-severe TBI, it is uncommon in mild TBI. If it occurs after a mild head trauma, then it usually suggests a pre-existing structural pathology [9, 10].

Third nerve palsy:
- It is associated with severe head injury.
- The site of injury is:
  - At exit from midbrain or an avulsion of nerve root
  - Subarachnoid part of third nerve
  - At SOF (superior orbital fissure):

    Uncal herniation due to traumatic supratentorial edema or hemorrhage can lead to compression of third nerve at tentorial edge or by PCA (posterior cerebral artery). Initially patient shows unilateral dilation of pupil with altered sensorium-Hutchinson pupil. Later on, complete third nerve palsy develops (Fig. 16.8).

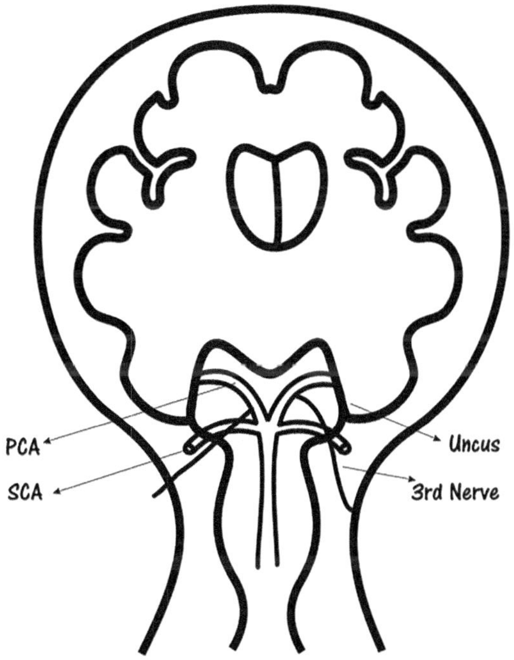

Fig. 16.8 Third nerve passing between posterior cerebral (PCA) and superior cerebellar artery (SCA) and can be compressed by herniated uncus

Retrospective review of 26 patients of traumatic third nerve palsy showed recovery of ptosis in 95%, EOM palsy in 83%, pupillary reaction recovery in 50% after a period of 14 months [11]. Aberrant regeneration can occur after resolution of palsy.

Clinically, patient presents with ptosis, dilated pupil, and abducted eye on affected side.

Treatment includes observation for 6 months to 1 year. Surgery is difficult to perform in third nerve palsy as many muscles are affected. It may require multiple procedures to achieve ocular alignment in primary position. Total third nerve palsy with no resolution cannot be corrected effectively surgically. If the involved eye is the only seeing eye, then LR is disinserted and sutured to lateral periorbita. Eye is fixed in primary position by suturing a piece of medial periorbita to medial rectus muscle. If partial resolution is there, then available muscles have to be noted and surgery is planned accordingly to give alignment in primary position and downgaze. Supra-maximal recession of lateral rectus with resection/plication of medial rectus may correct horizontal deviation. Spontaneous recovery is more frequently seen in unilateral than bilateral cases of traumatic third nerve palsy. In recent years, nasal transposition of lateral rectus to medial rectus has been tried with good results [12].

16.9 Fourth Nerve Palsy

- It is the commonest nerve to be affected on mild impact to the head.
- It is the thinnest, has longest course, and it runs along the free edge of rigid tentorium, hence more likely to be damaged during head trauma. Sometimes trauma reveals the already existing congenital fourth nerve palsy (Fig. 16.9). Old photographs of the patient and vertical fusional amplitude help to make the diagnosis of congenital fourth nerve palsy.

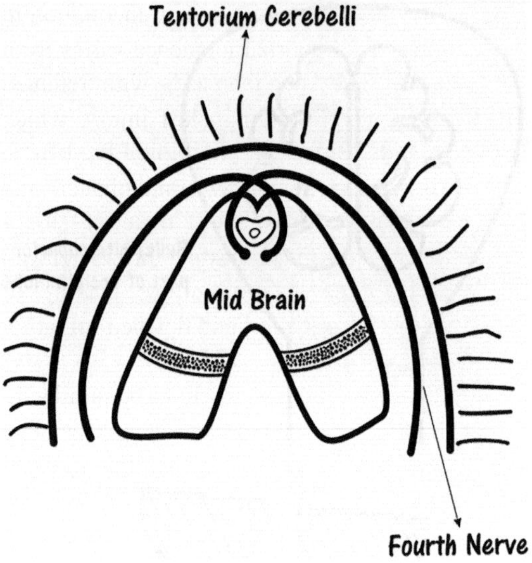

Fig. 16.9 Fourth nerve exiting from dorsal surface of midbrain, after decussation runs around the mid brain anteriorly, here it runs along the free edge of tentorium cerebelli

- It emerges from the dorsal surface of brain, damage at this site results in bilateral fourth nerve palsy.
- Clinically, patient complains of:
  - Vertical diplopia
  - Bielschowsky head tilt test +ve
- If extortion is more than 5°, then bilateral fourth nerve palsy should be suspected.
- One should wait for 6 months to 1 year for spontaneous resolution.
- If no resolution occurs by the end of 6 months to 1 year, then management is done on the basis of Knapp's classification. Recession/myectomy of ipsilateral IO is commonly performed surgery in fourth nerve palsy.
- If torsion of image persists after surgery, then Harada-Ito procedure is performed.

16.10 Sixth Nerve Palsy

- It is commonly involved in head injury especially skull base fracture. Dural entry point

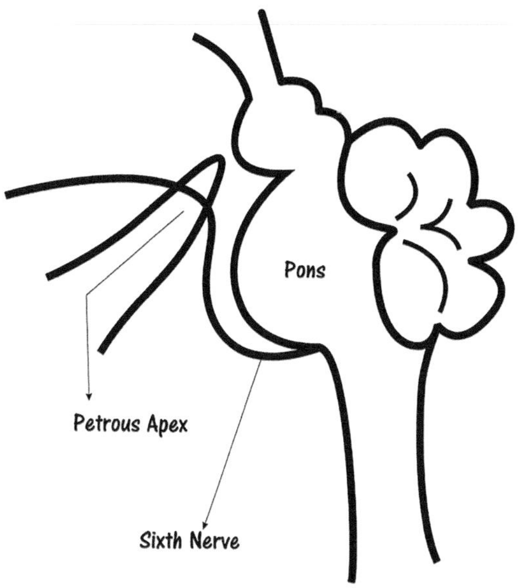

Fig. 16.10 Sixth nerve passing over apex of petrous bone after ascending along the clivus

and Petrous apex are the common sites of injury to this nerve (Fig. 16.10).

- Clinically, patient complains of horizontal diplopia.
- On examination, the eye on the affected side will be esotropic and shows abduction restriction.

16.11 Treatment

- Waiting for 6 months- 1 year is recommended, and partial/ complete recovery is seen more often in unilateral cases.
- Nonrecovery is seen in bilateral cases or in patients where the eye cannot move past the midline at the time of presentation.
- If on recovery, the eye moves up to mild line, then maximum recession of medial rectus and resection/plication of lateral rectus is performed.
- If on recovery, the eye does not move up to midline/minimal movement on abduction, then vertical recti transposition surgery with recession of MR is carried out.

  Patient with skull base fracture may have sixth and seventh nerve palsy together. Multiple cranial nerve palsy occurs when there is injury to orbital apex or cavernous sinus area.

16.12 Orbital Apex Injury

Third, fourth, and sixth cranial nerves along with ophthalmic division of Vth (Trigeminal) and optic nerve are involved.

16.13 Cavernous Sinus Injury

Third, fourth, and sixth cranial nerves along with ophthalmic and maxillary division of fifth nerve and sympathetic fibers are involved; optic nerve may be spared. Trauma to cavernous sinus may result in carotid cavernous fistula (CCF) high flow fistula. Clinically, this manifests as frozen globe, pulsatile proptosis, and arterialization of conjunctival vessels with audible bruit. CT/MRI shows enlarged Superior ophthalmic vein (SOV). CCF may become symptomatic immediately or may manifest after days or weeks of trauma. Treatment of CCF is selective embolization and detachable balloon occlusion.

16.14 Facial Nerve Palsy

Facial nerve injury is seen when there is fracture at skull base. Clinically there is lagophthalmos with exposure keratitis. Facial nerve when injured between seventh nerve nucleus and geniculate ganglion impairs lacrimation due to injury to parasympathetic fibers to lacrimal gland, which lie in this part of nerve (Fig. 16.11). Aberrant regeneration of this nerve may develop hemifacial spasm and crocodile tear. Crocodile tear results when parasympathetic fibers for salivary gland are misdirected to the lacrimal gland (Fig. 16.11). Treatment of crocodile tears depends on severity of lacrimation, which involves subtotal resection of the palpebral lobe of the lacrimal gland or botulinum injection into lacrimal gland.

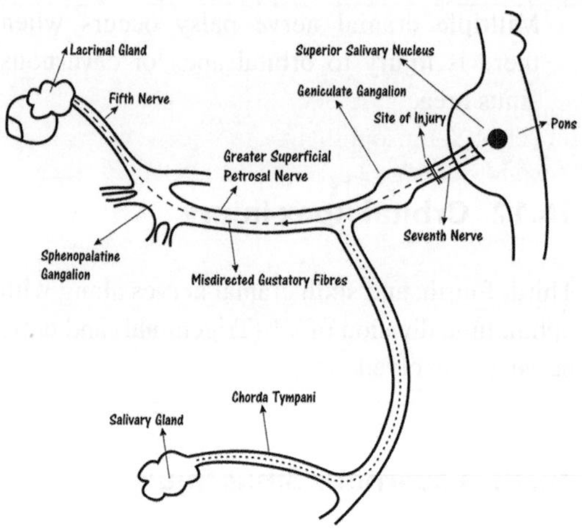

Fig. 16.11 Parasympathetic fibers destined for submandibular gland misdirected to lacrimal gland after trauma to seventh nerve

16.15 Convergence and Accommodative Insufficiency and Spasm

Most of the patients after head trauma have difficulty with convergence or accommodation. It is seen in mild head trauma. Near point of convergence is assessed by moving an object toward the patient's nose. The distance at which the patient experiences double vision or shows outward movement of one eye is noted. Normal near point of convergence is 10 cm. Convergence fusional amplitude is measured using a prism bar with base out. The prism through which the patient can no longer fuse the image of an object is noted. Normal convergence amplitude is 38 diopters at near and 14 diopters for distance. Centre for convergence and near reflex lie in rostral midbrain, this region is susceptible to injury in head trauma. In accommodative insufficiency, patient will have blurred vision for near, young patient may need plus lenses for reading. Accommodative insufficiency or slowness in changing focus from one object to another may be found in mild TBI cases. Vergence impairment is seen in 47–64% of patient who sustained mild TBI [13].

16.15.1 Convergence Insufficiency

Clinically, the patients with convergence insufficiency presents with the following symptoms:

- Headache, blurring of vision or sleepiness, loss of concentration, double vision on reading.
- Near point of convergence is remote.
- Convergence fusional amplitude decreased.
- Exophoria for near.
- Treatment of convergence insufficiency involves Base-out prism exercises or base-in prism on the glasses may be prescribed.

16.15.2 Divergence Insufficiency

The patient will be orthophoric for near and comitant esotropic for far. There will be diplopia on viewing distant objects. To make a diagnosis, there should be normal velocity of abducting saccades. Divergence insufficiency is rare following head trauma.

16.15.3 Spasm of Accommodation and Convergence

Spasm of near reflex convergence, accommodation, miosis, headache, and blurred vision are the presenting manifestations of this entity. Patient's eyes will be in convergence and abduction restriction is observed bilaterally. Cycloplegic drops should be used to give relief to the patient as 1% BD with full time use of bifocal. Slow tapering of cyclopentolate and bifocal use should be carried out till the patient has normal convergence response to near object with no corrective glasses.

16.16 Brainstem Injury

The injury to brainstem occurs when there is severe impact to the back of the head. Neuro-ophthalmic manifestations of brain stem injury are internuclear ophthalmoplegia, dorsal mid brain syndrome, skew deviation, and gaze palsy. These neuro-ophthalmic findings are less commonly seen in head injury.

16.16.1 Internuclear Ophthalmoplegia (INO)

This occurs when there is disruption of MLF (Medial longitudinal fascicle). There will be adduction deficit on the side of lesion with nystagmus of abducting eye. Skew deviation is a vertical imbalance of eyes and seen in trauma to brainstem.

16.16.2 Dorsal Mid Brain Syndrome

It includes

- Up gaze palsy.
- Light near dissociation of pupillary reaction.
- Convergency retraction nystagmus, lid retraction.
- It occurs following downward displacement of midbrain in head injury.

16.17 Supranuclear Disorders in TBI

In patient with mild TBI, there might be impairment in saccades, pursuit, and vestibulo-ocular reflex. Supranuclear movements of eyes are governed by frontal, parietal, and occipital lobes. Generation and execution of saccadic movements involve a wide variety of cognitive processes. Hence, eye movement testing has been used to assess high cognitive function- attention concentration, memory in case of TBI.

16.18 Saccadic Eye Movements

Voluntary saccades are generated at frontal eye field, while reflex saccades are controlled by parietal eye field. Pontine nuclei, cerebellum, basal ganglion, and superior colliculi also play a role in performing saccadic eye movements [14]. Anti-saccade, memory-guided saccades, and self-paced saccades were recorded in postconcussive syndrome and were found to be impaired. Kraus et al. found that eye movements were more sensitive than neuropsychological testing in recognizing persisting neurological abnormalities in postconcussion syndrome patients [15]. For testing of antisaccades, memory-guided saccades, self-paced and gap saccade consult review article on The Neuro-ophthalmology of head trauma written by Ventura et al. [1]

16.19 Pursuit Eye Movements

Pursuit eye movement is tested by asking the patient to follow on object, which is moved slowly (30° per second) from right to left and vice versa. It is generated at parietal-occipital-temporal (POT) area and controlled by frontal eye fields, pontine nuclei, and cerebellum.

16.20 Vestibulo-Ocular Reflex (VOR)

The VOR is tested by rapidly thrusting the patient's head from side to side with both of the examiner's hands, while asking the patient to fixate on examiner nose. Patient with impaired VOR due to damage to labyrinthine apparatus (in petrous fracture) cannot maintain fixation on examiner's nose on rapid head movement by the examiner. Peripheral vestibular nystagmus is usually horizontal or horizontal rotary is suppressed by visual fixation and short lasting. It can be made more obvious by using +10D lens in front of both eyes or by performing ophthalmoscopy in one eye, while other eye is being covered. Central origin vestibular nystagmus is vertical or rotational, increases on visual fixation, sustained and sometimes, associated with cerebellar signs of ocular dysmetria. Supranuclear movements are recorded with video oculography. Dysfunction of Supranuclear eye movements can be tested clinically at bed side.

Vascular injury in TBI can result in posttraumatic pseudoaneurysm or dissecting aneurysm of carotid/vertebral artery. Traumatic dissection of internal carotid artery presents as painful Horner syndrome. Head injury can exacerbate the preexisting migraine headache or a new-onset migraine headache may appear following head trauma; some patients of blast injury have photophobia and need dark glasses.

16.21 Conclusion

Neuro-ophthalmic trauma usually occurs in combat injuries and is mostly associated with systemic neurologic injuries. A close collaboration between neurologist and Ophthalmologist is required for proper evaluation of these cases. Optic nerve injury is associated with poor visual outcome. Testing of sensory and motor visual system is important to assess the damage and to decide the visual therapy. In war blast injury (concussion), visual system examination gives information about higher cognitive function like attention, memory concentration.

Acknowledgment We sincerely acknowledge our medical illustrator Mr. Amit Mohan for drawing Figs. 16.5, 16.6, 16.7, 16.8, 16.9, 16.10 and 16.11.

Conflict of Interest The authors have no conflict of interest.

References

1. Ventura RE, Balcer L, Galetta SL. The neuro-ophthalmology of head trauma. Lancet Neurol. 2014;13:1006–16.
2. Felleman DJ, Van Essen DC. Distributed hierarchical processing in the primate cerebral cortex. Cereb Cortex. 1991;1:1–47.
3. Steinsapir KD. Treatment of traumatic optic neuropathy with high dose corticosteroid. J Neuroophthalmol. 2006;26:65–7.
4. Levin LA, Beck RW, Joseph MP, Seiff S, Kraker R. The treatment of traumatic optic neuropathy, the international optic nerve trauma study. Ophthalmology. 1999;106:1268–77.
5. Chaon BC, Lee MS. Is there treatment for traumatic optic neuropathy? Curr Opin Ophthalmol. 2015;6:445–9.
6. Volpe NJ, Levin LA. How should patients with indirect traumatic optic neuropathy be treated ? J Neuroophthalmol. 2011;31:169–74.
7. Yu-Wai-Man P, Griffith PG. Surgery for traumatic optic neuropathy. Cochrane Database Syst Rev. 2011;6:CD006032.
8. Rodriguez A, Jose LA, Paez HJ. Post traumatic transient cortical blindness. Int Ophthalmol. 1993;17:277–83.
9. Kulkarni AR, Aggarwal SP, Kulkarni RR, Deshpande MD, Walimbe PB, Labhsetwar AS. Ocular manifestations of head injury: a clinical study. Eye (Lond). 2005;19:1257–63.
10. Zhang Y, Chen K, Liu B, Chen L. Incomplete oculomotor nerve palsy in the subarachnoid space caused by traumatic brain injury. Neurosciences. 2012;17:159–60.
11. Lin C, Dong Y, Lvl YM, Hau I. Clinical features and functional recovery of traumatic isolated Oculomotar nerve palsy in mild head injury with sphenoid fracture. J Neurosurg. 2013;118:364–9.
12. Saxena R, Sharma M, Singh D, Dhiman R, Sharma P. Medial transposition of split lateral rectus augmented with fixation sutures in case of complete third nerve palsy. Br J Ophthalmol. 2016;100:585–7.
13. Capo Aponte JE, Urosevich TG, Temme LA, Tarbett AK, Sanghera NK. Visual dysfunctions and symptoms during the sub-acute stage of blast- induced mild traumatic brain injury. Mil Med. 2012;177:804–13.
14. Liu GT, Volpe NJ, Galetta S. Neuro-ophthamology: diagnosis and management. 2nd ed. Philadelphia, PA: Elsevier; 2010. p. 551–4.
15. Krau MF, Little DM, Donnell AJ, Reilly JL, Simonian N, Sweeney JA. Oculomotor function in chronic traumatic brain injury. Cogn Behav Neurol. 2007;20:170–8.

17 Reconstruction of Eyelid Injuries in Military Trauma

V. Langer

17.1 Introduction

Ocular injuries in military conflict are very much different from civilian trauma. High-energy explosive blast injuries are sustained in 83% as compared with 3% in civilians [1]. Military injuries cause much greater damage to the eyes as compared to civilian trauma. In addition, ocular injuries in the military setting are associated with severe polytrauma in majority of cases. This appears to be uncommon in the civilian scenario. Isolated injuries to the eyelids are uncommon in military trauma. Indeed, it is a daunting challenge to treat these injuries, especially in the setting of polytrauma. If there are associated life-threatening injuries, and time is of essence, the severely damaged eye may often have to be sacrificed in the interest of saving life in these trying situations. These injuries are therefore best treated in a tertiary referral center with multidisciplinary approach and multiple operating teams if the vital eye has to be saved.

The eyelids are vital in protecting the globe. They form a barrier for the eyes against trauma, bright light, and help in maintaining the tear-cornea film. By the process of blinking, they also aid in pumping the tears toward the nasolacrimal duct system. To manage the reconstruction of the eyelids, it is important to have knowledge of the basic anatomical features of the eyelid, so as to restore it to as close to normal as possible to allow adequate functioning and aesthetics of the region and indeed the face.

17.2 Anatomy

Eyelids comprise skin, muscles, nerves, and blood vessels.

The normal eye has an elliptical shape with its horizontal palpebral fissure measuring 28–30 mm and vertical palpebral fissure measuring 10–11 mm at its widest points. The highest point of upper lid is just medial to the pupil in straight gaze and the lowest point of lower lid being just lateral to the pupil. The lateral canthus is approximately 2 mm higher than the medial canthus.

The eyelids are conveniently divided into two anatomical layers: the anterior (skin and orbicularis muscle) and the posterior lamellae (tarsal plate and the conjunctiva). A grey line is visible transversely along the middle of each lid margin, which marks the junction of these two lamellae. Just posterior to the grey line lies the mucocutaneous junction, at the Meibomian gland openings. The posterior edge of the lid margin is sharper compared to the anterior edge, which is rounded (Fig. 17.1).

V. Langer (✉)
Plastic and Reconstructive surgery, Ex Army Medical Corps India, Delhi, India

S. Waikar (ed.), *Ocular Trauma in Armed Conflicts*, https://doi.org/10.1007/978-981-19-4021-7_17

Fig. 17.1 Anatomy of eyelid

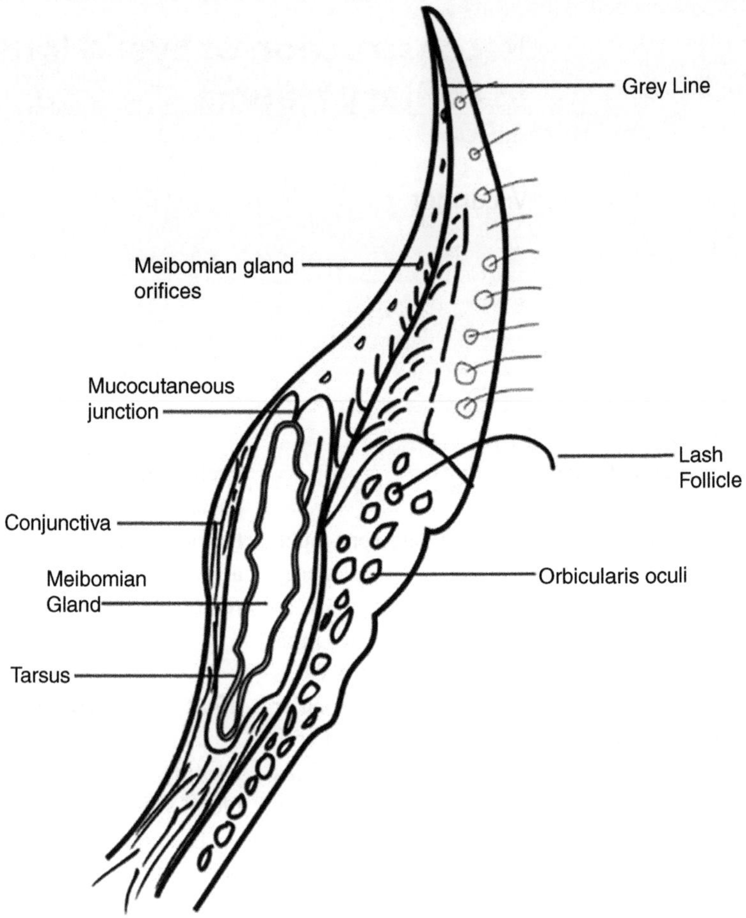

17.2.1 Skin

The skin of the eyelid is the thinnest in the body because of a weakened dermis and very few adnexal structures or sebaceous glands.

17.2.2 Orbicularis Oculi

The orbicularis oculi muscle acts as the main protractor of the eyelid, and is divided into orbital (helps in voluntary forced lid closure) and palpebral component (helps in involuntary closure). The orbital portion arises from the medial canthal tendon and laterally inserts into the zygoma. The palpebral portion is further subdivided into pretarsal and preseptal muscles. The pretarsal orbicularis is adherent to the anterior surface of the tarsal plate and attaches medially to the anterior and posterior lacrimal crests. It surrounds the lacrimal sac and aids in the lacrimal pump mechanism. The preseptal orbicularis is situated on top of the orbital septum originating medially from the anterior limb of the medial canthal tendon and from the posterior lacrimal crest. Laterally, both condense to form the lateral canthal tendon that inserts on Whitnall's tubercle.

17.2.3 Tarsal Plate

The tarsal plate is composed of dense fibrous tissue and forms the cytoskeleton of the lids. It is 28–29 mm long and 1 mm thick. The tarsus is 10 mm in height in the upper lid and 3.5–5 mm in the lower lid, narrowing medially and laterally.

These are attached to the orbital rim by the medial and lateral canthal tendons.

17.2.4 Medial and Lateral Canthal Tendon

The medial canthal tendon has an anterior and a posterior limb. The anterior limb inserts anterosuperiorly into the anterior lacrimal crest, while the posterior limb along with the deep head of the pretarsal orbicularis muscle inserts into the posterior lacrimal crest. The lateral canthal tendon also has an anterior component that inserts into the orbital rim, and the deeper component passes laterally deep into the septum orbitale to insert into the inner side of the lateral orbital rim.

17.2.5 Levator Palpebrae Superioris

Levator palpebrae superioris muscle elevates the upper eyelid. It takes origin at the orbital apex from the annulus of Zinn, and travels horizontally along the roof of the orbit to end vertically in an aponeurosis that inserts into the anterior surface of the tarsal plate, of which few fibers insert into the skin, to form the lid crease. The capsulopalpebral fascia is analogous to the levator aponeurosis in the lower lid and originates from the inferior rectus muscle encircling the inferior oblique muscle.

17.2.6 Blood and Lymphatic Supply

The upper lid is supplied by anastomosis of the superior branch of the medial palpebral artery, that is a branch of the ophthalmic artery, and superior branch of the lateral palpebral artery, that is a branch of the lacrimal artery. It has two vascular arcades, the marginal one that lies on the anterior tarsal surface, 2–3 mm from the lid margin, and a peripheral one lying on the anterior surface of the Muller's muscle, just superior to the superior tarsal border. The lower eyelid is supplied by the inferior palpebral artery, a branch from the ophthalmic artery and inferior branch of the lacrimal artery. It also receives a branch of the maxillary artery.

Most of the upper lid and the lateral half of the lower lid drains into the preauricular lymph node, while the medial portion of the upper lid and the medial half of the lower lid drain into the submandibular nodes along the lymphatics, which follow the angular and facial vessels.

17.3 Evaluation of Eyelid Defect

A proper preoperative assessment is paramount in meticulous eyelid reconstruction. So before surgery, we need to know the following:

1. If the defect is full-thickness with involvement of eyelid margin or an anterior lamellar defect alone
2. Size of defect – amount of lamella loss
3. Location—medial, lateral, or central
4. Medial or lateral canthus involvement
5. Lacrimal drainage system involvement
6. Age of the patient—laxity of lids
7. Condition of the opposite eyelid
8. Mobility of surrounding tissues

17.4 General Consideration for Lid Reconstruction

"When the eye is still present, reconstruction of an eyelid or even a part of it requires a minimum of three elements: an outer layer of skin; an inner layer of mucosa; and a semirigid skeleton interposed between them." Thus wrote the legend Mustarde`.

The goals of lid reconstruction are provision of adequate eye closure, preservation of the tear film, maintaining an unobstructed visual field, and to recreate an eye, which is cosmetically pleasing and normal to look at. Both the lamellae need to be replaced, skin–muscle lamina anteriorly and cartilagenous framework and smooth mucous lining posteriorly. One of the two lamellae needs to be reconstructed with a flap and the other lamella can then be replaced with a free graft/flap. A flap will help in providing vascular supply. However, there have been attempts to reconstruct the whole lower eyelid with a single thick flap [2]. The levator palpebrae superioris, orbicularis oculi, and inferior retractors must be repaired or an effort made to reconstruct them. Stable mucocutaneous lid margin with good apposition to globe should be achieved. Scars are hidden if incisions are made in, or parallel to, skin creases (relaxed skin tension lines or RSTLs) [3].These are present at right angles to the direction of action of the underlying muscle group. Curved scars are concealed better than straight scars. The upper lid crease is to be used for most skin incisions involving the upper eyelid [4]. Aim should be to achieve symmetry between the two eyes for better cosmesis. Overlapping of wound edges is to be avoided, wound margins are to be everted (Fig. 17.2), and depressed scars are avoided. This can be achieved by passing a suture loop, which is wider in the deeper layers than superficial. Sutures should be placed with knots on the skin to avoid corneal irritation (Fig. 17.3). At the end of the surgery, traction sutures may be placed to close the lids and to stabilize the graft/ flap during the healing phase.

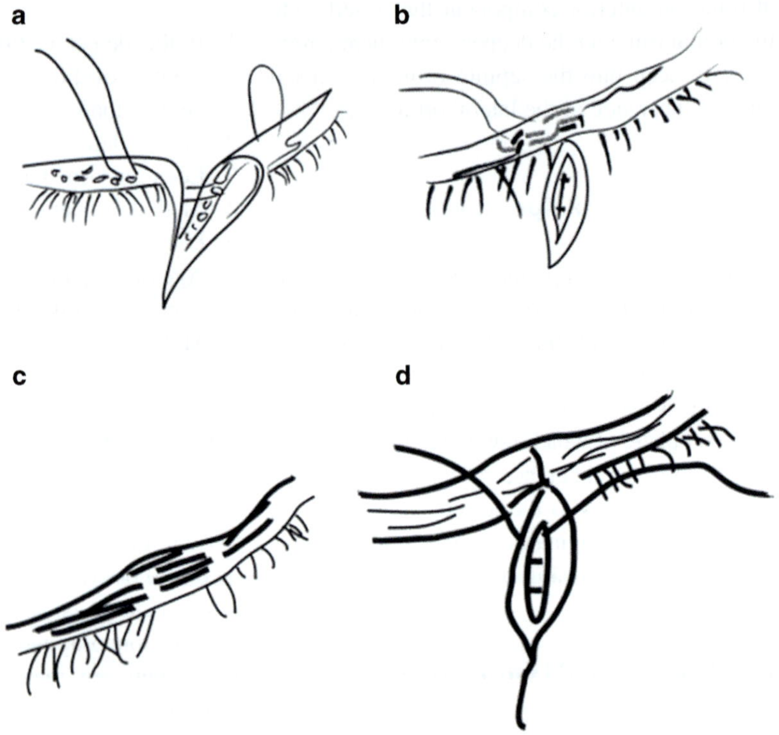

Fig. 17.2 (a–d) Suturing of lid margin

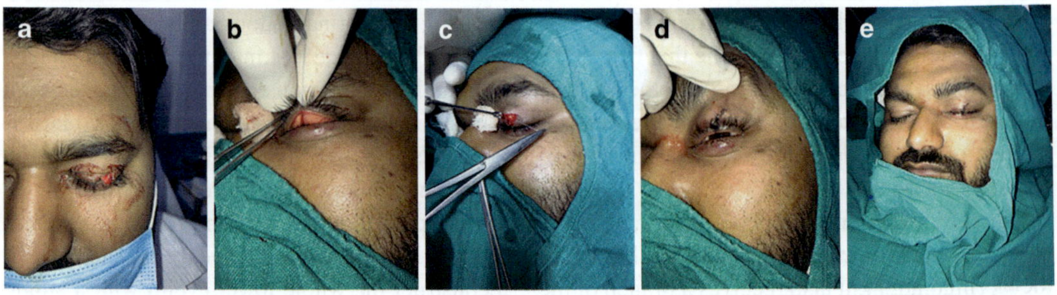

Fig. 17.3 (a–e) Suturing of lacerated wound of eyelid

17.5 Eyelid Reconstruction of Full-Thickness Lid Defects Involving Margin

ALGORITHM FOR RECONSTRUCTION OF FULL-THICKNESS EYELID DEFECTS

Upper Lid

DEFECT SIZE	TREATMENT
≤1/4	Primary closure ± Lateral canthotomy
> 1/4	Mustardé switch

Lower Lid

DEFECT SIZE	TREATMENT
Marginal <8 mm	Hughes tarsoconjunctival flap from upper lid
≤ ¼	Primary closure ± lateral canthotomy
Lateral half	Mustardé or Tenzel flap with chondromucosal graft (septum, split palate, upper lateral nasal cartilage)
Medial half	Nasojugal flap of Tessier with chondromucosal graft

Both Lids

TREATMENT
Forehead flap with chondromucosal or split palatal graft

17.6 Small Defect (Up to 25–50% of Lid Length)

Small defects (up to a third of the length of the eyelid) can be reconstructed by direct approximation, as the lid has an inherent stretch ability. The defect is managed by pentagonal wedge excision with direct closure. The defect is first converted into a pentagon with vertical sides covering height of tarsal plate and the two arms converging at the fornix like an inverted "V."

To approximate the tarsus, the use of the buried vertical mattress technique in a "far-far-near-near-near-near-far-far" pattern is preferred, originally described by Burroughs et al. [5]. The sutures are passed 3 mm from the cut edge and at 3 mm depth, coming back 1 mm from the cut edge and at 1 mm depth to complete the vertical mattress sutures. This is done using a 6–0 Vicryl suture. The eyelash line is then aligned with another simple interrupted 6–0 Vicryl suture, which is crucial for a good cosmetic outcome. Skin is then closed using 6–0 non absorbable sutures in an interrupted fashion.

If there is some tension (defects of size 33–50%), a lateral canthotomy and cantholysis of the upper crus of the lateral canthal tendon of corresponding lid can be done. The most important aspect of this repair technique is alignment of the lash line and eversion of the lid margin wound edges to prevent a notched appearance [5, 6].

17.7 Medium Defect (50–75% of Lid Length)

The Tenzel semicircular advancement was originally described in 1975 by RR Tenzel. The incision begins at the lateral canthus and curves superiorly and temporally in a semicircular fashion. This is followed by a lateral canthotomy and inferior cantholysis. A musculocutaneous flap is then dissected and advanced medially to cover the eyelid defect using buried vertical mattress technique as described by Burroughs et al. (Fig. 17.4). The vertical extent should not cross

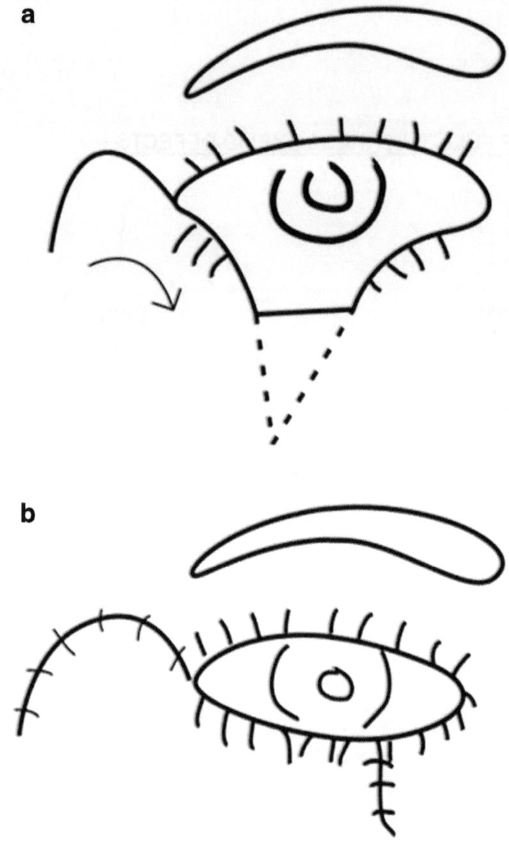

Fig. 17.4 (**a**, **b**) Tenzel's semicircular flap

the eyebrow for inferior eyelid defects and the flap should stay within the orbital margin or the arc as defined by the eyebrow [7]. The orbicularis oculi is sutured to the periosteum of Whitnall's tubercle to form the lateral canthal angle. The conjunctiva in the lateral fornix is dissected and advanced to the margin. Care should be taken to avoid damage to the lacrimal duct. Disadvantage of this reconstruction is that the lateral lid is devoid of cilia [8–10].

17.7.1 McGregor Flap

This incorporates a Z-plasty at the end of a Tenzel flap that will recruit more tissue from the vertical temporal area and provide horizontal tissue to the eyelid. This extension is known as McGregor flap and is useful for both the upper and lower eyelid reconstruction [11].

17.8 Large Defects(>75% of Lid Length)

17.8.1 Upper Lid

A reverse Tenzel semicircular advancement flap can be used for upper eyelid defects up to two-thirds of the eyelid length. For larger defect, lid-sharing procedure (Cutler-Beard), sliding tarsoconjunctival advancement flap, or a reverse Hughes flap is the norm.

17.8.2 Cutler–Beard Bridge Flap

It was first described in 1955 by NL Cutler and C Beard (Fig. 17.5). It is a two-stage full-thickness advancement flap from the lower eyelid [12]. A full-thickness (cutaneo-myo-conjunctival) incision is made 1–2 mm below the inferior portion of the tarsal plate. This preserves the tarsus and also avoids the inferior marginal arcade, maintaining the flaps vascularity. The two vertical limbs of the flap are inferiorly directed to the conjunctival fornix. The flap is then advanced under the bridge of the intact inferior eyelid margin. Complementary structures are sutured to each other using a 6–0 vicryl in an interrupted fashion. Few authors also describe the use of conchal/ nasal cartilage graft sutured to the remaining tarsus to provide rigidity. The skin is then closed using nonabsorbable suture. Dog ears at the lower end must be taken care of.

After 6–8 weeks, the pedicle is divided and the upper eyelid conjunctiva is advanced anteriorly onto the lid margin for 2 mm, to prevent any corneal erosions. The skin is incised 1–2 mm below the lid margin to compensate for retraction. Healing is slow because of lymphedema. Lower eyelid ectropion is common because of denervation. Upper eyelid entropion is a problem in many patients. Skin and lanugo hairs of the

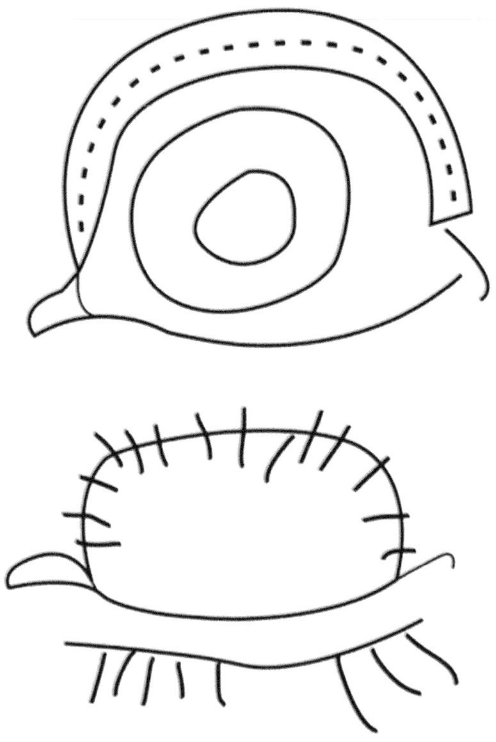

Fig. 17.5 Cutler Beard flap

new eyelid rub on the cornea, because the levator tends to pull the new posterior lamella more than the new anterior lamella. It is not suitable for monocular patients or infants because of risk of amblyopia. Adding to all of the above, the new lid margin lacks lashes.

17.8.3 Mustarde Lid Switch Flap

This flap transfers full-thickness lower lid, together with the lashes, into the upper lid defect (Fig. 17.6). The height depends on the height of the defect. At least 2 mm tissue is left between the flap and the lacrimal punctum. The flap is cut starting at the end opposite to the pedicle, taking care not to damage the vascular supply in the pedicle. A quarter of the lid length is marked from the lateral end of the defect [13]. This forms the hinge. The flap is marked on the medial side of the hinge. The size should be the size of the defect minus one-fourth of the lid length. The flap is incised full- thickness

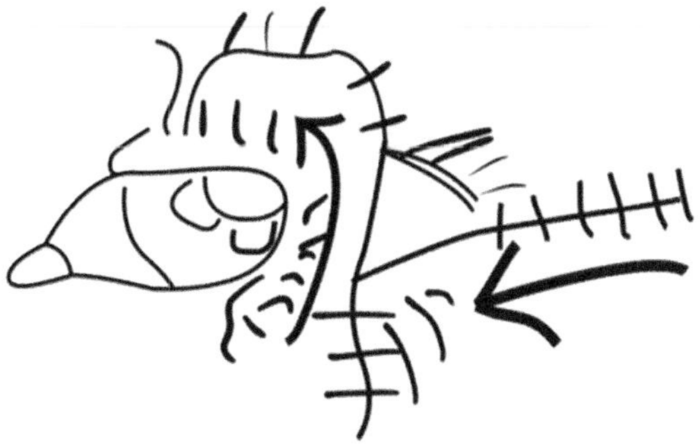

Fig. 17.6 Mustarde lid switch repair for upper eyelid

except at the hinge where it is stopped 4 mm from the lid margin [14].

The pedicle can be divided 2–3 weeks later. The exposed edges are freshened to allow accurate closure of the pedicle end of the flap to the upper lid. The upper lid is closed in layers as usual.

So, when neither of the above is preferred, a sliding tarsoconjunctival flap from the adjoining area / free tarsoconjunctival graft from the other lid is a good option for replacing the posterior lamella. The anterior lamella is fashioned with either a rotational flap (Fricke's flap, glabellar flap, or midline forehead flap) or using a full-thickness skin graft. This avoids the need for a two-staged procedure and limitations of lid-sharing procedures, while still achieving an aesthetically pleasing result and restoring function [15].

17.8.4 Glabellar Flap

The glabellar flap was first described by McCord and Wesley, and starts with an inverted V incision in the central forehead area between the eyebrows, which is partly closed as a Y and the rest of the flap is rotated into the adjacent medial canthal defect (Fig. 17.7). It is a combination of a V-Y and a rhomboid flap [16]. This is not an axial flap, so the length cannot be as long as a median forehead flap. The loose glabellar tissues are incised and undermined. The flap is rotated 90–120° into position. Good results occur,

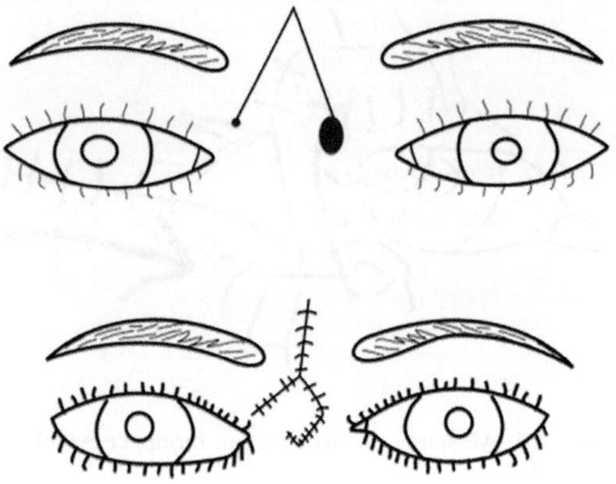

Fig. 17.7 Glabellar flap for medial canthal defect

because the thickness, color, and texture match well and the flap is single staged [17, 18]. The flap gives rise to an unnatural depth of the medial canthus, a bulky nasal bridge, and brings the eyebrows together. This flap is best used for small defects in the medial canthal area.

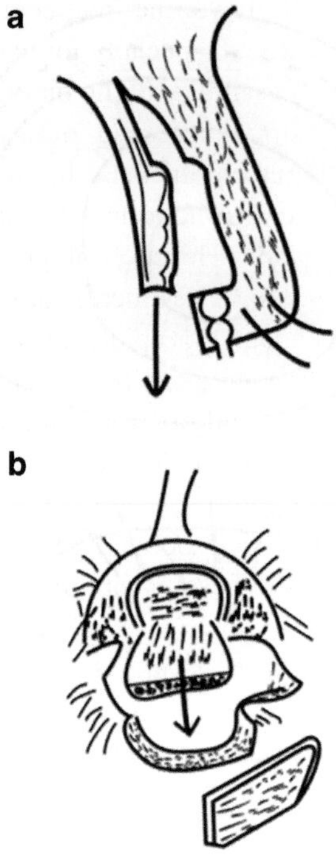

Fig. 17.8 (**a**, **b**) Hughes' tarsoconjunctival advancement flap for repair of lower eyelid posterior lamella

17.9 Lower Lid

Large defects of lower eyelid require different considerations than the upper lid. Here, the posterior lamella can be formed either by using Hughes flap or a free mucoperichondrial flap (nasal septum or palate) and the anterior lamella is formed using a myocutaneous advancement flap like Mustarde cheek rotation transposition flap, lateral or median forehead flap, Tripier flap, or a Fricke flap.

17.9.1 Hughes Tarsoconjunctival Flap

Wendell Hughes first described a tarsoconjunctival flap in 1937 [19], that was based on an earlier procedure described by Dupuy-Dutemps, who also described the dacryocystorhinostomy flaps [2]. It is also a two-staged lid-sharing procedure.

Regardless of the location of the lower eye lid defect, the flap is raised from the central part of the upper lid where the tarsal plate has the largest vertical dimension (Fig. 17.8). The leading edge of the flap is 4 mm superior to the eyelid margin, leaving a strip of tarsal plate for structural support. The vertical limbs of the flap are made perpendicular to the leading edge with the incision carried superiorly toward the fornix. The flap is then advanced across the palpebral aperture, and the edges are sutured to the remaining lower eyelid tarsus or canthal tendons using 6–0 Vicryl suture, and the leading edge is sutured to the conjunctiva using 8–0 Vicryl suture. It is a two-staged lid-sharing procedure that has similar problems like that of Cutler Beard flap. It may result in upper eyelid retraction; therefore, careful dissection of the levator muscle complex from the tarsoconjunctival flap is to be done before advancing to the lower eyelid defect. In some patients, conjunctiva will heal slightly over the edge of the new lid margin, which can create erythema as a result of drying of the conjunctiva. However, as compared to Cutler Beard flap, the results are better, as lashes in the lower lid are normally less appreciated.

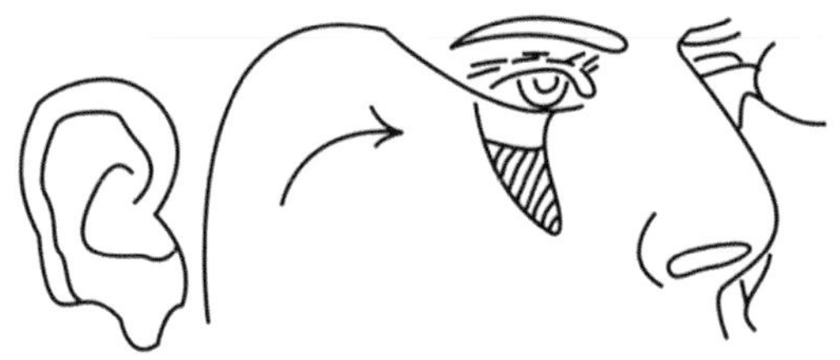

Fig. 17.9 Mustarde cheek rotation flap for large vertical lower eyelid defect

17.9.2 Mustarde Cheek Rotation Flap

This is a very useful flap for reconstructing the anterior lamella in larger vertical defects of lower lid. The flap is marked lateral to the defect extending to the lateral canthal area. It then curves upward and is carried down in front of the ear (Fig. 17.9).

Some quick tips include staying in the subcutaneous cheek plane ("fat up and fat down" when dissecting the flap) and using wide areas of undermining to allow the cheek to be rotated with minimal tension. In some patients, a small backcut or notch at the inferior extent of the incision helps in easy closure [20, 21]. The medial end of the defect should be vertical. This helps reduce a dog-ear. The medial end of the skin flap should be anchored to the medial wall of the orbit. Laterally too, it must be anchored to the lateral wall. Skin is closed using 6–0 nonabsorbable suture. Disadvantages of this type of reconstruction are lower lid retraction, dog-ear, dissection of a large area and possible hematoma formation, and sacrifice of the orbicularis of the lower lid. Lacrimal drainage has to be reconstructed in the second sitting. Also, the preauricular hairline gets distorted.

17.9.3 Fricke's Flap

It is a lateral forehead flap for large defect including the lateral canthus. It was first described by Jochim Fricke in 1829 [22]. The flap is incised along the curve of the eyebrow up to the medial end (Fig. 17.10). A laterally based skin flap above the eyebrow is raised and inserted into the defect as a single stage. The donor area is closed directly. Posterior lamella may now be constructed using a reverse Hughes tarsoconjunctival flap or free mucous membrane graft. After 2 weeks, the flap is divided.

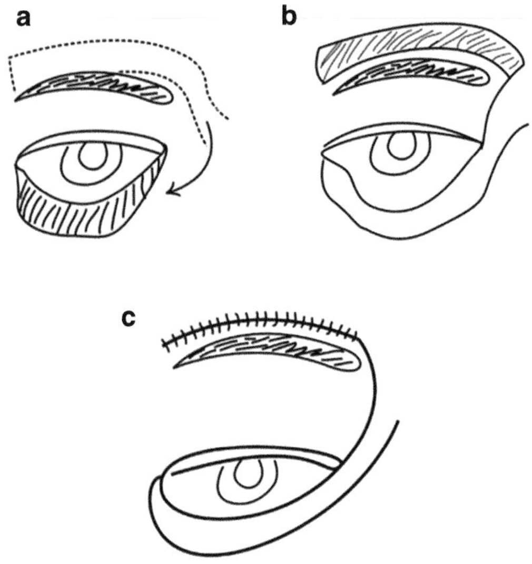

Fig. 17.10 (a–c) Fricke's flap for lower eyelid

Disadvantage is that thick skin hinders proper excursion of upper lid. Also, donor site results in a raised eyebrow as compared to the contralateral side.

17.9.4 Median Forehead Flap

The flap is raised from the center of the forehead depending on the width needed. The plane of dissection is superficial at the tip, but deepens as the dissection progresses, ideally incorporating the periosteum of the frontal bone 1.5–2 cm proximal to the base. The flap is rotated 120–180° into position covering the defect. A wide area of undermining is necessary to close the forehead wound. Up to 3 cm defect over the flap donor site can be closed primarily. The second-stage operation is performed 6 weeks postoperatively. The redundant tissues at the base of the flap are excised.

17.9.5 Tripier Flap

In 1889, Tripier first described the use of an innervated myocutaneous flap in the form of a bipedicle flap (with lateral and medial pedicles) from the upper lid, for reconstruction of a lower lid defect [23]. It is like a bucket handle and is possible only if there is lax skin available. It is mainly used in reconstructing narrow defects and lid margin.

17.10 Eyelid Reconstruction in Anterior Lamellar Defects

17.10.1 Primary Closure with or Without Undermining

Primary closure can be done in periocular areas that have redundant skin like the glabella, the upper lid skin fold, and the temporal region. There is normally less redundant skin in the lower eyelid and medial canthus. If required, tissue surrounding the defect must be undermined to decrease any tension in wound closure. When reconstructing the lower lid, any vertical traction on the eyelid is to be minimized by closing wounds to leave a vertical scar to avoid ectropion or lid retraction. Danger areas for the frontal branch of the facial nerve, viz., over the zygomatic arch and areas more than 1 cm lateral to the brow, should be avoided or the nerve safeguarded under loupe magnification.

17.10.2 Laissez Faire

It means healing by secondary intention. Fox and Beard were the first to describe it. It is applicable for relatively small medial canthal defects, as the region is concave and therefore, heals well [24]. Superficial defects of the eyelid or shallow anterior lamellar defects heal well by this method. In poor surgical candidates who are not fit for surgery, this option may be tried [24, 25].

17.10.3 Skin Grafts

Skin grafts are either full thickness (both epidermis and dermis without any subcutaneous fat) or partial thickness (entire epidermis and part of dermis). Full- thickness grafts provide better cosmesis and are, therefore, preferred in reconstruction in the periocular area, especially for the lower eyelid. However, when the areas are extensive and the nearby areas also have to be resurfaced, a split skin graft becomes the choice, as is so common in military trauma. Also, upper eyelids need thin and light tissue for resurfacing. Therefore, thin split-thickness skin grafts are preferred here for reconstruction. Donor sites for full-thickness skin grafts include upper eyelid skin, retroauricular skin, preauricular skin, and supraclavicular or upper arm skin. Grafts taken from the contralateral eyelid provide the best tissue match; however, the most practical donor site is retroauricular skin [6, 26].

Grafts for pretarsal defects need not be oversized; however, if being used in the medial canthal location or preseptal location, then the graft should be oversized by 10% and 30%, respectively, to prevent secondary contracture of the graft (F). After harvesting, full-thickness skin graft defatting has to be done to remove all fat. The graft is sutured at the recipient site using 4–0 silk, leaving the tails long. The tails of the silk sutures are then tied down over a xeroform petroleum gauze, which acts as a pressure dressing (bolster) and left in place for about 5–7 days for an adequate take. This is called a tie-over dressing. The stages of skin graft take are plasmatic imbibition (24–48 h), inosculation (third to fifth day) where donor and recipient capillaries are aligned, and revascularization where the graft is revascularized through "kissing" of capillaries.

17.10.4 Flaps

Myocutaneous flaps in the periocular area are formed of skin and orbicularis muscle. They have many advantages over free skin grafts. Flaps provide available local tissue for better match of

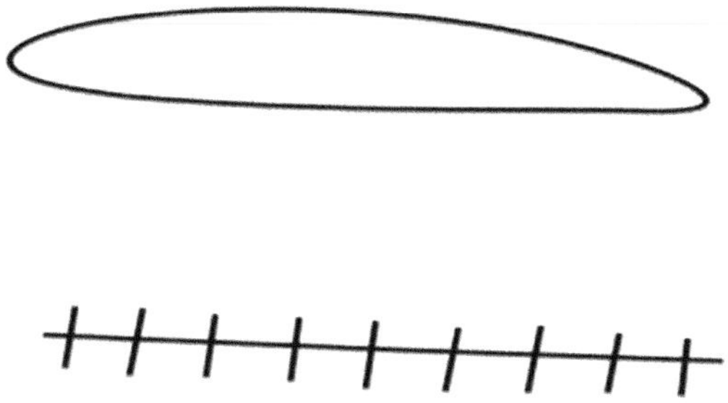

Fig. 17.11 Sliding flap

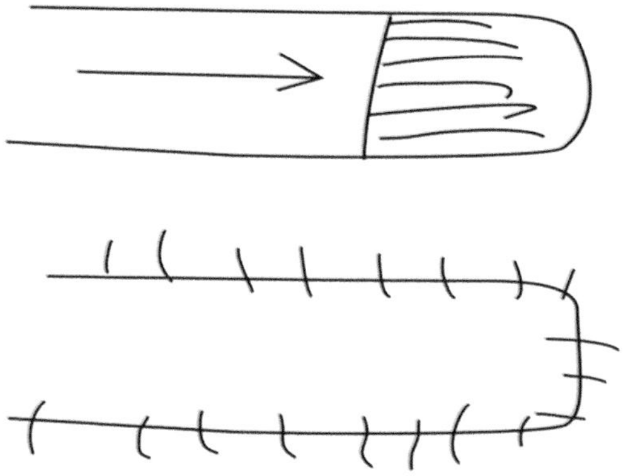

Fig. 17.12 Advancement flap

color and texture, near normal innervation, and coverage by vascularised tissue over bare bone and cartilage, with better function [27].

The various flaps used in periocular area can be divided into 5 types:

- Sliding flap: Undermining is done surrounding an ellipse to close the defect (Fig. 17.11) [3].
- Advancement flap: The surrounding skin is converted into a three sided flap, which is dissected and advanced along its own long axis to close the defect (Figs. 17.12, and 17.13). It can be single or a double advancement flap (H plasty).
- Rotation flap: These flaps are commonly used in the periocular area, where the adjacent skin is raised and rotated to fill the defect (Fig. 17.14).

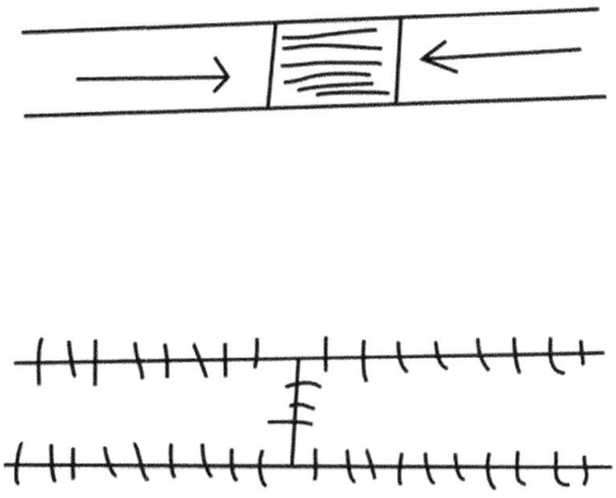

Fig. 17.13 Advancement flap

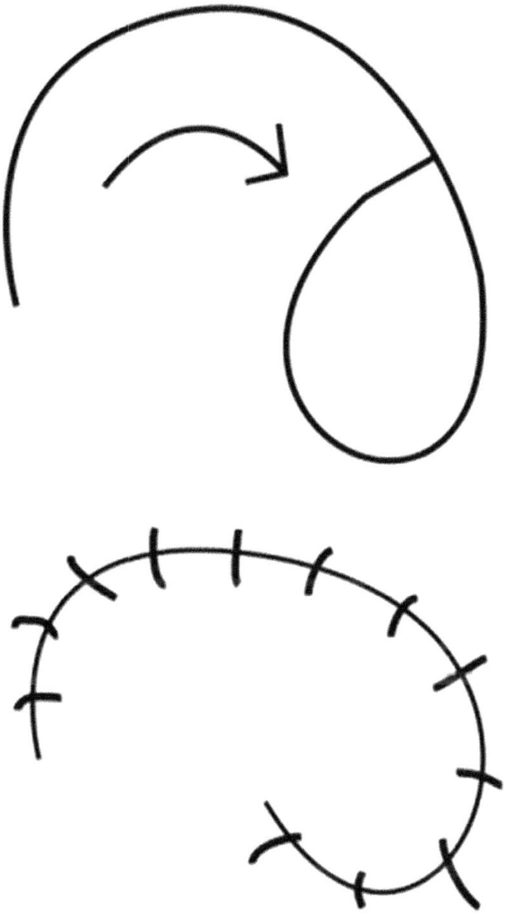

Fig. 17.14 Rotation flap

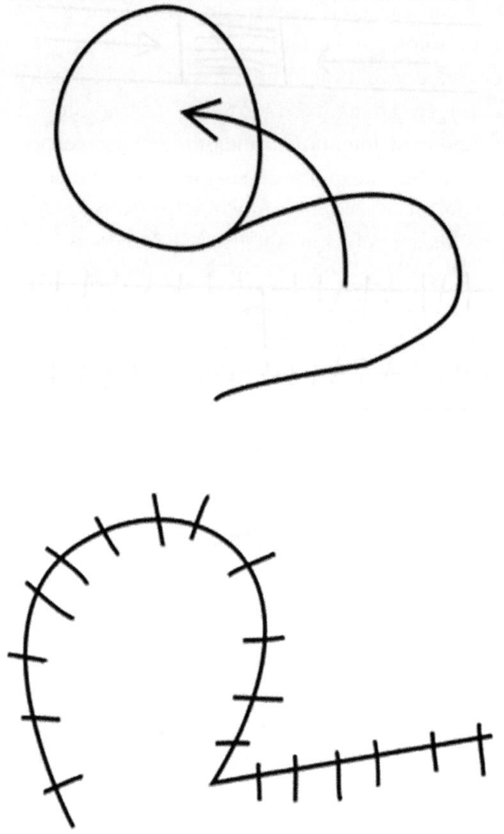

Fig. 17.15 Transposition flap

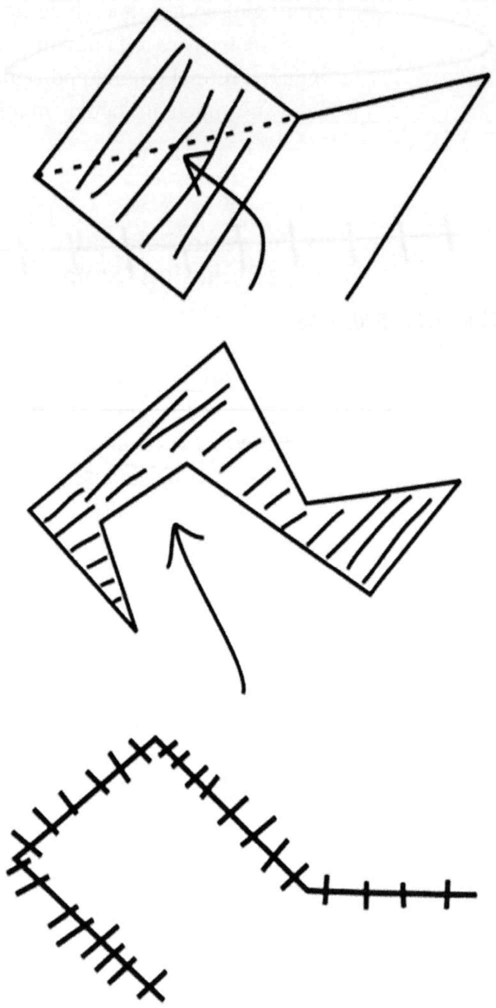

Fig. 17.16 Limberg Flap

- Transposition flap: In these flaps, the adjacent skin is raised to insert into the defect, but the flap donor site should be small so as to be closed primarily without tension on the flap (Fig. 17.15).

17.10.4.1 Special Transposition Flaps

(a) Limberg flap: Originally described by Alexander Limberg in 1946, it is one of the most useful flaps in periocular area [28]. A rhomboid defect is created with an equilateral parallelogram, and using the short diagonal, a triangular flap is drawn in a rhomboid shape, which can be transposed into the adjacent defect (Fig. 17.16).

(b) Bilobed flap: The bilobed flap was originally described by Esser in 1918 for reconstruction of defects of the nasal tip [29, 30]. This flap is widely used for circular defects of the nose, cheek, forehead, and medial canthal defects. It consists of 2 adjacent transposition flaps on a common pedicle, wherein the original defect is filled by the first larger flap and the second smaller flap fills in the defect left by the first. The angle between the two lobes can be varied from 30° to 120° (Fig. 17.17) [30].

17.10.5 Lateral Canthal Defects

Lateral canthus can be reconstructed by anchoring the remnant tarsal plate to a periosteal flap raised from the lateral wall of the orbit of a recommended 4 mm width. A fascial graft from deep temporal fascia or palmaris longus tendon can also be used instead and fixed to the lateral wall of the orbit via drill holes made in the bone. The fixation of the lateral tendon should be 3 mm above the level of medial canthus [31].

17.10.6 Medial Canthal Defects

Healing by secondary intention is sometimes recommended for skin defects in this area. If the underlying bone is exposed, a glabellar flap/median forehead flap can be transposed into the defect (Fig. 17.7). Medial canthus can be repaired in a similar fashion to that of the lateral canthus repair. Transnasal wiring may also be done in certain cases.

17.10.7 Canalicular Repair

Canalicular injury is commonly seen associated with lower lid avulsion. Most widely accepted approach is to find out the torn ends and place a well-tolerated stent temporarily in the system. Stents can be mono- or bicanalicular. In cases of unavailability, a 22 or 24 gauge IV cannula or a silicone rod can be put in situ.

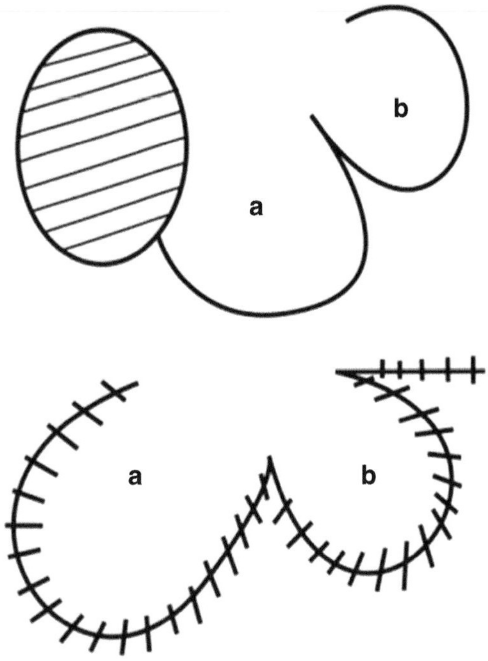

Fig. 17.17 (**a**, **b**) Bilobed flap

Identification of proximal end of canaliculus is done under high magnification. It appears paler than the surrounding area. Sterile saline can be poured in the wound and air bubbles watched for while injecting air from the canaliculus. Another method described is the use of flourescein dye injection from intact canaliculus coming out through the proximal cut end. Suturing is preferably done by fine microsutures over the stent under magnification (Figs. 17.18, 17.19, and 17.20).

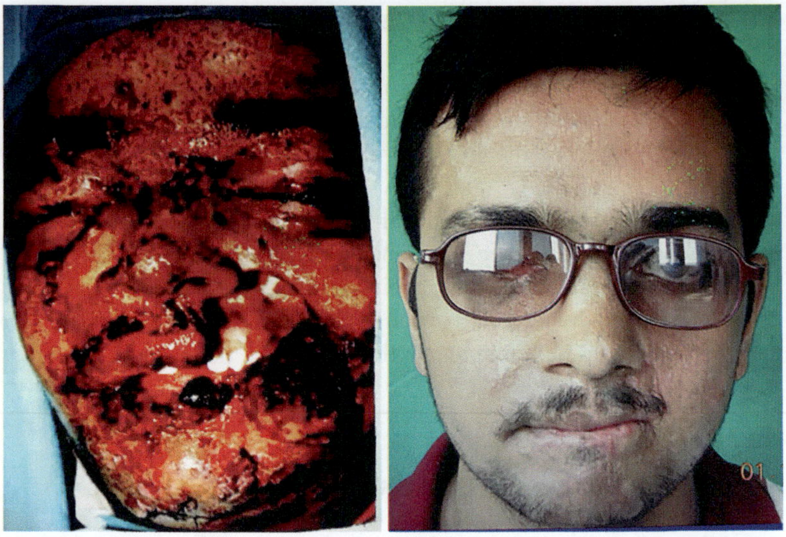

Fig. 17.18 Shrapnel injury, which resulted in this devastating injury to the face. Late post-operative picture following enucleation of right eye and eyelid repair (Courtesy: Department of Plastic and Reconstructive Surgery, Army Hospital (Research and Referral), New Delhi)

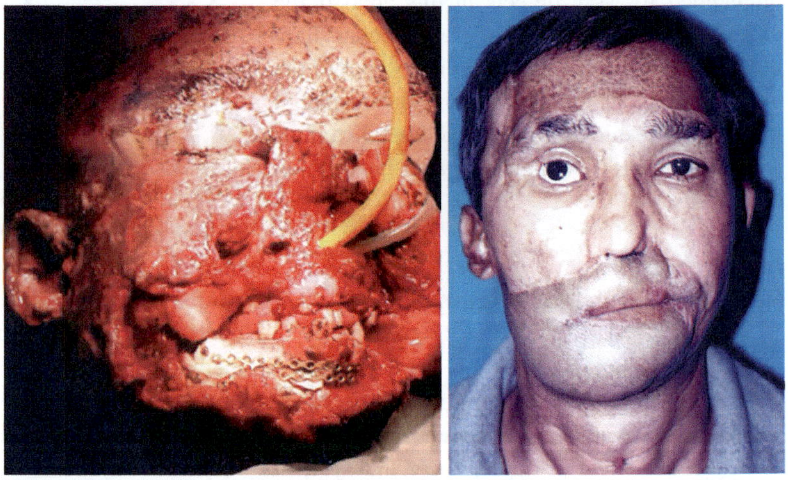

Fig. 17.19 Blast injury to face. Late postoperative result after split skin grafts, panfacial fractures reduction and fixation, enucleation of right eye, and multiple flaps to the face (Courtesy: Lt Gen P Bhargava, VSM (Retd) ex Senior Consultant Surgery and Reconstructive Surgery, Armed Forces Medical Service)

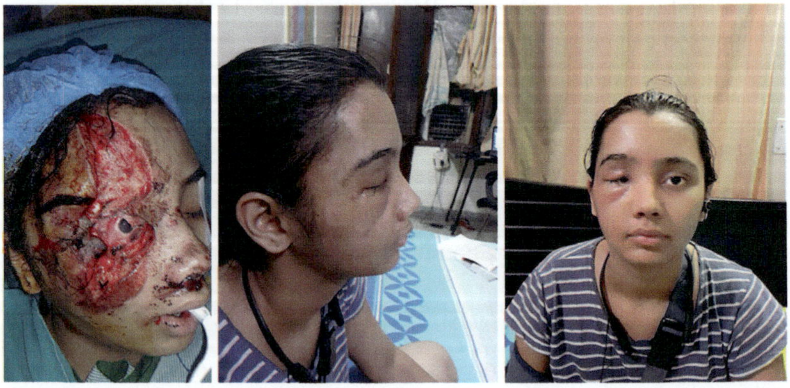

Fig. 17.20 Forehead wound, orbital fractures, and eyelid with canalicular injury. Early postoperative repair with local flaps, fracture reduction, and canalicular repair

Disclaimer Patient consent was obtained for Figs. 17.18, 17.19 and 17.20.

Acknowledgments We sincerely acknowledge Mr. Amit Mohan, Content Developer, Dept. of Telemedicine & Biomedical Informatics, Sanjay Gandhi Postgraduate Institute of Medical Sciences, Lucknow, for drawing Figs. 17.1, 17.2, 17.5, 17.6, 17.7, 17.8, 17.9, 17.10, 17.11, 17.12, 17.13, 17.14, 17.15, 17.16, and 17.7

References

1. Weichel ED, Colyer MH, Ludlow SE, Bower KS, Eiseman AS. Combat ocular trauma visual outcomes during operations Iraqi and enduring freedom. Ophthalmology. 2008;115(12):2235–45.
2. Porfiris E, Christopoulos A, Sandris P, et al. Upper eyelid orbicularis oculi flap with tarsoconjunctival Island for reconstruction of full-thickness lower lid defects. Plast Reconstr Surg. 1999;103:186–91.
3. Patrinely JR, Marines HM, Anderson RL. Skin flaps in periorbital reconstruction. Surv Ophthalmol. 1987;31:249–61.
4. Bowman PH, Fosko SW, Hartstein ME. Periocular Reconstruction. Semin Cutan Med Surg. 2003;22:263–72.
5. Morley AM, deSousa JL, Selva D, Malhotra R. Techniques of upper eyelid reconstruction. Surv Ophthalmol. 2010;55(03):256–71.
6. DiFrancesco LM, Codner MA, McCord CD. Upper eyelid reconstruction. Plast Reconstr Surg. 2004;114(07):98e–107e.
7. Tenzel RR, Stewart WB. Eyelid reconstruction by the semicircle flap technique. Ophthalmology. 1978;85:1164–9.
8. TenzelRR. Reconstruction of the central one half of an eyelid. Arch Ophthalmol. 1975;93(02):125–6.
9. Tenzel RR, Stewart WB. Eyelid reconstruction by the semicircle flap technique. Ophthalmology. 1978;85(11):1164–9.
10. Levine MR, Buckman G. Semicircular flap revisited. Arch Ophthalmol. 1986;104(06):915–7.
11. Chandler DB, Gausas RE. Lower eyelid reconstruction. Otolaryngol Clin N Am. 2005;38(05): 1033–42.
12. Cutler NL, Beard C. A method for partial and total upper lid reconstruction. Am J Ophthalmol. 1955;39(01):1–7.
13. Mustarde JC. Repair and reconstruction in the orbital region. 2nd ed. Philadelphia: Churchill Livingstone; 1991.
14. Tyers AG, Collin JRO. Eyelid reconstruction—anterior and posterior lamella combined. In: Colour atlas of ophthalmic plastic surgery. 4th ed. Amsterdam: Elsevier; 2018. p. 449–50.
15. Malik A, Shah-Desai S. Sliding tarsal advancement flap for upper eyelid reconstruction. Orbit. 2014;33(02):124–6.
16. Meadows AE, Manners RM. A simple modification of the glabellar flap in medial Canthal reconstruction. Ophthal Plast Reconstr Surg. 2003;19:313–5.
17. Maloof AJ, Leatherbarrow B. The glabellar flap dissected. Eye (Lond). 2000;14(Pt 4):597–605.
18. Field LM. The glabellar transposition "banner" flap. J Dermatol Surg Oncol. 1988;14(04):376–9.
19. Rohrich RJ, Zbar RI. The evolution of the Hughes Tarsoconjunctival flap for lower eyelid reconstruction. Plast Reconstr Surg. 1999;104:518–22.
20. Mustardé JC. The use of flaps in the orbital region. Plast Reconstr Surg. 1970;45(02):146–50.
21. Mustardé JC. Major reconstruction of the eyelids: functional and aesthetic considerations. Clin Plast Surg. 1981;8(02):227–36.
22. Wilcsek G, Leatherbarrow B, Halliwell M, FrancisI. The 'RITE' use of the Fricke flap in periorbital reconstruction. Eye. 2005;19:854–60.
23. Elliot D, Britto JA. Tripier's innervated myocutaneous flap1889. Br J Plast Surg. 2004;57(06):543–9.
24. Fox SA, Beard C. Spontaneous lid repair. Am J Ophthalmol. 1964;58:947–52.
25. Harrington JN. Reconstruction of the medial canthus by spontaneous granulation (laissez-faire): a review. Ann Ophthalmol. 1982;14(10):956–60, 963–966, 969–970.
26. Madge SN, Malhotra R, Thaller VT, et al. A systematic approach to the oculoplastic reconstruction of the eyelid medial canthal region after cancer excision. Int Ophthalmol Clin. 2009;49(04):173–94.
27. Nerad JA. Lid reconstruction. In: Techniques in ophthalmic plastic surgery. 1st ed. Amsterdam: Elsevier; 2010. p. 332.
28. Turan T, Kuran I, Ozcan H, Bas L. Geometric limit of multiple local Limberg flaps: a flap design. Plast Reconstr Surg. 1999;104:1675–8.
29. Iida N, Ohsumi N, Tonegawa M, Tsutsumi K. Simple method of designing a bilobed flap. Plast Reconstr Surg. 1999;104:495–9.
30. Sullivan TJ, Bray LC. The bilobed flap in medial canthal reconstruction. Aust N Z J Ophthalmol. 1995;23:42–8.
31. Subramanian N. Reconstruction of eyelids. Indian J Plast Surg. 2011;44(1):5–13.

18 Ocular Trauma in Armed Conflicts: Manifestations, Management, and Outcomes—Complex Case Scenarios

Pramod Bhende, Pradeep Susvar, and Kaushal Sanghvi

18.1 Introduction

Ocular munition injuries are an integral part of the war conflicts and pattern of such ophthalmic injuries depend on the specific ammunition used, which hit the eyeball. Conventional weapons such as mortars, rockets, sniper rifles, and automatic weapons causing severe penetrating ocular injury are well described in the literature [1]. Many eye injuries in a combat are due to fragmentary munitions. A small projectile due to an explosion that may be stopped by a flak vest, helmet, or heavy clothing may penetrate the eye easily even when from a great distance. Fragmentation injuries have accounted for a vast majority of eye injuries during recent major conflicts. Improvised explosive devices (IEDs) potentially cause splitting of the sclera and shredding the remnants of ocular tissues causing extreme difficulty to repair with almost no visual potential [1].

Open globe injuries and adnexal injury are the most frequent ophthalmic injuries reported in the literature related to armed conflicts [1]. Penetrating injuries and intraocular foreign bodies (IOFBs) are the most commonly encountered ocular injury in our day-to-day clinical practice [2]. It is one of the important ocular emergency, which needs immediate repair along with management of concurrent systemic injuries in the nearest located or the base (Armed Force) hospital. Open globe injuries and most of adnexal and facial injuries are primarily repaired in army hospitals, thereby achieving the primary objective of salvaging the globe. These patients who have undergone primary repair are then referred to tertiary care hospitals for further specific surgical interventions by appropriate subspeciality surgeons. Such cases warrant surgeries concurrently by different specialities like vitreoretina, glaucoma, cornea, and oculoplasty. Neurophthalmology and squint subspecialties also aid in the management in regard to the possible visual outcome and rehabilitation.

We have been managing such severely traumatized eyes in our tertiary care center since inception. The main objective would be timely appropriate intervention to achieve the best possible anatomical and visual outcome. We describe the study analysis of cases related to various ocular injuries due to armed conflicts, referred from military hospital to our center for further speciality management.

P. Bhende (✉) · P. Susvar · K. Sanghvi
Vitreoretinal Services, Medical Research Foundation (MRF), Sankara Nethralaya, Chennai, India
e-mail: drpb@snmail.org

S. Waikar (ed.), *Ocular Trauma in Armed Conflicts*, https://doi.org/10.1007/978-981-19-4021-7_18

18.1.1 Representative Cases

Case 1

A 38-year-old male lost his left eye vision from IED blast, 15 days back, sustaining a corneo-scleral injury. Scleral wound involving limbus was repaired at his base hospital and patient was referred to our center for further management. With visual acuity of counting fingers close to face(CFCF), left eye examination revealed multiple opacities and small foreign bodies on cornea and iris surface. Well-secured limbal and scleral wound was noted extending 4 mm temporally from 3'o clock. Aphakia was noted with blood and vitreous in anterior chamber (AC). Other eye was normal. Left eye had no view of fundus due to vitreous hemorrhage. Ultrasound B-Scan showed presence of Intraocular foreign body (IOFB) with attached retina, which was confirmed by CT scan also picking up orbital FB embedded in the lateral rectus muscle of the right eye. Oculoplasty expert evaluation suggested to observe this extraocular FB in his right orbit.

Patient underwent Vitrectomy with IOFB removal in the left eye. His vision improved to Snellen's 6/60 at 6 weeks follow-up. He had centrally placed multiple corneal scars, which were followed up over 3 months. Once the eye was stable post vitrectomy, penetrating keratoplasty (PK) was performed. Left eye developed secondary angle closure glaucoma, which was initially managed with IOP-lowering medication.

Three months later, he presented in emergency with complain of sudden onset of redness, pain, and decreased vision. Slit-lamp examination revealed presence of AC inflammation with hypopyon. AC tap smear for bacteria and fungus was initially negative. With clinical presentation, left eye was diagnosed as having endophthalmitis, possible fungal etiology. The patient was started on systemic and intravitreal voriconazole. Vitreous lavage was done on fifth day of infection. Over next 1 week, culture grew *Candida albicans*. Based on sensitivity, intravitreal amphotericin B was also added. Despite maximum antifungal by all routes, there was rapid worsening. B-Scan revealed exudates in vitreous cavity, total retinal detachment (RD) with diffuse choroidal thickening. Eventually by tenth day, eye was eviscerated for control of infection.

In short, early removal of IOFB helps in structural and functional improvement. PK should be contemplated preferably after stabilization of IOP for better graft survival. Regular and long-term follow-up is absolutely essential in cases of PK.

Case 2

35 -year-old male presented to us with a complaint of decreased vision in his right eye post perforating injury due to grenade blast. He underwent primary corneal tear repair at base hospital. On examination, his best-corrected visual acuity in right eye was CFCF. Anterior segment examination revealed sutured corneal tear with bullous keratopathy and aphakia. IOP with Tonopen was 26 mm of Hg. Patient was on two pressure-lowering medications. Synaechial angle closure was noted. Optic disc view was very hazy. Ultrasound B- Scan revealed attached retina in the right eye. Patient underwent trabeculectomy with mitomycin C for uncontrolled IOP due to traumatic angle closure glaucoma. With eye pressure under control with single IOP-lowering medication, he underwent PK 5 months later. His IOP remained well controlled with single IOP-lowering medication. With aphakic correction, vision improved to Snellen's 6/24, N18 at 6 weeks follow-up. Vision improved to 6/9, N8 after suture removal and with contact lens, 1 year post PK. Patient underwent medial rectus resection and lateral rectus recession for unresolved diplopia after prism trial. Patient remained stable till 6 years after surgery with aphakic correction. He underwent pars plana vitrectomy with scleral fixated intraocular lens (SFIOL) implantation with Ahmed glaucoma valve implantation and had stable vision. Patient lost to follow-up and came for evaluation after 8 yrs. At this last follow-up, he had failed graft with uncontrolled high IOP with advanced glaucomatous cupping and hand movement (HM) vision.

In short, post corneal tear repaired eyes do have higher risk of short-/long-term glaucoma, which necessitates early recognition, surgical intervention, if needed and long-term follow-up. PK with glaucoma is challenging situation and needs meticulous management. Improvement in the vision with early surgical interventions encourages the further vision rehabilitation procedures like squint corrections and IOL implantations.

Case 3

A 19-year-old soldier sustained penetrating injury due to grenade blast to his left eye and underwent primary corneal tear repair at his referral hospital. Post trauma, left eye developed secondary glaucoma and was managed locally with IOP-lowering medication. He was referred for further management.

Vision at the time of presentation was 6/6 in right eye and 6/36 in the left eye with aphakic correction. Anterior segment of the right eye was normal, the left eye had central corneal vascularized scar and aphakia. IOP in right eye and left eye were 12 and 15 mmHg respectively. In the left eye, quadrant synaechial angle closure was observed on gonioscopy; however, no glaucomatous disc damage was noted. He was medically managed with IOP-lowering medications. With two IOP-lowering medications, left eye IOP slowly increased to 26 mm of Hg with disc progression to cup disc ratio of 0.5 and early nasal depressed points noted on visual field. He underwent Ahmed glaucoma valve implantation with tube placement in anterior chamber in his left eye. On his last follow-up, left eye BCVA remained stable at 6/18 with contact lens and IOP 12 mm of Hg with single IOP-lowering medication.

The case again emphasizes the short- and long-term risk of glaucoma in cases of penetrating trauma and need for early recognition and intervention.

Case 4 (Fig. 18.1)

A 24-year-old male sustained injury to his left eye with sharp metal blade leading to lid lacera-

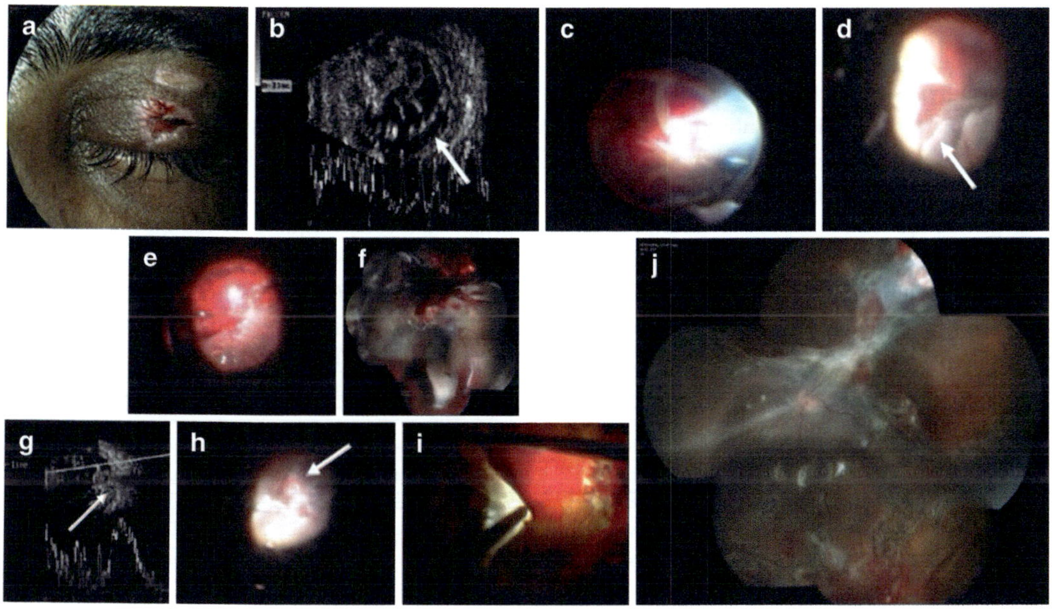

Fig. 18.1 Sequence of events observed in Case 4 of 24-year-old male sustaining perforating injury to left eye with sharp metal blade. (**a**) Repaired lid laceration. (**b**) Ultrasound showing vitreous hemorrhage and Hemorrhagic CD (arrow). (**c**) Intraoperative thick vitreous blood and (**d**) showing mounds of hemorrhagic CD (arrow) with RD noted after clearing the vitreous blood correlating ultrasound scan. (**e**) Retina attempted to flatten and displace the subretinal blood and choroidal mound to periphery under LPFC. (**f**) Montage photo of retina under silicone oil after first stage surgery (**g**) B scan done initially after the globe repair showing superior vitreoretinal incarceration (arrow) correlating with (**h**) intraoperative findings of retinal incarceration (arrow) after silicone oil removal in second stage surgery. (**i**) Evacuation of subretinal blood after reflecting the retina. (**j**) Fundus montage 3 months after second surgery with stable attached retina with extensive scarring

tion and globe perforation. On examination, right eye was normal. Left eye had vision of PL and inaccurate PR. There was severe lid edema with lid laceration of 4 × 2 mm and traumatic ptosis was noted. He also had subconjunctival hemorrhage, the posterior extent of which could not be made out. AC showed hyphaema inferiorly and finger tension was soft. Patient was taken up for lid tear repair and globe exploration. During globe exploration, posterior extension of scleral tear of about 8 mm from the superior rectus muscle was seen and was repaired.

Ultrasound B scan was done on day 1 post repair, which revealed RD, Hemorrhagic CDs with vitreous hemorrhage with vitreoretinal incarceration superiorly. Patient was started with topical and oral steroids to reduce the inflammation. PL was inconsistent and repeat ultrasound had minimal lysis of suprachoroidal blood. On day 5, the patient underwent choroidal drainage followed by lensectomy and vitrectomy. Intraoperatively along with thick vitreous hemorrhage, significant blood was noted behind the retina with persistent choroidal mounds all-round the periphery. Blood from subretinal space was maneuvered to periphery and evacuated by use of perfluorocarbon liquids (PFCL) and silicone oil was placed for temporary stabilization of retina. Second stage surgery was done 10 days later, where he was taken up for relaxing retinotomy along the area of retinal incarceration with aid of PFCL, endolaser and exchange of silicone oil. Vision was CFCF with retina attached at 6 weeks, IOP was low and oil was touching the corneal endothelium. On subsequent visit at 3 months vision in left eye was 2/60 with attached retina and silicon oil in situ.

This case emphasizes the early treatment with oral steroids to control inflammation and to prepare the eye for subsequent VR surgery after the primary repair. It is important to utilize the optimal time and the best opportunity available for a VR surgeon, to address the pathoanatomy as much as possible, before permanent structural changes ensue.

18.2 Sankara Nethralaya (SN) Experience

We reviewed records of patients referred from military hospital for armed-conflict-related injuries, which were primarily repaired and referred further to Sankara Nethralaya for second stage speciality surgeries. Data was collected from year 2003–2018.

Thirty patients (31 eyes) were managed exclusively in vitreoretinal department, of which 4 needed corneal intervention and 3 required oculoplasty procedures. Of those 30 patients, 8 required more than one subspeciality intervention which includes corneal, glaucoma, concurrently along with vitreoretinal surgery as combined or staged procedure.

We analyzed the details of these 31 eyes (30 patients) who underwent vitreoretinal surgeries in single and or multiple sitting and results are as follows. (Table 18.1).

Of the 30 patients, 16 (53.33%) patients were less than 30 years of age, 10 (33.33%) were between 31 and40 years, and 4 (13.33%) patients were more than 40 years. Right eye was involved in 15 and left eye in 14. One patient had bilateral injury.

The various modes of injury (Chart 18.1) were blast injury, splinter injury, weapon and cartridge injury, and recoil injury. Of the 31 injured eyes, blast injury was noted highest in the series, accounting for 16 (51.61%) eyes. Representative case of a pellet injury with double perforation is depicted in Fig. 18.2.

Table 18.1 Analysis of patients who underwent Vitreoretinal surgery

No of eyes	31 (30 patients)	
Study duration	15 years	
Type of injury	Penetrating	20
	Blunt	11
Zone involvement	Zone 1	24
	Zone 2	7
Primary repair for	Corneal tear	9
	Scleral tear	2
Interval between presentation and surgery		3–10 days
Follow-up	4 M-20 Years	

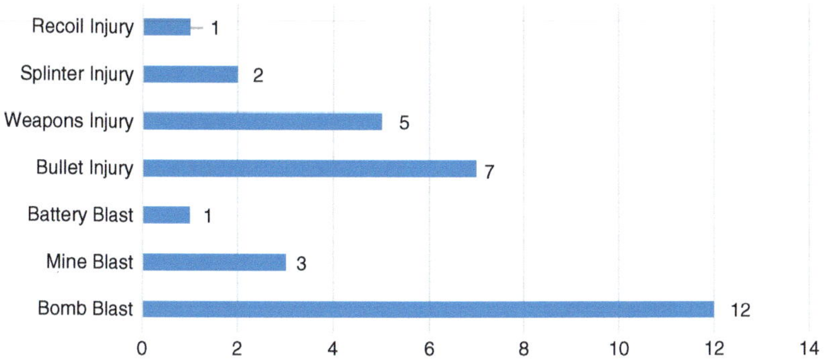

Chart 18.1 Mode of Injury

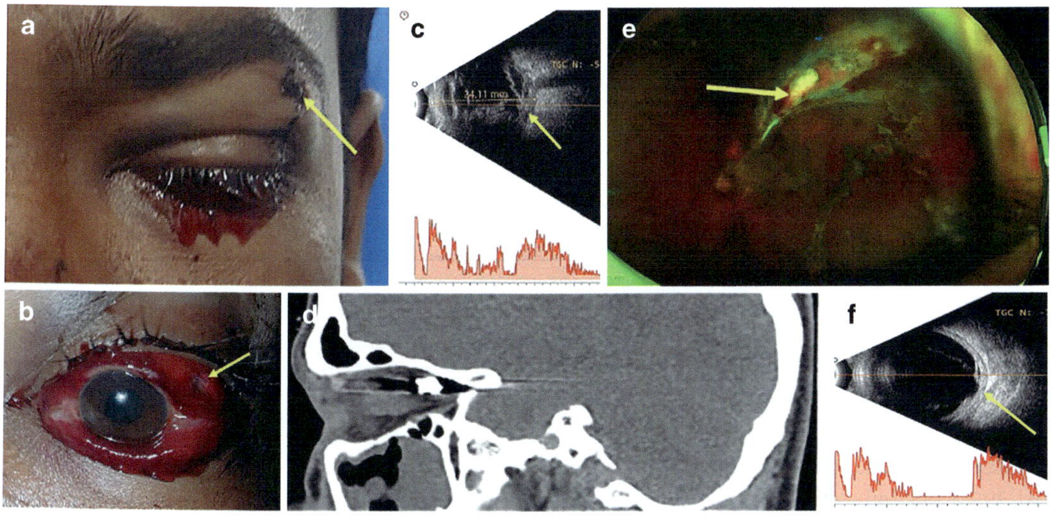

Fig. 18.2 Case of a pellet injury. Thirty year-old male sustained pellet injury to his left eye causing double perforation. Vision at presentation was PL+ but inaccurate PR. (**a**) Entry wound at upper lid. (**b**) Severe chemosis and subconjunctival hemorrhage (arrow showing the scleral entry). Cornea and lens was clear with round, centrally placed pupil. (**c**) USG showing scleral defect (exit wound) with vitreous incarceration (arrow) at perforation site. (**d**) CT scan showing pellet lodged in the superior orbit just above the optic nerve. The pellet was left behind in the orbit (**e**) Post surgery fundus photo (Optos) showing bare sclera and scarring at exit wound sight (**f**) corresponding B scan

Out of 31 eyes, 20 (64.51%) had penetrating trauma and 11 (35.48%) had blunt trauma.

Four patients (12.90%) had other bodily injuries which included shoulder injury due to bullet, amputation of right arm, sutured forearm wound and left leg fracture.

Twenty-eight patients (90.31%) had presenting complaints of diminution of vision. The BCVA in the affected eye was HMCF in 19 (61.21%) and PL positive with inaccurate PR in 12 (38.70%) eyes.

In 24 (77.41%) eyes, Zone 1 was involved and 7 (22.31%) eyes had zone 2 involvement.

Various anterior segment manifestations are shown in Chart 18.2.

Six eyes (19.35%) had an additional adnexal injury. Lid tear accounted for 5 (83.33%) eyes and eyebrow laceration in 1 (16.66%).

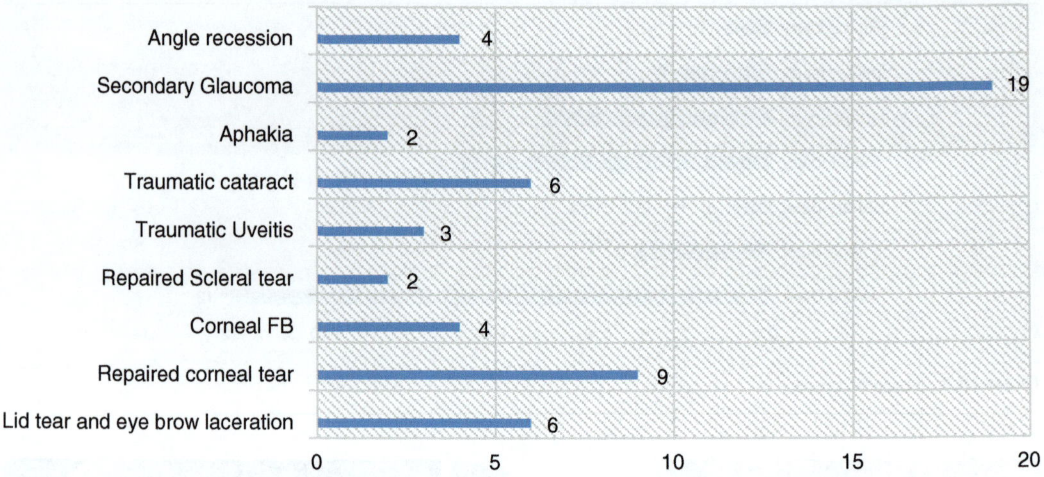

Chart 18.2 Anterior Segment Findings

Chart 18.3 Posterior segment findings

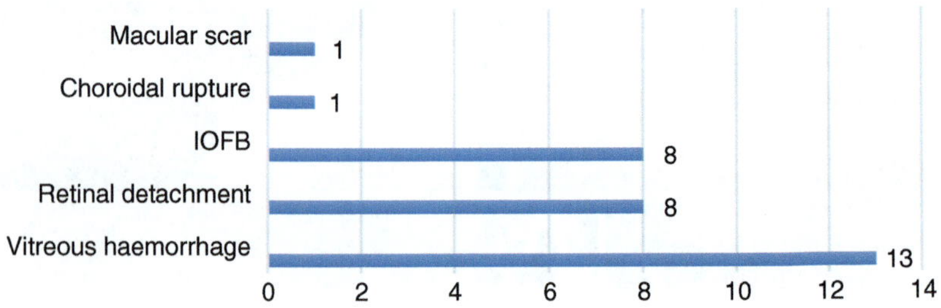

Secondary glaucoma was noted in 19 eyes (61.29%) but only 4 eyes (21.05%) had angle recession. Twelve eyes (63.15%) were successfully managed with antiglaucoma drugs. YAG PI (peripheral iridotomy) was done for 4 eyes (21.05%). %). 2 (10.5%) eyes required early trabeculectomy surgeries and one of the two had late second AGV surgery in our series.

Posterior segment involvement (Chart 18.3) was varied in their manifestation. Eighteen eyes (58.06%) had some fundus view to identify the pathology. Vitreous hemorrhage (VH) precluded fundus visualization in 13 eyes (41.94%).

Twenty-five (80.64%) eyes had USG B scan. IOFB were suspected in 12 of the 25 eyes (48%). RD with VH was noted in 4 eyes (16%), only VH in 7 eyes (28%) and VH with vitreous incarceration noted in 2 eyes (8%) (Fig. 18.3) Other investigations included CT scan done for 13 (41.93%) patients.

Out of 31 eyes (Table 18.2), vitrectomy was done in 30 (96.7%) eyes. Encirclage with 240 band was performed in 25 (80.64%). Lensectomy was done along with vitrectomy in 13 (43%) eyes. Per operative tamponade usage was needed in 19 eyes. Silicone oil was used in 16 eyes (51.61%), whereas C3F8 gas was used as an internal tamponade in 3 eyes (9.68%). Though FB was suspected on ultrasound in 12 eyes, only 8 eyes had actual CT scan confirmed IOFB and all underwent IOFB removal. One eye (3%) required sclera patch graft with vitrectomy and in one, iridodialysis repair was done. Vitrectomy with endolaser and phacoemulsification (PE) and IOL was done in one (3%) eye. Vitrectomy with SFIOL was done in one (3%) eye.

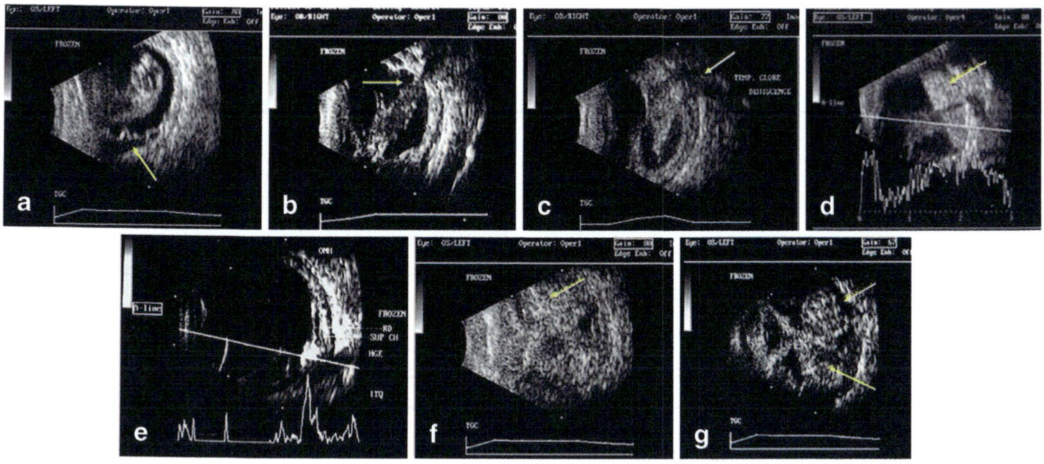

Fig. 18.3 Ultrasound B-scans of various intraocular findings observed in cases of armed conflicts, facilitating to take appropriate surgical decisions. (**a**) Vitreous hemorrhage with inferior RD (arrow). (**b**) Vitreous incarceration (arrow) at the scleral wound. (**c**) Vitreoretinal incarceration with post globe dehiscence (arrow) (**d**) Total RD pulled anteriorly toward repaired wound and layering of subretinal mobile blood (arrow) surrounding ONH at posterior pole (**e**) IOFB sitting on the retina and associated shallow RD. (**f**) Hemorrhagic CD with homogenous echoes (arrow) and no details to delineate retinal architecture (**g**) Clot lysis (arrows) noted in the same eye after a week of systemic and topical steroids

Table 18.2 Surgical intervention

Procedures performed	N
Vitrectomy	30
Lensectomy (along with vitrectomy)	13
240 band encirclage	25
Silicone oil injection	15
Gas(C3F8) tamponade	3
Vitrectomy with PE + IOL	1
Vitrectomy with SFIOL	1
Vitrectomy with scleral patch graft	1
Vitrectomy with IOFB removal	8

The average interval between presentation and surgery was 7 days (range: 3–10 days).

18.2.1 Surgery Outcome

All 3 eyes with gas tamponade had attached retina at 6 weeks. Fiffteen eyes having silicone oil were further studied. Silicone oil removal (SOR) was done in 8 eyes (53.33%) and had attached retina at last follow-up. 6 (40%) had retina re-detachment at 6 weeks follow-up. Of those 6 eyes, 2 (33.33%) underwent second VR surgery to stabilize the retina and had successful oil removal later, summing up of total 10 eyes (66.66%) having successful silicone oil removal.

Four eyes (26.66%) were left with silicone oil in situ, with no further intervention due to low IOP and corneal decompensation. One patient lost to follow-up.

To sum up, of 18 eyes that had internal tamponade (SIO and C3F8 gas), 13 eyes (72.22%) had attached retina and stable IOP (Fig. 18.4).

Silicone oil removal was combined with Epiretinal Membrane (ERM) removal in 2 eyes (15%), with PE + IOL in 2 eyes (15%), SFIOL in one eye (7.5%). Five eyes underwent SFIOL fixation with an average interval of 26 months from primary surgery. In 3 patients (14%) squint surgery was done 34 months (average) after primary surgery.

None of the eyes in our case series had acute endophthalmitis at presentation or in early post-operative period. But one case (Case 1) developed panophthalmitis at 6 months post vitrectomy necessitating evisceration.

Overall vision improved in 29 out of 31 eyes (93.54%). At 6 weeks postsurgery, BCVA was

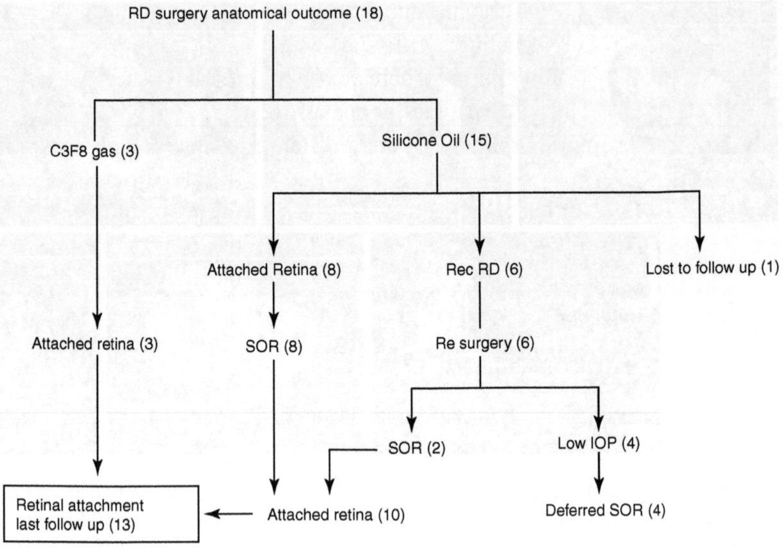

Fig. 18.4 Flow chart showing outcome in eyes with retinal detachment with internal tamponade

better than 6/24 in 8 eyes (25.8%) and in 23 eyes (74.2%), it was less than 6/60. Final BCVA was better than 6/24 in 12 eyes (38.7%), and in 19 eyes (61.3%), it was less than 6/60.

Average duration of follow-up was 7 years (57 months), ranging from 4 months to 20 years.

18.3 Discussion

Ferenc Kuhn, in an editorial, quotes the paraphrase of Leonid Trotsky: "You may not be interested in war or terrorism, but they are interested in you." War injury in any nation is a painful one, with important implications for all ophthalmologists, that regardless of whether they expect to see such conflicts in their own clinical practice [3]. They can be of any munition related or ammunition specific injury. Circumstances leading and the mode of injury are highly variable and also unpredictable. The specific characteristics of the armed injuries make them unique and challenging for an ophthalmic surgeon. Wide spectrum of the ocular tissue damage, presence of various types of foreign bodies entrapped in various ocular structures, threat of severe infection due to contamination during the injury, are the salient characteristics of such armed force-related ophthalmic injuries. This highlights the characteristic pathomechanism of the war field injuries, which differentiates from other common vitreoretinal pathologies. The ophthalmologist's role in this scenario is to treat the injured eye in a best possible way and to provide feedback for those who make policy decisions. One of the observations made in war injuries was relative low compliance to protective eyewear among the soldiers, leading to devastating consequences [1, 2].

Multiorgan injuries specially to major vital organs, prioritize the stability for life-threatening management at the base hospital first, then toward the management of the ophthalmic trauma [1]. The process of transport from the front lines can take from days to weeks, depending on the severity of ocular and systemic injuries and concomitant demands on Air force resources [3]. Primary repair of the eye is an essential and emergency surgery required to salvage the globe in any ophthalmic trauma, once the patient is systemically stable. There is general consensus with supported evidence that eyes with no light perception due to trauma should not be abandoned, much less enucleated during primary repair [3]. In rare circumstances, primary repair of the globe can be combined with management of systemic injury under care of multispecialty setup under general anesthesia. Primary repair of the eyeball structurally facilitates the injured eye to undergo further visually rehabilitating surgeries. These second stage interventions ideally should be comprehensive in nature to handle the tissue-specific damage at one single point of time. Speciality or tertiary eye care centers have a unique advantage of having subspecialty trained surgeons under one roof, who help in managing these cases with holistic and best possible care. Most commonly encountered expert opinions needed are from vitreoretina, cornea, glaucoma, and oculoplastic subspecialties based on our experience in managing these armed conflicts patients. Managing and operating such eyes with the best possible interventions ultimately helps to have a reasonable ambulatory vision and a long-term stability in these severely injured eyes.

Systematic clinical evaluation of these eyes is of paramount importance to plan the treatment strategies. Detailed history of mode of the injury, baseline best-corrected visual assessment, thorough slit-lamp examination for noting every positive as well as negative findings, complete dilated fundus examination of both eyes need not be underrated in the injury scenario. Anterior segment and posterior segment clinical photography, Ultrasound B-Scan (Fig. 18.3), and CT scan, probably, are absolute necessary investigations for every injured eyes. They help to document ocular and periocular damage, IOFB status, diagnosis of the vitreoretinal pathology, and planning the management. This is essential for both clinical management and medicolegal perspectives. Electrodiagnostic VEP tests are again helpful in decision making and medicolegal purpose. Single or combined surgeries with different subspecialities and staging of the procedures are based upon the thorough evaluation from all specialities leading to a consensus for surgical management.

We enumerate the highlighting issues of each of the subspecialities in handling such injured eyes.

18.3.1 Anesthesia-Related Issues and Management

Traumatic eyes in acute setting warrant surgeries under general anesthesia (GA). The reasons for operating under GA are as follows: (a) multidisciplinary interventions leading to prolonged surgical duration time, (b) history of recently operated eyes, (c) presence of inflammation/infection, (d) blow-out fracture of orbital walls, (e) "open sky" "situations" if corneal graft is planned, (f) inability of the patient to lie down flat if associated skeletal fracture with plaster of paris cast is present, and (g) due to associated mental stress and anxiety following injury and anticipated surgery (Fig. 18.5). A smooth induction/intubation and extubation must be aimed for safe surgery. Fiber-optic intubation is attempted in case of any associated fracture of facial bones with restricted mouth opening.

However, GA might be contraindicated due to the presence of any associated systemic conditions like fractured ribs, skull/facial bone fracture, etc. In such situation, regional anesthesia under systemic sedation with IV Dexemedetomidine infusion would be safer choice. One of the main relative contraindications for proceeding with regional anesthesia would be possible extrusion of ocular contents through gaping of previous primary surgical

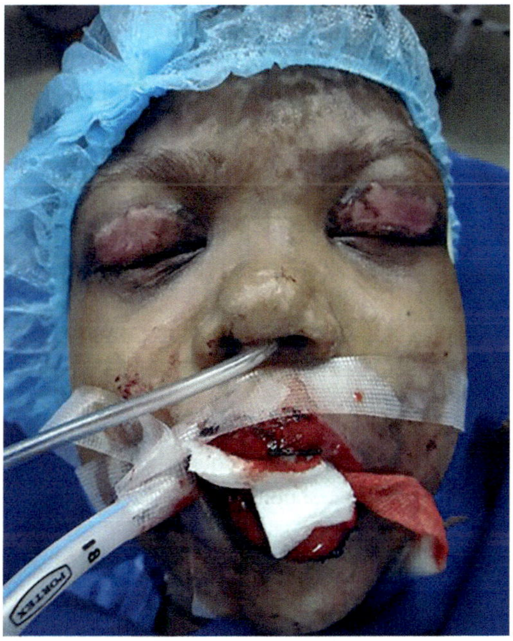

Fig. 18.5 Photo depicting difficult induction of anesthesia and intubation in a case of facial injury requiring intraocular surgery

wound repair site. Hence, a careful combined peri-retrobular block or a fractionated sub-tenon block with longer acting local anesthetic agents like 0.5% Bupivacaine or 0.75% Ropivacaine is recommended in such cases [4].

18.3.2 Vitreoretinal Issues in Acute Trauma Settings and Its Management

18.3.2.1 Timing of the VR Surgery

Most common vitreoretinal situation encountered, requiring secondary intervention after a primary repair are - dislocated and subluxated lens/IOLs, vitreous incarceration at the corneoscleral repaired site, vitreous hemorrhage, retinal detachment, retinal incarceration, hemorrhagic choroidal detachment (CD), IOFB and macular holes.

The healing sequalae of the vitreous and retina in post penetrating injury setting varies depending on the severity of the injury but is highly unpredictable [6]. Aim of surgery is to address all the issues related to vitreoretinal damage noted after the primary repair. Timing of the second surgery after primary repair is well explained by Kuhn [5]. We in our center also follow similar pattern of timing of surgery in handling these post repaired eyes. In post primary repaired eyes, infection, IOFB and hemorrhagic CD are the three important determinants to time the surgery. Intraocular infection with or without IOFB are the true emergencies which warrant immediate surgery to save the eye.

Hemorrhagic CDs require minimum time gap of 5–7 days before taking up for surgery in order to wait for clot lysis to occur. Topical and oral steroids post primary repair helps to reduce inflammation and tissue oedema for a safe second surgery. One should be ready to operate as soon as resolution of inflammation and clot lysis signs are noted on serial B-Scans. In our experience, we could address and manage most of the steps of the VR procedures, completing the surgery in a single sitting. Rarely, situation forced us to operate in a staged manner depending on the intraoperative difficulties. Such intraoperative situations posing difficulty are as follows: difficult visualization due to cornea-related issues, continuing intraocular bleeding thereby causing difficulty in tissue delineation, inflamed retina and choroid, persisting or increasing hemorrhagic choroidal detachment. These factors prevent completion of the planned VR surgical steps at one sitting. A brief gap of 1–2 weeks sometimes resolves such issues and helps in the successful completion of the procedure (Case 4).

In an essence, ideally, the ultimate vitreoretinal procedure is expected to be completed by maximum 3–4 weeks by which time otherwise optic nerve damage and vitreoretinal tissue scarring would progress toward irreversible and irreparable damage [6]. Delayed referral, comorbid situations, periocular infections from injured cornea, lacrimal system, and lids are some of the reasons we have encountered for postponing the surgery beyond 4 weeks' timeline.

18.3.2.2 Intraocular Foreign Body (IOFB) Related Issues

IOFBs should ideally be removed at the time of primary repair if there is a VR surgeon and setting available. Early removal of a foreign body has been thought to decrease the risk of endophthalmitis and proliferative vitreoretinopathy (PVR). Visualization compromised due to corneal wound integrity and other factors are realistic situations faced in majority of such penetrating injuries, which compels a VR surgeon to defer the concomitant IOFB removal during primary repair. With the literature favoring for early removal of IOFB, we in our setup make an attempt to perform concomitant IOFB removal during primary repair provided adequate fundus visualization is possible. In true sense, post traumatic endophthalmitis with IOFB is an indication for an urgent vitrectomy and IOFB removal. Despite a frequent debate for optimal timing, in most situation, IOFB removal is done as early as possible once the globe is secured in primary repair and media is clear enough for surgical intervention. Difficulties arise when there is a large exit wound, which may have a risk of fluid leak and hypotony. One may have to wait for a few days for scleral scar to form at exit wound

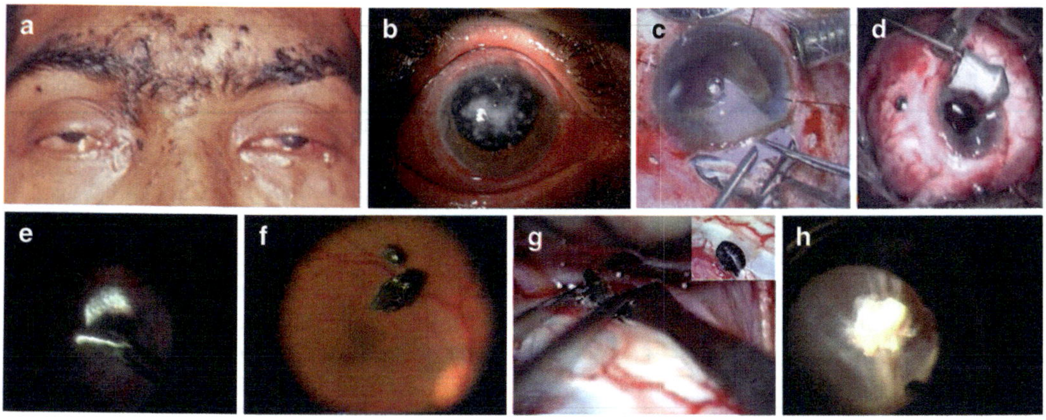

Fig. 18.6 Ocular foreign bodies observed and removed from various routes. (**a**) Multiple small FBs over the upper face involving medial canthus area and cornea following a blast (**b**) Multiple corneal FBs in the visual axis with clear cornea in the periphery. (**c**) Large intraocular glass piece removed via limbal route. (**d**) Large bullet removed from vitreous cavity (open sky) after corneal trephining. The surgery was completed using temporary keratoprosthesis (**e**) Large irregular intraocular metallic FB following blast. (**f**) Intraoperative multiple FB fragments sitting on the retina (following mine blast) (**g**) Transscleral removal of ocular coat impacted FB (**h**) Intraoperative photo of encapsulated pellet stuck to detached mobile retina

site before attempting a safe IOFB removal. Various modes of IOFB impaction and routes adopted for its removal are shown in Fig. 18.6. The time interval to reach definitive subspecialty care is often delayed because of the location of the patient when injured.

18.3.2.3 Endophthalmitis-Related Issues

Post injury endophthalmitis is not uncommon in war settings. The reported incidence varies from 2% to 16%. The risk increases with retained IOFB, especially following blast injury, which typically is associated with multiple FBs. FBs in these settings can be highly contaminated and may include dust, non-metallic material, shrapnel, etc. The management may get further delayed due to associated co-morbidities, leading to increased risk of infection and delayed initiation of specific treatment.

Although clinical features may be similar to postoperative endophthalmitis, diagnosis can delayed or masked due to overlapping signs of infection and inflammation induced due to trauma. Clues for suspected infection are, out of proportion pain or visual loss, purulent discharge, exudates or hypopyon in anterior chamber, associated vitritis, retinitis, or retinal periphlebitis. There is a high prevalence of polymicrobial infection containing Gram negative species. Thorough clinical evaluation with high index of suspicion is needed for early diagnosis.

Although overall prognosis is poor, early vitrectomy, with simultaneous management of associated posterior segment pathologies, aggressive topical, intravitreal and systemic antibiotics can help salvage few of these eyes.

18.3.3 Glaucoma Issues and Management

Reported incidence of glaucoma post penetrating trauma varies from 2.7% to 25%. [7–9] Glaucoma can occur because of various mechanisms. Intraocular pressure spike can be due to inflammation, hyphaema, retained lens particles, subluxated cataract causing pupillary block, and ghost cell glaucoma in early posttrauma period and synechial angle closure, epithelial ingrowth or fibrous down growth, inflammation secondary to retained foreign body in later period. Correct measurement of intraocular pressure is possible only after primary repair. Angle recession (AR) is one important finding to be assessed as baseline evaluation. Though AR is established finding in the literature in blunt trauma, surprisingly we noted it in only 4 eyes in our series. Aqueous suppressants are the drug of choice for IOP control. Prostaglandin analogues are avoided in immediate post trauma period to minimize risk of worsening of inflammation. Two-third of the patients can be managed with medical treatment, while rest requires surgical intervention. Surgical intervention requires a combined approach, lowering of IOP along with treatment of primary cause for IOP spike. Patients with glaucoma secondary to lens-related etiology usually require lensectomy, vitrectomy with or without SFIOL along with trabeculectomy. None of our cases required immediate combined glaucoma surgery along with VR surgery. Implantation of IOL in combined VR glaucoma surgeries depend on the anterior segment integrity and capsular support. Post-vitreoretinal surgery conjunctival scarring is an issue, so combined retina and glaucoma surgery is preferable. Those who already underwent vitreoretinal intervention earlier with conjunctival scarring need glaucoma valve implantation. Silicone oil in a single chambered eye is a contraindication for glaucoma surgery. In eyes with extensive surface damage an Ahmed glaucoma valve can be placed at the first sitting with a pars plana tube placement. In aphakic silicon oil filled eye with poor prognosis, diode cyclophotocoagulation or endo-cyclophocoagulation is preferred. IOP control post cyclophotocoagulation is unpredictable. Though glaucoma and vitreoretinal intervention can be done as combined approach, we prefer two stage approach if cornea procedure is planned for the case. We usually prefer corneal surgery after glaucoma surgery. Watertight wound closure and adequate control of inflammation are the important measures taken to prevent the failure of the surgery.

18.3.4 Corneal Issues and Management

Open globe injuries, which have undergone corneal tear repair, can pose problems for retinal visualization due to either corneal edema, sutures causing corneal distortion, wound gape (tissue loss), wound infiltrate, or closely situated sutures. Ideally, it is preferable to complete VR procedure without keratoplasty. This would be facilitated by wide angle viewing system which helps in visualizing the vitreous cavity intraoperatively and allow to complete the surgery. Further PK could be planned based on the stability of the globe.

One of the challenges in the treatment of open globe injuries is coexistence microbial keratitis with impending vitreoretinal emergencies. Usually microbial keratitis presenting either before or after wound repair is managed prior to retinal intervention. Polymicrobial keratitis due to wound contamination is very common and is particularly challenging to manage in wound-related infiltrates and can hamper or delay managing coexisting retinal emergencies.

Very commonly, suture-related infiltrates are seen in healing corneal wounds that are managed by selective suture removal followed by corneal scraping. Loose sutures that are removed are plated on liquid/solid media, and wound is treated medically. In the event of wound dehiscence that occurs after suture removal, it is managed by either tissue adhesives, BCL, or resuturing. Microbial keratitis that are unresolving or associated with impending retinal emergencies are managed by temporary keratoprosthesis followed by penetrating keratoplasty at the end of retinal surgery. None of the eyes in our series had coexistent corneal infection during VR procedure. One case in our series developed fungal endophthalmitis 3 months after PK, progressing to panophthalmitis necessitating evisceration.

It is imperative to perform detailed slit lamp examination to enable prior management of wound or suture related infiltrate, if needed. When there is a need for immediate retinal intervention either for retinal detachment, vitreous hemorrhage or endophthalmitis, combined approach with corneal surgeon is to be planned. Clean wounds with either tight or loose sutures are corrected by proper suturing techniques enabling completion of retinal surgery [10]. Tissue adhesives with bandage contact lens, corneal patch grafts, Tenon patch graft and amniotic membrane may sometimes be necessary for corneal wound or tissue reconstruction although these may sometimes hamper visualization of the interior part of the globe. Temporary keratoprosthesis improves the visualization of fundus during V R surgery and helps surgeon to address retinal pathologies more completely.

In the rare event of complete blood staining of cornea presenting along with an indication for immediate retinal intervention, the approach is to plan temporary keratoprosthesis assisted vitrectomy followed by penetrating keratoplasty at the end of surgery. Temporary keratoprosthesis significantly enhances the fundus view to complete combined corneal and vitreoretinal procedures.

Most of these injured eyes having silicone oil in situ tend to have low IOP on long term, eventually leading to corneal decompensation and band shaped keratopathy. The timing of removal of silicon oil however should be decided based on the intraocular pressure, retinal status and visual outcome. None the less, we have noted successful VR procedures having maintained normal IOP with oil tamponade. In the event of successful outcome of retina surgery with failed first graft, an optical keratoplasty can be performed at the time of silicone oil removal. During optical keratoplasty, IOL can be secured to correct aphakia at the same sitting, if needed. The choice of the IOL depends on the availability of the support.

Endoscopic vitrectomy is an adjunct to microincision VR surgery for operating on eyes with opaque cornea and other anterior segment opacities. Endoscope helps in providing a clear view to perform vitrectomy in select traumatised eyes where delay in surgery due to hazy media or non-availability of donor cornea for simultaneous penetrating keratoplasty can lead to severe PVR [11]. Depending on the salvageability of the retinal architecture during the endoscopic visualization, surgeon can accordingly plan PK in same sitting after vitrectomy depends on the availability of the donor cornea and the anticipated visual outcome. This would avoid unnecessary use of precious donor cornea.

Patients with bilateral ocular injuries with severe anterior segment and posterior segment damage might need permanent keratoprosthesis for visual rehabilitation.

Eyes with a good blink reflex and a moist surface such as those with silicone oil induced keratopathy might be good candidates for the Boston Type 1 keratoprosthesis. Eyes with extensive lid/adnexal damage or bilateral limbal damage with posterior segment pathology might need a Boston type 2 or Modified Osteo-odonto keratoprosthesis (MOOKP) [12]. The posterior segment pathology is addressed prior with a temporary keratoprosthesis and penetrating keratoplasty to assess the visual potential and subsequently a Type 2 Boston or MOOKP is performed for restoring useful vision [13].

18.3.5 Oculoplasty-Related Issues and Management

Adnexal injuries range from simple skin abrasions, lid lacerations, orbital foreign bodies, orbital cellulitis, retrobulbar hemorrhage, traumatic nasolacrimal duct obstruction to orbitofacial fractures. These injuries can occur in isolation or in association with intraocular injuries. Orbit and adnexal interventions in most situations are performed as a second stage procedure. They are planned once the eye is stabilized with regards to cornea, retina and IOP. Oculoplastic procedures are done for both functional and cosmetic indications.

Lid laceration when present can be repaired along with the intraocular surgery or at a later date. Orbital foreign bodies are common post war trauma and are most often inorganic in nature. High velocity injuries have small external wounds. Thus a low threshold of suspicion needs to be maintained to look for possible orbital foreign bodies. Metallic foreign bodies appear as hyperdense structure with multiple streak artifacts radiating from it. CT scan gives information about the location, size of the foreign body, any associated fractures or globe injuries, thus acting as a map which aids in their easy removal. Metallic intra-orbital foreign bodies not associated with any complications are better treated conservatively (Fig. 18.2).

Surgical removal is indicated for larger foreign bodies invading the adjacent sinuses and cranial cavity, contaminated objects and foreign bodies causing ocular motility restriction or optic nerve dysfunction. Anteriorly located foreign bodies can be removed if required due to their easy access. Surgical management is tailored to suit each patient based on the location of the FB. Quite often, a multidisciplinary approach may be needed.

Traumatic nasolacrimal duct obstruction when present requires intervention prior to elective vitreoretinal surgeries. External dacryocystorhinostomy (DCR) with or without intubation can be performed.

Orbital fractures are not considered to be an emergency and surgery can be delayed until completion of intraocular procedures. Most patients tend to have associated facial fractures, and combining surgery with maxillofacial surgeon's help to achieve a better cosmetic outcome.

Oculoplasty intervention also includes prosthetic implants for patients having phthisical eyes. This is important since most of these patients are young and in the productive age group. Improving the appearance helps restore their confidence and thus the quality of life.

18.4 Conclusive Remarks

1. Multiorgan life-threatening injuries are common in war settings. Open globe injuries and adnexal injury are frequent ophthalmic injuries during armed conflicts.
2. Blast injury is one of the most common causes with wide spectrum of tissue damage, presence of multiple FBs (nonmetallic, more common) entrapped in various ocular tissues with high risk of polymicrobial contamination.
3. Prompt primary repair, at peripheral center or at base hospital, to restore anatomical integrity is a crucial step in the management. If necessary, primary repair can be combined with management of systemic injuries.
4. No light perception is not a contraindication for primary repair. Primary enucleation should be avoided as far as possible.
5. Multi-subspecialty approach at tertiary care center is needed for better subsequent management.
6. Loss of vision and vitreous hemorrhage are the commonest presenting features.
7. Due to obvious reasons, majority of these eyes need general anesthesia for the surgery, which needs expertise on the part of anesthesiologist due to associated facial injuries. A smooth induction, intubation, and extubation are must for the safe surgery. Regional anesthesia with sedation can be used in exceptional situations.
8. Majority of eyes need vitrectomy along with one or more additional procedures.
9. Polymicrobial keratitis is not uncommon, and its management is challenging.
10. Intraocular infection, with/without IOFBs, needs urgent intervention.
11. Most patients need systemic antibiotic therapy along with topical antibiotics.
12. Due to trauma setting and high risk of PVR, there is a need for prolonged internal tamponade. Silicone oil is a preferred option.
13. Post trauma glaucoma can be of early or late onset. There is a need for close IOP monitoring. Aqueous suppressants are the drugs of choice and surgery for IOP control, if needed, is targeted at primary cause for IOP spike.
14. Eyes with uncontrolled IOP more commonly need drainage implant due to trauma-related conjunctival scarring.
15. In eyes with hazy cornea, temporary keratoprosthesis gives adequate visualization for vitrectomy. Penetrating keratoplasty can be performed at the end of surgery.
16. Corneal transplant, if needed, should be delayed till ocular inflammation subsides and IOP stabilizes.
17. Boston keratoprosthesis or MOOKP can be an option in hypotonous eyes with corneal opacity when there is need to retain silicone oil.

18. Functional/cosmetic orbital and adnexal intervention is usually done as a second procedure once the eye condition is stabilized.
19. Prolonged regular follow-up is essential, especially for those undergoing corneal and glaucoma procedures.
20. Ocular war injuries are serious and vision threatening but timely and staged approach can help to achieve good functional and anatomical outcome, especially in this working age group patients.
21. At the end, the ophthalmologists' role in this scenario is also to provide feedback for those who make policy decisions apart from treating the injured eye in a best possible way.

Acknowledgment Our sincere acknowledgments to our colleagues working in Sankara Nethralaya, Chennai: Dr. Jaichandran VV, (Dy Director, Anesthesialogy Dept); Dr. Trupti S Patil (Sr. Glaucoma consultant); Dr. Meena Lakshmipathy (Sr. Cornea Consultant); Dr. Bhaskar Srinivasan (Sr. Cornea Consultant); Dr. Kirthi Koka (Sr Consultant Oculoplasty) for their expert inputs in writing the subspecialty-related discussion.

References

1. Mader TH, Carroll RD, Slade CS, George RK, Phillip Ritchey J, Page S, Neville. Ocular war injuries of the Iraqi insurgency, January–September 2004. Ophthalmology. 2006;113:97–104.
2. Thach AB, Ward TP, Dick JSB 2nd, Bauman WC, Madigan Jr WP, Goff MJ, Thordsen JE. Intraocular foreign body injuries during operation Iraqi freedom. Ophthalmology. 2005;112:1829–33.
3. Kuhn F. Ocular trauma: from epidemiology to war-related injuries. Graefes Arch Clin Exp Ophthalmol. 2011;249:1753–4.
4. Niemi-Murola L, Immonen I, Kallio H, Maunuksela EL. Preliminary experience of combined peri- and retrobulbar block in surgery for penetrating eye injuries. Eur J Anaesthesiol. 2003;20:478–81.
5. Kuhn F. The timing of reconstruction in severe mechanical trauma. Ophthalmic Res. 2014;51:67–72.
6. Winthrop SR, Cleary PE, Minckle DS, Ryan SJ. Penetrating eye injuries: a histopathological review. Br J Ophthalmol. 1980;64:809–17.
7. Razeghinejad R, Lin MM, Lee D, Katz LJ, Myers JS. Pathophysiology and management of glaucoma and ocular hypertension related to trauma. Surv Ophthalmol. 2020;65:530–47.
8. Girkin CA, Mc Gwin G Jr, Morris R, Kuhn F. Glaucoma following penetrating ocular trauma: a cohort study of the United States eye injury registry. Am J Ophthalmol. 2005;139:100–5.
9. Osman EA. Glaucoma after open globe injury. Saudi J Ophthalmol. 2015;29:222–4.
10. Vlasov A, Ryan DS, Ludlow S, Coggin A, Weichel ED, Stutzman RD, Bower KS, Colyer MH. Corneal and Corneoscleral injury in combat ocular trauma from operations Iraqi freedom and enduring freedom. Mil Med. 2017;182(S1):114–9.
11. Al Sabti K, Raizada S. Endoscope-assisted pars plana vitrectomy in severe ocular trauma. Br J Ophthalmol. 2012;96:1399–403.
12. Iyer G, Srinivasan B, Agarwal S, Ravindran R, Rishi E, Rishi P, Krishnamoorthy S. Boston type 2 keratoprosthesis—midterm outcomes from a tertiary eye care centre in India. Ocul Surf. 2019;17:50–4.
13. Iyer G, Srinivasan B, Agarwal S, Talele D, Rishi E, Rishi P, Krishnamurthy S, Vijaya L, Subramanian N, Somasundaram S. Keratoprosthesis: current global scenario and a broad Indian perspective. Indian J Ophthalmol. 2018;66:620–9.

Ocular Manifestations and Management Strategies in CBRN Warfare

19

J. K. S. Parihar and Ashwini K. S. Parihar

19.1 Introduction

CBRN is an acronym referring to Chemical, Biological, Radiological, and Nuclear-related incidents and weapons in which any of these four hazards have presented themselves. It also highlights persistent threat from a variety of CBRN agents that can be used to kill or incapacitate the military/paramilitary forces and the undefended civilian targets. These hazards may be the consequences of any Accidental, Occupational, Industrial Disaster, and Warfare or linked with Terrorist activities as well. CBRN disasters are invariably involving large population in the vicinity. The quantum and extent of various systemic involvements of such threats are directly linked with the severity and duration of the exposure and contamination as well as distance from the epicenter of the disaster [1–6]. CBRN is likely to affect all exposed parts of the body including Eyes, Skin, & Respiratory system. The impact of such injuries and contamination also affects cardiac, neurological, and other systems of the body. Ocular Injuries in CBRN engage huge spectrum of ophthalmic involvement and invariably present in all types of agents whether nuclear, chemical, radiological, or biological [1–5] . Incidence of ocular involvement is 20–50 times higher as compared to other part of the body because of posture, selective exposure and could be affected by the exposure to small particles even of very short duration [6, 7]. Severity of ophthalmic involvement is dependent upon the toxicity of chemical/biological agents, their, impact, duration, depth, and the area of involvement [7, 8]. In addition to immediate and acute symptoms, delayed clinical sequelae of CBRN are also considered as a big health and environmental hazard. Hence, CBRN disasters or warfare are not only health hazards but also equally impose significant challenges on socioeconomic, political, and environmental framework of the community [8–10].

The present deliberation will be restricted to the review of broad outline of various systemic involvements of CBRN with emphasis on ocular manifestations and their management and recommendations on the prevention or minimizing the impact of CBRN on ocular status.

19.2 Chemical Warfare and Eye Injuries

The term Chemical warfare (CW) applies to the use of toxic properties of chemical substances as weapons [1, 2]. Despite Geneva Protocol of 1925 and Chemical Weapons Convention 1993 on

J. K. S. Parihar (✉)
Ophthalmology, Major General (retd), Armed Forces Medical Services (Medical Research, Health and Trg, Education), Delhi, India

A. K. S. Parihar
Index Medical College, Indore, MP, India

S. Waikar (ed.), *Ocular Trauma in Armed Conflicts*, https://doi.org/10.1007/978-981-19-4021-7_19

international prohibition on use of chemical weapons, the chemical formulated weapons or devices have been used in various military operations by several countries or deliberate release of these Chemical warfare agents (CWA) did take place in recent past to inflict death or harm on human beings. The era of first as well as of Second World War and post world war period has witnessed several occurrences of use of chemical agents as weapons [1, 2]. Chlorine gas was used in the First World War in 1915 during the conflict between combined forces of Belgium and Germany against the French and British troops [11]. Sulfur mustard gas was also used in First World War [11, 12]. Germans conducted several studies between September 1939 and April 1945 on non-volunteers in concentration camps by deliberate exposure of mustard gas and lewisite to investigate the most effective treatment of chemical burns. During the post second world war period, chemical weapons were used by Iraqi forces during the Iran-Iraq war of 1980–1988. This decade long war had witnessed about 200,000 deaths and 400,000 casualties of whom more than 60,000 Iranian military and Kurdish civilians had vulnerable exposure to sulfur mustard gas and other chemical agents like tabun [13, 14]. In addition to the use of chemical agents in conventional warfare, there have been multiple and small area-specific incidences of accidental or deliberate release of chemical gases in the civil vicinity. Among them, accidental leakage of methyl isocyanate gas in 1984 in Bhopal led to massive loss of human lives, livestock, and the environment. On 20 March 1995, Japan had faced deliberate release of Sarin gas (Neuro toxic synthetic organophosphorus compound) in Tokyo subway by a domestic terror outfit. This act of terrorism had resulted in the killing of 13 people, whereas about 5500 civilians faced various kinds of injuries including around 1000 people with temporary vision problems. In the same manner, the deliberate release of domestic anthrax strain by an unidentified group in USA in 2001 killed five politicians and media workers. Another unfortunate occurrence took place in Russia on 23rd October 2002 when an undisclosed chemical agent was released by the Russian special forces to counter local terror act in Moscow theatre hostage crisis, which accidentally killed 129 hostages. Later on, the chemical agent was speculated to be an opiate derivative KOLOKOL. However, Russian authorities had never disclosed the use of any chemical agent.

Use of tear gas by law enforcement agencies to control mob protests is gradually increasing all over the world. Tear gas agents are undoubtedly very effective and minimize the risk of physical injuries to both demonstrators and law enforcement personnel during any civil agitation [15].

Few scientific data are available on the adverse impact of tear gas agents on humans as well as to identify minimal titrated concentration of the tear gas, well within the bracket of health safety measures. Certain studies on the subject have specified that health of humans is highly vulnerable to tear gas agents specially in children, elderly individuals, women as well as in any person having comorbidities like cutaneous, respiratory, and cardiovascular involvements [16–18].

19.3 Classification of Chemical Warfare Agents

Based on physiological action, chemical agents are classified as follows:

19.3.1 Types

Nerve agents: GA-Tabun, GB- SARIN,GD-SOMAN, Vx.

Vesicants or Blister agents (Alkylating & Arsenical agents): Mustards (HD), Lewisite (L).

Choking Agents (Asphyxiants): Phosgene (CG), Diphosgene (DP), Chloropicrin (PS).

Blood agents: Hydrogen cyanide (AC), Cyanogen chloride (CK), Arsine (SA).

CNS Depressants: BZ, Tetrahydrocannabinols,

CNS Stimulants: LSD.

Riot control agents: They are also known as Tear agents, e.g., CS.

Vomiting agents: Diphenylchloroarsine (DA), Adamsite (DM), DC.

Defoliants.
Plant growth regulators.
Soil sterilants.

19.3.2 Common Properties and Clinical Presentation of Exposure of Chemical Warfare Agents to Human Body

On the basis of their chemical properties, these agents may be classified as asphyxiants, respiratory irritants, vesicants, and acetyl cholinesterase (AChE) inhibitors. Immediate and initial assessment of it, is based on the smell and other physical properties, which suggests probable chemical exposure due to accidental leakage or deliberate release of chemical agents as a tool of the warfare [8, 19]. Specific properties of common chemicals or gases used in warfare are as follows:

Sulfur Mustard (H) produces Garlic or mustard smell and slow exposure may take 4–12 h to produce symptoms.

Nitrogen Mustard (HN) produces fishy smell and slow exposure may take one to 6 h to produce symptoms.

Lewisite (L) has Geranium smell with immediate symptoms.

Phosgene oximes (CX) (CCI2==NOH) cause immediate onset of symptoms, in low concentration spreads smell of freshly mown hay, whereas pungent, acrid, and disagreeable smell if outbreak is having higher concentration.

Ophthalmic & general presentation and management guidelines of chemical injuries:

19.3.3 Nerve Agents

Nerve agents used in chemical warfare include Tabun (GA), Sarin (GB), Soman (GD), and organo-phosphorus compounds (OP) that bind Cholinesterase [12]. On exposure, common generalized and early presentation is running nose, increased salivation, tightness in chest, and breathing difficulties. Late symptoms include headache, drooling, dizziness, excessive sweating, and general weakness [12]. Ophthalmic presentation invariably comprises of Irritational Blepharospasm, ocular pain, and photophobia [8, 12]. The features of Conjunctivitis or Keratoconjunctivitis are also seen [14, 15]. Delayed changes are like any other chemical injuries such as lid burns, corneal perforation, symblepharon, and signs of anterior segment derangements [20].

Treatment: In addition to general line of systemic management of nerve agent toxicity by Atropine and Pralidoxime Chloride (2-PAM Cl), ocular management remains on the line of any alkali injuries [20].

19.3.4 Vesicants or Blister Agents

The vesicant agents include Sulfur mustard (HD), Nitrogen mustard (HN), the arsenical vesicants such as lewisite (L) (this may well be used in a mixture with HD), and the halogenated oximes whose properties and effects are very different from those of the other vesicants [21]. Alkylating agents disrupt DNA replication, whereas Arsenical lewisite liberates HCl, a highly acidic content of having pH less than 1.3 [21, 22].They act on the eyes, mucous membrane, lungs, skin, and blood-forming organs. Vesicants burn and blister the skin or any other part of the body they come in contact with [21, 22].

19.3.5 Arsenical Vesicants

19.3.5.1 Lewisite: BAL (Dimercaprol)

The arsenicals possessing the AsCl2 group are endowed with vesicant properties. Upon contact, pain and blepharospasm occur instantly within 2–10 min of exposure. Edema of the conjunctiva and lids follow rapidly and close the eye within an hour. Inflammation of the iris is usually evident by this time. After a few hours, the edema of the lids begins to subside, while haziness of the cornea develops and iritis increases. Mild conjunctivitis due to arsenical vesicants heals in a few days without specific treatment [22].

The corneal injury, which varies with the severity of the exposure, may heal without residual effects, induce pannus formation, or progress to massive necrosis. After heavy exposure, hypopyon may ensue, terminating in necrosis, depigmentation of the iris, and synechiae formation. Necrosis and sloughing of both bulbar and palpebral conjunctiva may follow.

19.3.6 Mustard Agents (Sulfur Mustard (H) and Nitrogen Mustard (HN)

Mustard agents are highly cytotoxic and abundant warfare chemicals [8]. Sulfur mustard and nitrogen mustard forms have been used as chemical weapons in recent past. They are in use as chemotherapeutic agents in dermatology practice also. Nitrogen mustard is more toxic as compared to Sulfur mustard; however, the influence of Sulfur mustard remains for a longer period in environment, hence preferred as a chemical weapon. They produce incapacitating short- and long-term ocular injuries as major manifestations of mustard toxicity, affecting up to 90% of those exposed [9]. Mustard agents lead to severe inflammation in exposed surfaces of body such as skin, nasal mucosa, eyes, and respiratory tract due to their ability to develop severe metabolic interaction with the wet and mucosal surface of these tissues and organs [10].

Mustard gases are known to produce delayed-onset changes in human body even after 1–30 years following exposures, as studied after Iraq-Iran war [12, 14].

19.3.7 The Most Common Ocular Presentations

Mustard gases primarily affect ocular tissues. Photophobia, Blurred vision, Spasm of the eyelids along with swelling, and edema of skin and pupillary constriction are the noted presentations [8–10]. After several hours, the corneal epithelium begins to form vesicles and slough [8–10, 12]. Signs of anterior uveitis may also be observed. Late sequelae include decreased corneal sensation, recurrent corneal abrasions, corneal scarring with thinning, and formation of neovascularization. Due to chemical injury, loss of limbal vessels and stem cell deficiency is not an uncommon feature. Conjunctival scarring leads to fibrosis and loss of goblet cells; hence, moderate-to-severe dry eyes and keratinization of conjunctiva are most frustrating outcomes of these chemical injuries [23–27]. In addition, cataract and neovascular glaucoma are also evident as delayed sequelae. Such changes invariably lead to progressive and irreversible visual loss [14, 20].

19.4 General Guidelines for Initial Management

To date, no specific antidote and treatment is available to reduce such ocular damage due to exposure to vesicants or blister agents. Systemic antibiotics may be used to combat infection. The systemic use of morphine may be necessary for control of pain. General ophthalmic management is on the line of management of any chemical injury. Use of local analgesics may increase corneal damage and are not recommended. Treatments include use of protective gear, removal of victims from contaminated areas, and copious ocular irrigation (The eyes can be flushed with copious amounts of water, or, if available, isotonic sodium bicarbonate (1.26%) or saline (0.9%)). It is recommended to refrain from covering the eyes with a bandage; however, dark or opaque goggles should be used to protect ocular photophobia and spasm.

Atropine sulfate eye ointment should be instilled to obtain and maintain good mydriasis in all cases with corneal erosions, iritis, cyclitis or with marked photophobia or miosis. Antibiotic ophthalmic ointment should be applied to the lid margins to help prevent their sticking together. Dimercaprol eye ointment may diminish the effects of lewisite if applied within 2 min of exposure. Its value is questionable if applied later than this.

19.5 Choking Agents (Asphyxiants). Phosgene (CG), Diphosgene (DP), Chloropicrin (PS)

19.5.1 Halogenated Oximes

Dichloroformoxime is the most irritant compound; it is commonly known as phosgene oximes, symbolized by CX. In low concentrations, phosgene oximes severely irritate the eyes, causing corneal lesions and blindness. There is no specific treatment available against exposure of Halogenated oximes. The eyes should be flushed immediately using water or isotonic sodium bicarbonate solution if available [22].

19.5.2 Tear Gas

The major riot-control agents (RCAs) in use include 2-chlorobenzylidene malononitrile (CS), oleoresin capsicum (OC, pepper spray), dibenz [*b,f*]-1,4-oxazepine (CR), and 2-chloro-1-phenylethanone, CN and Mace (CN) [15]. Tear gas agents readily react with mucosal surfaces of eyes, nose, and respiratory tract due to their electrophilic properties [16, 18]. They are known to damage and deplete intrinsic lining fluid of epithelial cells, alter cellular mitochondrial structural proteins as well as derange tissue metabolism, thereby leading to enzymatic malfunction and mucosal edema [15, 18]. Oleoresin capsicum (OC, pepper spray) is a mixture of several compounds extracted from chilli peppers where capsaicin is being used as the predominant ingredient. Pepper spray was initially used as an animal repellent in the early 1960s [15, 17]. However, Pepper spray is now most preferred choice as an aerosol ingredient RCA.

19.5.3 Systemic Adverse Effects of RCA

Spectrum of symptoms and severity of RCAs may vary according to the concentrations of tear gas agents (CS or OC) used as well as on the duration and proximity to the exposure to such agents. Extremes of the age as well as existing comorbidities in the affected individuals are important contributing factors. These manifestations may range from very minor to severe involvement of cutaneous and mucosal surfaces including skin burns and dermatitis, mild-to-moderate respiratory involvement, and, in extreme and rare situations, severe reactive airways dysfunction syndrome and pulmonary edema may also be seen [15, 16]. Various cardiovascular effects like transient hypertension, cardiac arrhythmias are not uncommon [17, 18]. In very rare and extreme cases, even cardiac arrest may take place due to precipitation of sensory–autonomic reflexes, anxiety, pain, or psychological distress. Other noted systemic involvements following tear gas exposures are nausea, vomiting, diarrhea, and hematemesis due to irritation of the gastrointestinal tract as a sequelae of ingestion of RCA compounds like CS.

However, in most of the situations, the impact of RCA gets resolved within a short duration once affected person is removed from the affected environment [15].

19.5.4 Ocular Effects of Tear Gas Substances

Ocular involvement depends upon the duration and proximity to the exposure. Severe ocular injuries may be seen in case of exposure to tear gas from a very close distance [15, 16]. Intense lacrimation, blurred vision, lid edema, conjunctival chemosis, and corneal edema are very common sequences [15, 16] .Concussion injuries due to direct burst of teargas on face may lead to even open globe injuries [15, 27]. Deranged ocular surface due to chemical injury may manifest delayed changes like formation of symblepharon, and pseudopterygium. Recurrent trophic keratopathy, cataract and glaucoma are not uncommon delayed manifestations following tear gas exposure [15, 16].

19.5.5 Ocular Management

No specific antidote is required. These cases are managed on the basis of general guidelines of ophthalmic management of acute chemical injuries of mild-to-moderate nature.

19.6 General Guidelines to Be Followed by Mass Population in Case of Chemical Strike

19.6.1 When Protective Equipment Is Available

Wear various items of IPE.

Non essential personnel, not in immediate combat zone, to remain under cover.

Food and water to be kept under cover.

NAPS tablets to be taken when ordered.

Alarm system and chemical sentries must be deployed on upwind.

Protective glasses having properties of high Impact resistance, antifog, shatterless, side shields or SIPE (Soldier Integrated protection Ensemble) may be used if available.

19.6.2 When Protective Equipments Are Not Available

Close your eyes and control breathing. Use a wet cloth or towel on face to cover eyes and respiratory tract.

Get under cover. Lie flat on the ground in case of vapor contamination if cover not available, use Personal raincoat to cover the complete body to avoid liquid contamination. Hang blanket or sheet as a curtain at the entrance of the shelter for an air lock cover.

Do not eat, drink and smoke in a chemically contaminated environment.

Various studies on chemical warfare survivors with ophthalmologic complications have demonstrated that delayed keratitis, corneal vascularization, thinning, and epithelial defect invariably lead to a highly complicated and frustrating health-related quality of life [28]. The surgical management of chemical injuries of eyes including stem cell and corneal transplantation have very poor outcome in the long term [28–31]. Over and above a complex spectrum of multisystem engagement following chemical warfare leads to grossly affected quality of life compounding with socio psychological issues and needs further assessment and more research to improve overall management [12].

19.7 Biological Warfare: Ophthalmic Manifestations, Prevention and Management

The term Biological warfare defines the intentional use of biological toxins or infectious agents such as bacteria, viruses and fungi, with the intent to kill or incapacitate humans, animals or plants in an act of war [3–5].Biologics have been used as a hidden weapon in different era including in the recent past.The Indian history and mythology has depicted ample evidence of application of biologics during ancient warfare. Various kingdoms and regimes have used many agents notably Tularaemia, Anthrax, Brucellosis, Botulism, Small pox, etc. on various occasions. In the ancient history, the well-known attempt of the use of biological warfare agent was during the fourteenth century medieval siege of Kaffa, Feodosiya and Ukraine. In this incident, the Tartars (Mongols), who attacked Kaffa, tossed dead and dying plague victims into the city in an attempt to spread the disease.

The importance of biological weapons was significantly advanced in the present century due to several wars and multiple threats. Biologics and chemical weapons were used by all major armed forces during world war one and two [1, 3]. British, US, Soviet, German and Japanese armed forces had developed weapons of Anthrax, Tularaemia, Brucellosis, Botulism and other biologics. The most notorious program of biological warfare was conducted by the secret Imperial Japanese Army units during World War Two. The army unit based at Manjuri conducted research on fatal experiments on prisoners, and produced biological weapons for combat use. In 1940, the Japanese Air Force bombed Ningbo with ceramic bombs full of fleas carrying the bubonic plague. Infamous German human experiments by medical professionals in human concentration camps are glaring example of bioterrorism and biological warfare. From about Feb 1942 to April 1945 several experiments were conducted at the Dachau concentration camp in order to investigate immunization for Malaria, Epidemic jaundice and on other diseases, without consent and forcefully, on several thousands of population so as to enhance medical facilities in the German Armed Forces. Most of the individuals died in the experiments. However biologics have been used even after Second World War despite the fact that chemical, biological and radiation warfare are globally banned by international agencies under various treaties. Biological weapons have the peculiarity of being masked and silent weapons that can be unexpected and may attack silently on unprepared enemy [4, 5]. It is very difficult to identify biologics as a military threat as the early symptoms of any biologics will be very similar to any common illnesses at large scale [4, 5]. The small amount of biological agents can produce maximum loss. In the form of epidemics they act as a grave public health problem and invariably lead to massive destruction which continues on its own. Over and above, the treatment of such diseases is very difficult specially for uncommon organisms.The accessibility to the biologics, scientific expertise to handle and mass produce them and deliver in the proper size for dissemination as aerosol are also important factors to use them as bio weapons.Hence Biologics can be used as a source of mass destruction or morbidity in a fashion of endemic or epidemics before the problem, agent or source can be recognized.The accidental release of anthrax from a military testing facility in the former Soviet Union in 1979 and possession of anthrax, Botulinum toxin and aflatoxin in Iraq in 1995 pointed out to research and development of these agents in spite of the 1972 Biological Weapons Convention. World has witnessed HIV terrorism In 2008, three HIV-positive Dutch men were convicted of grievous bodily harm by a Netherlands court for purposely infecting a dozen men at drug parties over the course of 2 years by drugging and then injecting them with a "cocktail" containing the infected blood of all three men. Though there is no direct evidence of COVID-19 pandemic as a deliberate act or accidental outbreak but facts remain that this pandemic has shaken- up the entire globe in last 1 year with significant mortality and huge blow to the global economy. Viruses like Small pox, Ebola, Bacteria Bacillus anthracis (Anthrax) and toxins like Staphylococcal Enterotoxin and Botulinum Toxin, Tularaemia and Plague have been identified as potential military biologics and used by several countries during first and Second World War as well as during conflict in Middle East in recent past [3, 4]. Biologics and chemical warfare are becoming a big threat to mankind and their misuse in future by terrorist outfits as Bioterrorism cannot be ruled out [32, 33].

19.8 Biological Weapons: Classification and Methods of Delivery of Biological Agents

19.8.1 Classification of Biological Agents (Microorganisms or their Toxic Products)

Lethal or Nonlethal effects.

19.8.2 These Agents Can Be Transmitted from One Man to Another Causing Large Number of Casualties

Lethal Transmissible: Small Pox, Plague, and Cholera.

Lethal Nontransmissible: Anthrax, Yellow Fever and Epidemic Typhus.

Nonlethal Transmissible: Influenza, Typhoid.

Nonlethal Nontransmissible: Dengue Fever, Q fever.

Antianimal Agents: Cattle Plague, New Castle Disease, Hog Cholera, Psittacosis, African swine fever, Foot and mouth disease.

Antiplant Agents: Bioherbicides like Pucciniagraminis against wheat, Pyrioeulariaoryzal against rice.

19.8.2.1 Methods of Delivery

Aerosol method: Aerosols are fine particles of liquid or solids suspended in gaseous medium and very difficult to detect them by physical senses. Biologics can penetrate shelters, bunkers along with the wind [34].

Vectors: Mosquito, flies, fleas, ticks, and mites. They can readily attack human beings as well as are capable of ensuring the persistence of biological agents [35].

Explosive munitions: Like aircraft bombs and artillery shells [36].

Clandestine action: Either by aerosol method or by poisoning food or water resources.

19.8.2.2 Systemic Involvements of Biologics

Clinical spectrum of biologics will vary according to the organism used.Hence the presentation will be exactly like disease per se and will be very difficult to identify as a tool of biological warfare [32, 33].

19.8.2.3 Ophthalmic Manifestations

The eye is particularly vulnerable to any kind of exposure. Ophthalmic manifestation may signal the first indication of contact. Most common and initial general presentation invariably reflects generalised ocular pain, redness, irritation, watering and painful blepharospasm [34, 35, 37]. Whereas inflammation, iritis, decreased visual acuity, inflammation, uveitis and Corneal Ulceration may be evident as signs of potential exposure to biological agents [34, 35, 37].

19.8.2.4 Specific Ophthalmic Manifestations

Botulism

Clostridium botulinum is a Gram-positive, rod-shaped, anaerobic, spore-forming, motile bacterium, which produces the neurotoxin Botulinum. Ophthalmic manifestations may reflect the anticholinergic effects of the neurotoxins or a deficit at the neuromuscular junction.

Ocular Manifestations

Accommodation paresis with blurred vision.

Dry eye symptoms with impairment of lacrimation.

Oculoparesis or ophthalmoplegia manifests as diplopia. Nystagmus maybe there.

Blepharoptosis is common.

Mydriasis and poorly reacting pupils [37].

Management

Rigorous supportive care is essential and vital in the management of Botulism.

Recently, FDA approved a Heptavalent Antitoxin to treat Botulism. Botulism immune globulin intravenous (human) (BIG-IV; also called BabyBig) is FDA-approved for the treatment of infant botulism caused by C Botulinum type A or type B [37].

Anthrax

Bacillus anthracis is a large endospore form ing, aerobic, gram-positive nonmotile bacteria. It produces a black, eschar like cutaneous lesion after cutaneous inoculation, giving rise to the name anthrax, which in Greek means "coal " [38].

Ocular Manifestations

Eyelid necrosis leading to corneal drying and without appropriate ocular treatment, in turn, leads to corneal scarring and ulceration with vision loss.

Proptosis, Preseptal, and Orbital cellulitis.

Toxic optic neuropathy [38].

Management

Symptomatic treatment.

Drug of choice: Systemic Antibiotics.

Quinolone antibiotics or Doxycycline.

Clindamycin may be added for its Antiexotoxin effect.

Smallpox

Smallpox is caused by the infection with one of two virus variants, variola major and variola minor. Variola virus belongs to the genus Orthopoxvirus, the family Poxviridae. The virus was found to have high mortality rate of 20–35% among unvaccinated individuals.

The last naturally occurring case was diagnosed in October 1977 and the WHO certified the global eradication of the disease in 1980.

Ocular Manifestations

Eyes are affected in 10% of cases [39]. Eyelid and conjunctival infections are more common. Corneal ulcers with the tendency of corneal perforation, intraocular infection and inflammation are also common ocular presentations. However Optic nerve inflammation, glaucoma as well as Periorbital and orbital inflammation are seen as infrequent ocular involvements. Small pox can lead to blindness due to corneal complications, glaucoma or optic neuritis [39, 40].Immunization may affect eyes with similar complications as of primary disease and is known as Ocular Vaccinia [39].

Management

Topical antiviral therapy.

Topical steroids.

Topical and oral antibiotics.

Vaccinia-immune globulin (VIG) only recently has become available for the treatment of complications of smallpox vaccination.

19.8.2.5 Tularaemia

Caused by *Francisella tularensis*, a highly infective bacterium

Also known as rabbit fever

Spread by arthropod vectors

Causes fever, lymphadenopathy, skin ulcers, pneumonia, sepsis, etc. [35]

Ocular Manifestations

Oculoglandular Tularaemia is characterized by symptoms of photophobia, lacrimation, and rarely vision loss associated with the clinical signs of periorbital oedema and follicular conjunctivitis. Conjunctival chemosis, corneal epithelial defects, and ulceration is not uncommon presentation [41].

Management

General preventive measures include protection against Ticks.

No vaccine is currently available.

Streptomycin is the Drug of Choice.

19.8.2.6 Early Detection and Prevention of Effects of Biological Agents

The Following actions are useful for early detection and prevention of severe and mass complications:

19.8.2.7 Early Detection and Warning

Early detection is very difficult in field conditions. Hence, high order of suspicion is very crucial for early detection of biological warfare. Following occurrences or events should be kept in mind to arouse suspicion:

- Low flying aircraft that produces mist or spray
- Functioning of any kind of spray device
- Finding of bomblets that appear to have no immediate effect
- Unusual types of bomblets found in the area
- Swarms of insects arising suddenly
- Preventive measures against biological threats:
  - Vaccination if available
  - Wearing of individual protective equipment (IPE)
  - Use of collective protective shelters
  - Food and water hygiene
  - Control measures for vectors

Challenges

The threat of use of biological warfare agents in a terrorism-related issue or in a warfare situation is real and looming before us. The highly unpredictable nature of any event involving biological warfare agents has given rise to the need for developing rapid and accurate detection systems [42, 43]. The bioterrorist events are difficult to predict and prevent; in the case of a release, accurate easy and deployable detection systems are needed to minimize the damage and to prevent further spread of these agents. The intentional release of spores of Bacillus anthracis in the US postal service proved the need for these detection platforms. Although many such detection systems are under development and are at various stages of evaluation, a single system to detect all the known bio warfare agents is going to be a real challenge [42–44].

19.9 Radiological Warfare

The term Radiological warfare defines any kind of warfare or act of terror against legalized institutions where intentional use of radiological sources are used as a weapon to infuse radiation poisoning or contamination within target location [45]. Though conventional high fission thermonuclear atomic weapons are technically the tools of radiological warfare, however as per the convention and practice, the Radiological warfare differs from nuclear warfare. In contrast to Nuclear weapons, radiological weapons are invisible weapons, low to moderate in intensity and very slow to trigger the impact of radiation [45]. Radiation warfare produces less mortality as compared to the nuclear warfare but have more and chronic morbidity [46]. Despite such variation from the nuclear weapons, the radiological warfare can induce mass destruction in a targeted location. It is very difficult to identify the radiological attack or deliberate leakage of radiological material at an early phase. Over and above, human senses are not able to detect them and use of specific survey instruments are essential to identify radiation exposure [45].

Radiological weapons may attack a smaller target with precision in the same manner as it was allegedly conducted by Russian Federal Security Services(FSB) on 01 Nov 2006 to inflict radiation poisoning to Alexander Litvinenko an activist by using radioactive polonium-210. Despite international restrictions, other than conventional high fission thermonuclear weapons, various kinds of low intensity radiological weapons like radioactive "dirty bomb" or radiological dispersal device (RDD) have been developed by many countries since 1964 onwards. In these devices conventional explosives are used to facilitate spread of radiation by external or internal sources of contamination in a large area. The impending threat of misuse of RDD or Radioactive materials readily accessible from medical institutions, laboratories, industries and food irradiation plants by antinational terror outfits cannot be underestimated [46, 47]. The deliberate release of low intensity radioactive materials from Alpha, beta, gamma and X-rays sources may raise multiple short and long term medical issues like intra cellular damage to exposed skin,ocular and mucous membrane of nasal and respiratory tract [48] . The higher incidence of haematopoietic disorders and various kinds of malignancies, genetic, hereditary & carcinogenic mutations as well as neuropsychological disorders cannot be ruled out [46, 47, 49].

19.9.1 Effects of Radiation on Ocular Tissue of Humans and Animals

Threshold values of Radiation exposure: The quantity and impact of radiation exposure is assessed as follows:

Gray (Gy): SI unit of absorbed radiation dose (equal to 1 J/kg).
1 Gray = 100 Rad (Radiation Absorbed Dose)

Sievert (Sv): SI unit of equivalent dose, effective dose, and operational dose quantity (equal to 1 J/kg).
1 Sievert = 100 REM (Radiation Equivalent in Man) [50]

19.9.2 Ocular Radiation Injuries

Ophthalmic manifestations of radiation injuries are invariably seen at the earliest due to the most obvious reason of being exposed and highly delicate tissue. These changes are visible at all phases of exposure including acute and immediate, intermediate as well as delayed irreversible blinding complications [51].

Ocular manifestations of radiation will be varying according to the intensity, duration and type of the radiation exposures. Intense heat generated due to radiation is known to produce acute and severe involvement. Infrared exposure is clubbed with glass blowers cataract, whereas microwave exposure may lead to the formation of anterior and posterior subcapsular cataract. UV – Long term and prolonged exposure to sunlight is associated with delayed changes due to Ultraviolet ray's exposure [51].

Threshold values of Radiation exposure for detectable Lens Opacities as assessed by ICRP (International Commission on Radiological Protection for Occupational Hazards):

Acute single exposure: 0.5–2 Sv (50–200 REM).

For highly fractioned or protracted exposure: 5 Sv (500 REM).

Annual dose of yearly highly fractioned or protracted exposure: >0.1 Sv (>10 REM per year).

19.9.3 Acute Onset of Radiation Induced Manifestations

Intense heat generated through radiation exposure is linked to acute symptoms and illness. Excessive lacrimation, conjunctival edema, and chemosis along with corneal epithelial erosions, perforation and melting of cornea, and sloughing of anterior capsule of the lens are not uncommon. Acute radiation induced retinal edema and optic neuritis are also known immediate ocular manifestations [51].

19.9.4 Intermediate and Delayed Onset Post Radiation Ocular Changes

Intermediate changes are associated with Radiation induced Cataract and Radiation Retinopathy [52, 53].Where as conjunctival scarring, talengectasia, loss of collagen tissues and dry eyes are seen as delayed adnexal and ocular surface disorders [53]. Other late sequelae include corneal scarring and neovascularization, severe refractory neovascular glaucoma. Altered ERG, altered photoreceptors (rods and cones), Optic Atrophy, CRAO, CRVO, CNVM, Vitreous haemorrhage and tractional retinal detachment are most significant irreversible blinding complications of radiation injuries [52, 53]. Various kind of ocular changes like punctate keratitis, acute choroiditis with fluffy edges, iris atrophy, glaucoma, cataract, temporary choroid pallor with constriction of retinal vessels, atrophy of choroid and retina and retinal changes simulating hypertensive retinopathy may also manifest as complications of Radiotherapy [52–54].

The ocular manifestations of radiation induced injuries may be earliest to occur [50, 51]. Our role as ophthalmologists is vital in making a prompt diagnosis and instituting immediate management. The incidence of radiation exposure in medical and industrial setup can be minimized by the regular use of protective eye wear. It is recommended that radiological exposure to human body should be restricted up to 5 Sv per year in regular practice so as to ensure minimal adverse impact on the human body including lenticular and retinal changes in the eye [50].

19.10 Nuclear Warfare and Its Impact on Health Status

Nuclear warfare is a severe and most violent form of radiological warfare however differs from latter as a convention of high fission thermonuclear atomic weapons [6]. In contrast to Radiological weapons or intentional release, nuclear weapons are visible weapons and trigger an immediate impact of a very high intensity radiation energy and blast explosion resulting in a massive and lethal mass destruction [6]. Such kind of occurrences may be intentional or accidental. The United States of America had dropped a nuclear bomb (Code named "Little Boy") on Hiroshima, a military hub of Japan on 06 Aug 1945 at 8.15 am. This nuclear bomb detonated 15,000 tons of TNT and destroyed almost 9 square km area. Another nuclear bomb was dropped by USA on Nagasaki around 300 km away from Hiroshima on 9 Aug 1945 at 11.02 am. This Plutonium bomb (code name Fat Man) weighed approximately 4400 kg (10,000 pounds) and produced a blast of around 22 kt. This nuclear explosion had wiped out more than 30% of Nagasaki city within no time. These two nuclear explosions produced mass destruction of environment and human lives [6]. Around 2,26,000 people were killed and millions were injured as a consequence of nuclear bombing. The entire affected land has converted into waste land. Even after 75 years post explosion, the delayed socio economic, environmental and health issues like severe genetic mutations and very high prevalence of chronic diseases and malignancies are still visible in the affected population [7]. There have been numerous occasions of accidental or deliberate leakage of nuclear radiations as consequences of nuclear test or Nuclear Reactor fall out (1986) in the recent past. Another major and accidental nuclear disaster took place at Chernobyl (erstwhile Soviet Union / Ukraine) on 26 April 1986 when number four reactor in the Chernobyl Nuclear power plant had a steam explosion and burned due to faulty design or improper operation of the plant. This explosion had resulted in death of more than 100 people as well as complete destruction of environment and plants. The impact of explosion is still visible in the surrounding areas even after 35 years of post explosion period. It is estimated that this entire affected area will remain uninhabited upto next 20,000 years.

19.10.1 Basic Effects of Nuclear Explosion

Radiation effects of nuclear explosion may be limited to the circle of 10–20 km. This explosion can be visualized even from a distance of 50 km. It is estimated that nuclear blast can lead to flash blindness upto 5.9 km and retinal burns up to 21 km away, from the epicenter of explosion. Delayed medical, genetic mutations and other environmental effects of nuclear explosion may continue to progress from months to several years [6, 7, 55].

Blast wave: It is produced because of high temperature and pressure released following nuclear detonation. Within a fraction of a second, the heat from the fireball causes a high-pressure wave to develop and move outward producing the blast effect. The blast impact generates shock wave that rapidly travels away from fireball as a torsional moving thunder comprising of highly compressed air.

Thermal radiation: It is electromagnetic radiation. It produces burn injuries.

Radiation: This is in the form of alpha, beta, gamma and neutron. They can penetrate the body and cause damage.

Blast, thermal radiation, and massive ionizing radiation produce near total destruction within a very short spell of time following nuclear detonation.

Residual radioactive material is propelled into the upper atmosphere following a nuclear blast. Fall out particles vary in sizes from 1000th of a mm to several mm. Radioactive particles blown in air fall in the form of dust and mix with soil and stay there for a long time.

19.10.2 Effects of Nuclear Radiation on Human

Most of the deaths occurred in initial 3 months due to thermal injuries and super lethal ionizing radiation exposure [55]. Delayed effects are due to multiple effects of ionizing radiation.

Early effects of nuclear radiation
Radiation sickness
Prodromal syndrome
Bone marrow death
Gastrointestinal death
CNS death

19.10.3 Long-Term Effects of Nuclear Explosion on Human Body

Hematopoietic changes, genetic mutations, carcinogenesis, infectious diseases and infertility are noted involvements. Leukemia, Skin and Lung Cancer are more frequently seen in nuclear explosion survivors [7, 55–60] .

19.10.4 Ocular Injuries in Blast and Thermal Effects

Can affect all components of the visual system [61, 62]. Quantum of impact on ocular tissues depends upon severity of exposure to the blast wave, and thermal and nuclear radiation. In addition to the direct impact of nuclear explosion, multiple penetrating and perforating ocular injuries are also seen as a consequence of direct penetration of flying debris into the eye due to the force of blast wave [61, 62]. Most noted ocular injuries are lid burns, closed or open globe injuries with retained intraocular foreign body as well as fracture of the orbit. Shock wave induced optic nerve injuries are also not uncommon. Most of the injuries are pan systemic injuries where orbit and ocular injuries are seen as a part of multisystem injuries [61].

Thermal radiation induced visible light produces Flash-blindness in people who are looking in the direction of the explosion. It is estimated that A1-megaton explosion can cause flash blindness at distances as great as 21 km on a clear day.

Direct impact of thermal and nuclear radiation is known to produce its effect on lids, adnexa and ocular tissues. Lid burns, conjunctival edema, and chemosis, corneal epithelial erosions, perforation and necrosis are seen as acute events in most of the cases [61, 62]. Xerosis, conjunctival telangiectasia and scarring, cataract formation,secondary glaucoma, and radiation-induced chronic uveitis are delayed ocular surface and anterior segment changes [63, 64]. Whereas Optic Atrophy, CRAO, CRVO, CNVM, vitreous hemorrhage, and tractional retinal detachment are seen as delayed posterior segment involvements [7, 52, 53, 63].

19.11 Conclusion

The CBRN attacks are always without any warning. CBRN weapons differ from conventional weapons in terms of their capabilities to produce immediate, massive and unpredictable damage. The triad of flash, extreme heat and strong winds is very lethal. The pattern of casualties can simulate conventional warfare or specific to CBRN. They invariably generate severe disruption of the logistics, and other basic amenities and civil administration, health and other essential system thus producing tremendous psychological impact on the affected population. Hence, medical support in NBC operations to the maximum possible extent is very crucial.

As a consequence of delayed effects of radiation damage to hematopoietic, gastrointestinal, or neurovascular system, genetic mutations and carcinogenesis appear months to years after the exposure.

There is no specific guide line to manage ophthalmic manifestations of CBRN. Each and every ophthalmic manifestation has to be treated as per the standard protocol of ophthalmic surgery.

Undoubtedly, the real presentation and impact of CBRN will be beyond any imagination.

References

1. Smith KJ, Skelton H. Chemical warfare agents. Their past and continuing threat and evolving therapies. Part I. Skinmed. 2003;2:215–21.
2. Tuorinsky SD, Sciuto AM. In: Tuorinsky SD, editor. "Medical aspects of chemical warfare" in textbooks of military medicine. Washington, DC: Office of the Surgeon General; 2008. p. 339–70.
3. Bhalla DK, Warheit DB. Biological agents with potential for misuse: a historical perspective and defensive measures. Toxicol Appl Pharmacol. 2004;199(1):71–84. https://doi.org/10.1016/j.taap.2004.03.009. PMID: 15289092.
4. Janik E, Ceremuga M, Saluk-Bijak J, Bijak M. Biological toxins as the potential tools for bioterrorism. Int J Mol Sci. 2019;20:1181. https://doi.org/10.3390/ijms20051181.
5. Whellis M. Biotechnology and biochemical weapons. Nonprolif Rev. 2002;9:48–53. https://doi.org/10.1080/10736700208436873.
6. The Committee for the Compilation of Materials on Damage Caused by the Atomic Bombs in Hiroshima and Nagasaki. Hiroshima and Nagasaki: the physical, medical, and social effects of the atomic bombings. New York: Basic Books; 1981.
7. Mabuchi K, Fujiwara S, Preston DL, et al. Atomic-bomb survivors: long term health effects of radiation. In: Shrieve DC, Loeffler JS, editors. Human radiation injury. Philadelphia: Lippincott Williams & Wilkins; 2011. p. 89–113.
8. Ghasemi H, Ghazanfari T, Yaraee R, Soroush MR, Ghassemi-Broumand M, Poorfarzam S, et al. Systemic

and ocular complications of sulfur mustard: a panoramic review. Informa Health Care. 2009;28:14–23.
9. Safarinejad MR, Moosavi SA, Montazeri B. Ocular injuries caused by mustard gas: diagnosis, treatment, and medical defense. Mil Med. 2001;166:67–70.
10. Solberg Y, Alcalay M, Belkin M. Ocular injury by mustard gas. Surv Ophthalmol. 1997;41:461–6.
11. William F. Hughes mustard gas injuries to the eyes. Arch Ophthalmol. 1942;27:582–601.
12. Berens C, Hartmann E. The effect of war gases and other chemicals on the eyes of the civilian population. Bull N Y Acad Med. 1943;19:356–67.
13. Kadar T, Dachir S, Cohen L, Sahar R, Fishbine E, Cohen M, et al. Ocular injuries following sulfur mustard exposure—pathological mechanism and potential therapy. Toxicology. 2009;263:59–69.
14. Ghasemi H, Ghazanfari T, Ghassemi-Broumand M, Javadi MA, Babaei M, Soroush MR, et al. Long-term ocular consequences of sulfur mustard in seriously eye-injured war veterans. Cutan Ocul Toxicol. 2009;28:71–7.
15. Schep LJ, Slaughter RJ, McBride DI. Riot control agents: the tear gases CN, CS and OC—a medical review. J R Army Med Corps. 2013;161:94–9.
16. Gray PJ, Murray V. Treating CS gas injuries to the eye. Exposure at close range is particularly dangerous. BMJ. 1995;311:871.
17. US Marine Corps. Flame, riot control, and herbicide operations. Washington, DC: U.S. Marine Corps; 1996.
18. Anderson PJ, Lau GS, Taylor WR, et al. Acute effects of the potent lacrimator O-chlorobenzylidenemalononitrile (CS) tear gas. Hum Exp Toxicol. 1996;15:461–5.
19. Mandel M, Gibson WS. Clinical manifestations and treatment of gas poisoning. J Am Med Assoc. 1917;69:1970–1.
20. Rajavi Z, Safi S, Javadi MA, Jafarinasab MR, Feizi S, Moghadam MS, et al. Clinical practice guidelines for prevention, diagnosis and management of early and delayed-onset ocular injuries due to mustard gas exposure. J Ophthalmic Vis Res. 2017;12(1):65–80. https://doi.org/10.4103/jovr.jovr_253_16. PMCID: PMC5340066 PMID: 28299009.
21. Saladi RN, Smith E, Persaud AN. Mustard: a potential agent of chemical warfare and terrorism. Clin Exp Dermatol. 2006;31:1–5.
22. Goswami DG, Agarwal R, Tewari-Singh N. Phosgene oxime: injury and associated mechanisms compared to vesicating agents sulfar mustard and lewisite. Toxicol Lett. 2018;293:112–9. https://doi.org/10.1016/j.toxlet.2017.11.011. Epub 2017 Nov 12.PMID: 29141200
23. Baradaran-Rafii A, Eslani M, Tseng SC. Sulfur mustard-induced ocular surface disorders. Ocul Surf. 2011;9:163–78.
24. McNutt P, Hamilton T, Nelson M, Adkins A, Swartz A, Lawrence R, et al. Pathogenesis of acute and delayed corneal lesions after ocular exposure to sulfur mustard vapour. Cornea. 2012;31:280–90.
25. Mann I. A study of eighty-four cases of delayed mustard gas keratitis fitted with contact lenses. Br J Ophthalmol. 1944;28:441–7.
26. Javadi MA, Yazdani S, Sajjadi H, Jadidi K, Karimian F, Einollahi B, et al. Chronic and delayed-onset mustard gas keratitis: report of 48 patients and review of literature. Ophthalmology. 2005;112:617–25.
27. Javadi MA, Jafarinasab MR, Feizi S, Karimian F, Negahban K. Management of mustard gas-induced limbal stem cell deficiency and keratitis. Ophthalmology. 2011;118:1272–81.
28. Kadar T, Dachir S, Cohen M, Gutman H, Cohen L, Brandeis R, et al. Prolonged impairment of corneal innervation after exposure to sulfur mustard and its relation to the development of delayed limbal stem cell deficiency. Cornea. 2013;32:e44–50.
29. Javadi MA, Yazdani S, Kanavi MR, Mohammadpour M, Baradaran-Rafiee A, Jafarinasab MR, et al. Long-term outcomes of penetrating keratoplasty in chronic and delayed mustard gas keratitis. Cornea. 2007;26:1074–8.
30. Feizi S, Javadi MA, Jafarinasab MR, Karimian F. Penetrating keratoplasty versus lamellar keratoplasty for mustard gas–induced keratitis. Cornea. 2013;32:396–400.
31. Jafarinasab MR, Feizi S, Javadi MA, Karimian F, Soroush MR. Lamellar keratoplasty and keratolimbal allograft for mustard gas keratitis. Am J Ophthalmol. 2011;152:925–32.
32. Sidwell RW, Smee DF. Viruses of bunya and Togaviridae families: potential as bioterrorism agents and means of control. Antivir Res. 2003;57(1–2):101–11. https://doi.org/10.1016/s0166-3542(02)00203-6. PMID: 12615306.
33. Blazes DL, Lawler JV, Lazarus AA. When biotoxins are tools of terror. Early recognition of intentional poisoning can attenuate effects. Postgrad Med. 2002;112(2):89–92, 95–6, 98. https://doi.org/10.3810/pgm.2002.08.1278.
34. Atlas RM. The medical threat of biological weapons. Crit Rev Microbiol. 1998;24(3):157–68. https://doi.org/10.1080/10408419891294280. PMID: 9800098
35. Katz L, Orr-Urteger A, Brenner B, Hourvitz A. Tularaemia as a biological weapon. Harefuah. 2002;141:78–83, 120.PMID: 12170560.
36. Agarwal R, Shukla SK, Dharmani S, Gandhi A. Biological warfare—an emerging threat. J Assoc Physicians India. 2004;52:733–8. PMID: 15839453.
37. Caya JG. Clostridium botulinum and the ophthalmologist: a review of botulism, including biological warfare ramifications of botulinum toxin. Surv Ophthalmol. 2001;46(1):25–34. https://doi.org/10.1016/s0039-6257(01)00227-2. PMID: 11525787
38. Bratisl PM, Listy L. Bacillus anthracis as a biological warfare agent: infection, diagnosis and countermeasures. Bratisl Med J. 2020;121(3):175–81. https://doi.org/10.4149/BLL_2020_026. PMID: 32115973.
39. Wallin A, Luksiene Z, Zagminas K, Surkiene G. Public health and bioterrorism: renewed threat

of anthrax and small pox. Medicina (Kaunas). 2007;43(4):278–84. PMID: 17485954.
40. Henderson DA. Smallpox: clinical and epidemiologic features. Emerg Infect Dis. 1999;5(4):537–9. https://doi.org/10.3201/eid0504.990415. PMID: 10458961 .PMCID: PMC2627742.
41. Gok SE, Celikbas AK, Baykam N, Buyukemirci AA, Eroglu MN, Kemer OE, Dokuzoguz B. Evaluation of tularemia cases focusing on the oculoglandular form. J Infect Dev Ctries. 2014;8(10):1277–84. https://doi.org/10.3855/jidc.3996. PMID: 25313604.
42. Franz DR, Jahrling PB, McClain DJ, Hoover DL, Byrne WR, Pavlin JA, Christopher GW, Cieslak TJ, Friedlander AM, Eitzen EM Jr. Clinical recognition and management of patients exposed to biological warfare agents. Clin Lab Med. 2001;21(3):435–73. PMID: 11572137.
43. Gooding JJ. Biosensor technology for detecting biological warfare agents: recent progress and future trends. Anal Chim Acta. 2006;57:185–93. https://doi.org/10.1016/j.aca.2005.12.020.
44. Pohanka M, Skladal P, Kroca M. Biosensors for biological warfare agent detection. Def Sci J. 2007;57:185–93. https://doi.org/10.14429/dsj.57.1760.
45. Hansen CL Jr. Radiological warfare. JAMA. 1961;175:9–11. https://doi.org/10.1001/jama.1961.03040010011003. PMID: 13711318.
46. Hagby M, Goldberg V, Becker S, Schwartz D, Bar-Dayan Y. Health implications of radiological terrorism: perspectives from Israel. J Emerg Trauma Shock. 2009;2(2):117–23. https://doi.org/10.4103/0974-2700.50747.
47. Timins JK, Lipoti JA. Radiological terrorism. N J Med. 2003;100(6):14–21. quiz 22-4. PMID: 12854429.
48. Yehezkelli Y, Dushnitsky T, Hourvitz A. Radiation terrorism—the medical challenge. Isr Med Assoc J. 2002;4(7):530–4. PMID: 12120466.
49. National Research Council, Committee to Assess Health Risks from Exposure to Low Levels of Ionizing Radiation. Health risks from exposure to low levels of ionizing radiation: BEIR VII Phase 2. Washington, DC: National Research Council; 2005.
50. International Commission on Radiological Protection. ICRP publication 103: the 2007 recommendations of the international commission on radiological protection. Oxford: Elsevier; 2007.
51. Pascu RA. Effects of optical radiation in ocular structures. Oftalmologia. 2007;51(3):23–40. PMID: 18064950.
52. Ainsbury EA, Bouffler SD, Dorr W, Graw J, Muirhead CR, Edwards AA, Cooper J. Radiation cataractogenesis: a review of recent studies. Radiat Res. 2009;172(1):1–9. https://doi.org/10.1667/RR1688.1. PMID: 19580502.
53. Choshi K, Takaku I, Mishima H, et al. Ophthalmologic changes related to radiation exposure and age in adult health study sample, Hiroshima and Nagasaki. Radiat Res. 1983;96(3):560–79.
54. Stefan C, Timaru CM, Iliescu DA, Schmitzer S, De Algerino S, Batras M, Ramhormozi JH. Glaucoma after chemical burns and radiation. Rom J Ophthalmol. 2016;60(4):209–15. PMID: 29450351.PMCID: PMC5711283.
55. Schull WJ. Effects of atomic radiation: a half-century of studies from Hiroshima and Nagasaki. New York: Wiley; 1995.
56. Kodama Y, Pawel DJ, Nakamura N, et al. Stable chromosome aberrations in atomic bomb survivors: results from 25 years of investigation. Radiat Res. 2001;156(4):337–46.
57. Finch SC, Hrubec Z, Nefzger MD. Detection of leukemia and related disorders. Hiroshima and Nagasaki research plan. Hiroshima: Atomic Bomb Casualty Commission; 1965.
58. Richardson D, Sugiyama H, Nishi N, et al. Ionizing radiation and leukemia mortality among Japanese atomic bomb survivors, 1950–2000. Radiat Res. 2009;172(3):368–82.
59. Iwanaga M, Hsu W-L, Soda M, et al. Risk of myelodysplastic syndromes in people exposed to ionizing radiation: a retrospective cohort study of Nagasaki atomic bomb survivors. J Clin Oncol. 2011;29(4):428–34.
60. Preston DL, Ron E, Tokuoka S, et al. Solid cancer incidence in atomic bomb survivors: 1958–1998. Radiat Res. 2007;168(1):1–64.
61. Ritenour AE, Baskin TW. Primary blast injury: update on diagnosis and treatment. Crit Care Med. 2008;36(7 Suppl):S311–7. https://doi.org/10.1097/CCM.0b013e31817e2a8c. PMID: 18594258.
62. Wang H-CH, Choi J-H, Grene WA, Plamper ML, Cortez HE, Chavko M, Li Y, Dalle Lucca JJ, Johnson AJ. Pathophysiology of blast-induced ocular trauma with apoptosis in the retina and optic nerve. Mil Med. 2014;179(8 Suppl):34–40. https://doi.org/10.7205/MILMED-D-13-00504. PMID: 25102547.
63. Miller RJ, Fujino T, Nefzger MD. Lens findings in atomic bomb survivors. A review of major ophthalmic surveys at the atomic bomb casualty commission (1949–1962). Arch Ophthalmol. 1967;78(6):697–704.
64. Cogan DG, Martin SF, Kimura SJ. Atom bomb cataracts. Science. 1949;110(2868):654.

20 Classification Systems for Ocular Trauma

B. Rajesh Babu

20.1 Introduction

Ocular injuries are increasingly becoming a major preventable cause of blindness and low vision especially among persons in the productive age group. These blinding injuries cause significant socioeconomic impact among the sufferers [1]. According to the WHO, there are 55 million eye injuries causing restriction of daily activities, of which 1.6 million go blind every day [2]. Eye injuries impact not only the individual, but also the country's health-care system and community [3, 4].

Military combat-related ocular trauma has increased in the last 40 years with the emergence of more powerful explosives with higher fragmentation power and poor acceptance of eye protection among combat soldiers [5]. The use of body armor leads to increased survivability in explosions, but the head and face are exposed to combat risks. Eye trauma results in visual loss that leads to loss of career, forcing lifestyle changes and permanent disfigurement [5].

Trauma can result in a wide spectrum of tissue lesions of the eye and adjacent tissues, ranging from the relatively superficial to vision threatening.

B. Rajesh Babu (✉)
Akash Institute of Medical Sciences and Research, Bangalore, Karnataka, India

The understanding of the pathophysiology and management of eye injuries have evolved over the last 50 years. It is critical that a standardized classification system of terminology and assessment be used by both ophthalmologists and nonophthalmologists when describing and communicating clinical findings [6, 7].

A standardized system of classification is essential for better communication and analysis of the results of medical and surgical interventions in ocular trauma [7].

The Ocular Trauma Classification group [8] classified mechanical injuries of the eye into open globe and closed globe injuries. The classification system was based on four specific variables that have been of prognostic significance for final visual outcome: Type of injury, grade of injury (based on visual acuity (VA) at the initial examination), presence of relative afferent pupillary defect (RAPD), and the zone of injury. The zone of injury was defined by the location of the most posterior aspect of the globe opening. Zone I injuries occur when the break in the globe was isolated to the cornea or corneoscleral limbus (Fig. 20.1). Zone II injuries are those that involved anterior 5 mm of the sclera: 5 mm extension into the sclera is chosen as a landmark as it has been hypothesized that wounds located in this zone would not extend posteriorly beyond the pars plana (Fig. 20.1). Zone III injuries are those that extended full thickness into the sclera more than 5 mm posterior to the corneoscleral limbus

S. Waikar (ed.), *Ocular Trauma in Armed Conflicts*, https://doi.org/10.1007/978-981-19-4021-7_20

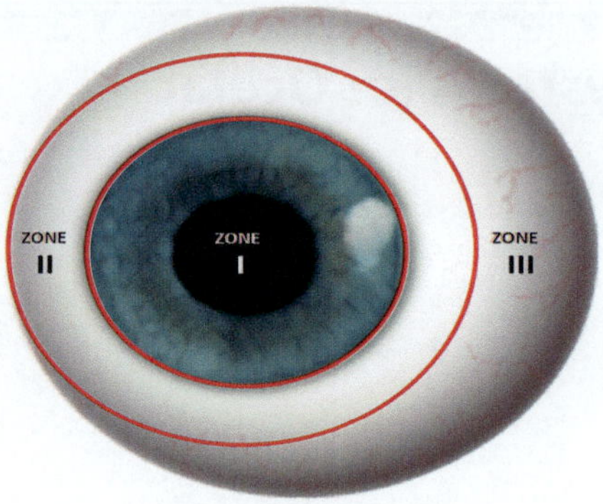

Fig. 20.1 Zones for open-globe injury

(Fig. 20.1). Though, the zone of injury was often determined at the time of the initial examination, the exact extent of the injury may be more accurately determined at the time of surgical intervention [9].

Numerous examples from older literatures are characterized by the lack of definitions, with obvious implications. The use of standard terminologies enables us to score the severity of eye injuries using the ocular trauma score (OTS) facilitating the conduct of clinical trials comparing the outcomes of various interventions and communicating the findings unambiguously between ophthalmologists.

It is important to have clarity about terminologies like penetrating or nonpenetrating injury, whether it was due to sharp or blunt [10–13] object, rupture or contusion, or both.

20.2 Birmingham Eye Trauma Terminology

The *Birmingham Eye Trauma Terminology* (BETT) (Table 20.1) was created by Kuhn et al. in 1996 to provide both a clear definition of all injury types and placing the injuries within a comprehensive framework [6, 8]. BETT provides a clear, consistent, and simple understanding of standard eye trauma terminology by providing a clear definition for all injury types and places each injury type within a comprehensive framework [8]. The terminologies use the entire globe as the tissue of reference, thereby avoiding confusions. BETT has been endorsed by several organizations including the American Academy of Ophthalmology, International Society of Ocular Trauma, Retina Society, United States Eye Injury Registry and its 25 international affiliates, Vitreous Society, and the World Eye Injury Registry. It is mandated by several journals such as Graefe's Archives, Journal of Eye Trauma, Klinische Monatsblätter, and Ophthalmology [8].

Table 20.1 Terms and definitions in Bett [8]

Term	Definition and Explanation
Eyewall	*Sclera and cornea* *Although technically the eyewall has three coats posterior to the limbus, for clinical and practical purposes, violation of only the most external structure is taken into consideration*
Closed-globe injury	No full-thickness wound of eyewall
Open-globe injury	Full-thickness wound of the eyewall
Contusion	There is no (full-thickness) wound *The injury is due to either direct energy delivery by the object* (e.g., *choroidal rupture) or the changes in the shape of the globe* (e.g., *angle recession)*
Lamellar laceration	Partial-thickness wound of the eyewall
Rupture	Full-thickness wound of the eyewall, caused by a blunt object *Because the eye is filled with incompressible liquid, the impact results in momentary increase in IOP. The eyewall yields at its weakest point (at the impact site or elsewhere;* e.g., *an old cataract wound dehisces even though the impact occurred elsewhere); the actual wound is produced by an inside-out mechanism*
Laceration	Full-thickness wound of the eyewall, caused by a sharp object *The wound occurs at the impact site by an outside-in mechanism*
Penetrating injury	Entrance wound *If more than one wound is present, each must have been caused by a different agent* Retained foreign object(s) *Technically a penetrating injury, but grouped separately because of different clinical implications*
Perforating injury	Entrance and exit wounds Both wounds caused by the same agent

20.3 Classification of Ocular Trauma

A committee of thirteen ophthalmologists from seven different institutions met to discuss the standardization of ocular trauma classification [7]. They classified ocular trauma based on the BETT [8] and features of eye injury at initial examination.

Only mechanical trauma to eye (globe) was considered in this classification. Injuries due to thermal, electrical, and chemical causes were not included in their protocol for classification [7, 8]. A general classification of ocular trauma is described in Table 20.2.

The mechanical trauma to eye (globe) was further subdivided into open- and closed-globe injuries (Fig. 20.2), because these have different pathophysiological and therapeutic implications [7]. This system classifies both open-globe and closed-globe injuries according to four separate variables: type of injury, based on the mechanism of injury; grade of injury, defined by visual acuity in the injured eye at initial examination; pupil, defined as the presence or absence of a relative afferent pupillary defect in the injured eye; and zone of injury, based on the anteroposterior extent of the injury [7]. Closed-globe injury is classified using the highest zone of injury details of which are described in Table 20.3. The ocular trauma score as described by Kuhn by assigning a raw point for initial visual acuity and then subtracting the appropriate raw points based on each diagnosis of globe rupture, endophthalmitis, perforating injury, retinal detachment, and RAPD [14] (Table 20.4). Multiple studies [15–18] indicate that the higher zones of injury and correspondingly lower ocular trauma scores had a poorer prognosis for good visual recovery. Higher ocular trauma scores indicate better visual prognosis at 6 months.

An appropriate classification of ocular trauma not only allows uniform assessment and communication across the world but also helps in interpretation, documentation, and correlation in multicentric studies. It also provides indicators for prognostication and also helps policy makers to draw meaningful conclusions and take appropriate actions.

Table 20.2 General classification of ocular trauma

Local	Nonmechanical	Chemical Thermal-Radiation-induced Ultrasonic Barometric
Mechanical	Adnexal	1. Palpebral 2. Conjunctival 3. Orbital 4. Lacrimal
	Global	1. Structural (a) Anterior segment (corneal, scleral, uveal, pupillary, ciliary body, and lenticular) (b) Posterior segment (Scleral, Retinal, vitreous, choroidal, optic nerve)
		2. Pathological (a) Closed-globe injury • Contusion • Lamellar • Laceration • IOFB • Dislocation of lens (b) Open-globe injury • Rupture • Penetration • Perforation • IOFB (c) Destructive globe injury • Traumatic evisceration • Traumatic enucleation • Full-thickness laceration greater than 1/3 globe circumference

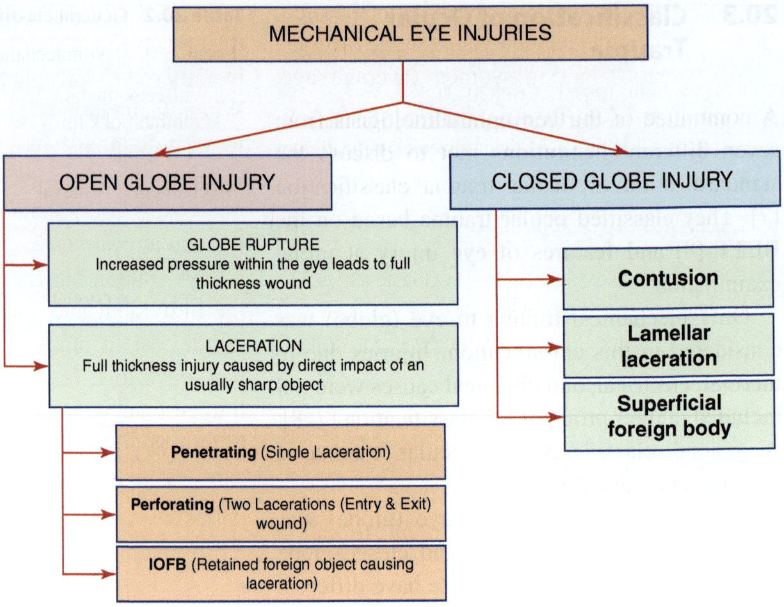

Fig. 20.2 Classification of mechanical eye injuries

Table 20.3 Open-globe injury classification

Type	Grade (visual acuity)	Pupil	Zone (see Fig. 20.1)
(a) Rupture (b) Penetrating (c) IOFB (d) Perforating (e) Mixed	(a) >20/40 (b) 20/50 to 20/100 (c) 19/100 to 5/200 (d) 4/200 to light perception (e) NLP (no light perception)	(a) Positive, relative afferent pupillary defect in injured eye (b) Negative, relative afferent pupillary defect in injured eye	I. Cornea and limbus II. Limbus to 5 mm posterior into sclera III. Posterior to 5 mm from the limbus

Table 20.4 Ocular trauma score

Variables	Raw points
Initial vision	
NPL/enucleation/evisceration	60
LP/HM	70
1/60–5/60	80
6/60–6/15	90
6/12 or better	100
Negative points	
Rupture	−23
Endophthalmitis	−17
Perforating injury	−14
Retinal detachment	−11
RAPD	−10

OTS Score 1–5
1—Raw points 0–44
2—Raw points 45–65
3—Raw points 66–80
4—Raw points 81–91
5—Raw points 91–100

References

1. Shukla B, Agrawal R, Shukla D, Seen S. Systematic analysis of ocular trauma by a new proposed ocular trauma classification. Indian J Ophthalmol. 2017;65(8):719–22.
2. Negrel AD, Thylefors B. The global impact of eye injuries. Ophthalmic Epidemiol. 1998;5(3):143–69.
3. Thylefors B. Epidemiological patterns of ocular trauma. Aust N Z J Ophthalmol. 1992;20(2):95–8.
4. Wong TY, Klein BE, Klein R. The prevalence and 5-year incidence of ocular trauma. The Beaver Dam Eye Study. Ophthalmology. 2000;107(12):2196–202.
5. Blanch RJ, Scott RA. Military ocular injury: presentation, assessment and management. J R Army Med Corps. 2009;155(4):279–84.
6. Kuhn F, Morris R, Witherspoon CD, Heimann K, Jeffers JB, Treister G. A standardized classification of ocular trauma. Graefes Arch Clin Exp Ophthalmol. 1996;234(6):399–403.

7. Pieramici DJ, Sternberg P Jr, Aaberg TM Sr, et al. A system for classifying mechanical injuries of the eye (globe). The Ocular Trauma Classification Group. Am J Ophthalmol. 1997;123(6):820–31.
8. Kuhn F, Morris R, Witherspoon CD, Heimann K, Jeffers JB, Treister G. A standardized classification of ocular trauma. Ophthalmology. 1996;103(2):240–3.
9. Knyazer B, Levy J, Rosen S, Belfair N, Klemperer I, Lifshitz T. Prognostic factors in posterior open globe injuries (zone-III injuries). Clin Exp Ophthalmol. 2008;36(9):836–41.
10. De Juan E Jr, Sternberg P Jr, Michels RG. Penetrating ocular injuries. Types of injuries and visual results. Ophthalmology. 1983;90(11):1318–22.
11. Kylstra JA, Lamkin JC, Runyan DK. Clinical predictors of scleral rupture after blunt ocular trauma. Am J Ophthalmol. 1993;115(4):530–5.
12. Meredith TA, Gordon PA. Pars plana vitrectomy for severe penetrating injury with posterior segment involvement. Am J Ophthalmol. 1987;103(4):549–54.
13. Liggett PE, Gauderman WJ, Moreira CM, Barlow W, Green RL, Ryan SJ. Pars plana vitrectomy for acute retinal detachment in penetrating ocular injuries. Arch Ophthalmol. 1990;108(12):1724–8.
14. Kuhn F, Maisiak R, Mann L, Mester V, Morris R, Witherspoon CD. The ocular trauma score (OTS). Ophthalmol Clin N Am. 2002;15(2):163–5, vi.
15. Fujikawa A, Mohamed YH, Kinoshita H, et al. Visual outcomes and prognostic factors in open-globe injuries. BMC Ophthalmol. 2018;18:138. https://doi.org/10.1186/s12886-018-0804-4.
16. Han SB, Yu HG. Visual outcome after open globe injury and its predictive factors in Korea. J Trauma. 2010;69(5):E66–72.
17. Yalcin Tok O, Tok L, Eraslan E, Ozkaya D, Ornek F, Bardak Y. Prognostic factors influencing final visual acuity in open globe injuries. J Trauma. 2011;71(6):1794–800.
18. Yu Wai Man C, Steel D. Visual outcome after open globe injury: a comparison of two prognostic models--the ocular trauma score and the classification and regression tree. Eye (Lond). 2010;24(1):84–9.

21 Imaging in Eye Injury

Manab J. Barman, Kasturi Bhattacharjee, and Hemlata Deka

- Introduction
- Various Imaging modalities
- Imaging in specific conditions

Ocular injuries are increasingly being recognized among the most important causes of ocular morbidity and vision loss. According to World Health Organization report, eye injuries result in complete blindness in about 1.6 million people and unilateral blindness or vision loss in almost 19 million people each year [1]. The overall prevalence of trauma-related eye injuries is approximately 2–6%, with as many as 97% of cases resulting from blunt trauma [2].

Physical examination of the globe may be challenging during acute trauma due to hemorrhage, presence of surrounding soft-tissue swelling, and other associated injuries. There are often difficulties related to the patient cooperation caused by other injuries, anxiety, or altered state of consciousness. While comprehensive knowledge of injury is crucial in the management of ocular trauma, ocular imaging modalities add valuable information for management as well prognostication.

In general, conventional ultrasonography, ultrasound biomicroscopy, optical coherence tomography, retinal angiography, and fundus autofluorescence are useful in the diagnosis and monitoring most of the cases of ocular injuries in an Ophthalmic trauma setting. Plain x-ray, computerized tomography (CT), and Magnetic Resonance Imaging (MRI) are helpful in some complicated injuries of orbit, optic nerve, and ocular adnexa.

21.1 Various Imaging Modalities

A detailed discussion on the technical aspect behind different imaging modalities is beyond the scope of this chapter; however, knowledge of the basic principles is useful for understanding the applications of these imaging modalities.

M. J. Barman (✉)
Vitreo Retina Service, Sri Sankaradeva Nethralaya, Guwahati, Assam, India

K. Bhattacharjee
Oculoplasty, Aesthetics and Reconstructive Surgery, Sri Sankaradeva Nethralaya, Guwahati, Assam, India

H. Deka
Medical Retina Service, Sri Sankaradeva Nethralaya, Guwahati, Assam, India

S. Waikar (ed.), *Ocular Trauma in Armed Conflicts*, https://doi.org/10.1007/978-981-19-4021-7_21

21.1.1 Ultrasonography

Ultrasound is noninvasive, nonionizing, and relatively inexpensive imaging technique. Ultrasound frequencies in the 2–50 MHz range are usually used for medical purpose. Higher the frequency, more is the resolution but with lower depth of tissue penetration.

The use of ultrasound for diagnostic imaging of the eye originates with the work of Mundt and Hughes (unidirectional amplitude modulated -A-scan, 1956) and Baum and Greenwood (two-directional cross-sectional brightness -B-scan, 1958) [3, 4].·Amplitude modulation (A-scan), displays the intensity of the echo as a vertical spike plotted against the echo's time delay, which is equivalent to the distance from the transducer. Brightness modulation (B-scan) displays two-dimensional real-time, cross-sectional images. Usually both the A-scan and B-scan complement each other. Conventional ophthalmic ultrasonography (USG) uses a 7.5–12 MH probe. It is useful in outlining soft tissue abnormalities of the eye and orbit and also helps in detecting intraocular foreign bodies (IOFBs) in the presence of opaque media. It is relatively contraindicated in open-globe injury prior to primary repair, as it may lead to further trauma and wound contamination. If ultrasound examination is indicated in such cases, it should be performed with extreme caution to avoid further trauma and risk of infection to the eye.

21.1.1.1 Ultrasound with Tissue Harmonic Imaging

Fundamental frequency is the original frequency of an acoustic beam emitted from the transducer. Harmonic waves are integer multiples of the fundamental frequency. The second harmonic wave (twice the fundamental frequency) with elimination of the fundamental frequency by imageprocessing techniques is currently used for tissue harmonic imaging (THI). The THI provides improved contrast resolution, improved lateral resolution, improved imaging of deeper tissue, improved signal-to-noise ratio, and artifact reduction [5].

21.1.2 Ultrasound Biomicroscopy (UBM)

Conventional ultrasound B-Scan alone has its limitation in imaging the anterior segment structures of the eye due to lower frequency. This led to a shift toward alternate imaging modalities like ultrasound biomicroscopy (UBM). The first practical Ultrasound biomicroscopy (UBM) system was developed by Foster and Pavlin in the early 1990s. UBM uses high-frequency (35–50 MHz) acoustic waves to produce high-resolution, cross-sectional images of the anterior segment anatomy and pathology to a depth of approximately 5 mm [6].

Currently available UBM machines provide lateral and axial physical resolutions of approximately 50 μm and 25 μm, respectively. The scanner produces 256 vertical image lines in a 5 × 5 mm field at a scan rate of 8 frames/s. The real-time image is displayed on a monitor and can be recorded for analysis.

21.1.2.1 Conventional Ophthalmic B-Scanner (10 MHz) Versus Ultrasound Biomicroscopy (UBM)

Characteristic	Conventional B-Scanner	UBM
Frequency (MHz)	10	50
Aperture (mm)	10	6
Focal length (mm)	30	12
F-ratio	3	2
Axial resolution (μm)	150	30
Lateral resolution (μm)	450	60
Depth of field (mm)	9.6	0.85
Attenuation in water (dB/mm)	0.02	0.55

21.1.3 Scheimpflug Imaging

Scheimpflug system images the anterior segment. It uses a camera perpendicular to a slit beam, creating multiple optical sections of the cornea and lens. The images are digitized and creates 3-dimensional virtual model of the anterior segment. Approximately 25,000 data points are used to calculate topographic corneal thickness, corneal curvature, anterior chamber angle, volume, and depth.

21.1.4 Optical Coherence Tomography (OCT)

Developed with the work of Adolf Fercher and colleagues, Optical coherence tomography (OCT) is the imaging device based on the principle of low-coherence interferometry. It is typically employing near-infrared light that penetrates into the scattering medium and captures two- and three-dimensional images of tissue morphology in near-microscopic resolution. OCT provides high-depth resolution (10–12 μm), cross-sectional tomographs, enabling detailed imaging of the anatomical structures of the retina.

First-generation, Time-domain OCT technology (TD-OCT, 1991) systems acquired approximately 400 scans per second and required mechanical acquisition of a depth scan resulting in slow imaging speed and poor image quality. Fourier domain OCT (FD-OCT) is the second-generation OCT that used spectral information to generate scans without the need for mechanical scanning of the optical path length. With introduction of Spectrometer-based FD-OCT, the spectral domain OCT (SD-OCT, 1995), that could capture the whole depth information simultaneously, there was significant improvement in image quality and imaging speed. Further improvements in OCT technology, like enhanced depth imaging (EDI), Spectralis, or the Swept source technology (SS-OCT), facilitated rapid scanning and enhanced visualization of deeper structures as well better followability and reproducibility. More recently, both spectral domain and swept source OCT have been used to generate OCT angiography (OCT-A) images for imaging the microvasculature of the retina and the choroid without using dye.

In case of posterior segment trauma, OCT helps in monitoring various macular and chorioretinal morphological changes with high accuracy and precision. It is comfortable to the patient due to its noncontact and noninvasive nature.

Anterior segment OCT imaging (ASOCT, 1994) was first described by Izatt et al. using the same wavelength of light as posterior segment OCT (830 nm) [7]. Later development of OCT imaging of the anterior segment with a longer wavelength of 1310 nm provided better penetration through sclera as well as optimal imaging of the angle structures. ASOCT can achieve axial resolution in the range of 3–20 μm.

21.1.5 Fundus Autofluorescence (FAF)

Fundus autofluorescence (FAF) imaging is in vivo mapping of ocular fluorophores, mostly lipofuscin (LF) and melanolipofuscin granules in the retinal pigment epithelium (RPE). As photoreceptor function is dependent on normal RPE function, any compromise in RPE health may lead to accumulation of the toxic fluorophores and other byproducts and eventually cell death [8]. It is noninvasive and simple method for assessing changes in the integrity and metabolism of retinal cells using confocal scanning laser ophthalmoscope (cSLO) or a near infrared (NIR)-AF system.

21.1.6 Fluorescein and Indocyanine Green Angiography

Fluorescence occurs when a molecule is excited by light of certain wavelength that raises it to a higher energy state and then allows it to release energy to bring back to its original state. This technique was used in fluorescein angiography by Mac Lean and Maumenee to evaluate ocular circulation. Fluorescein angiography (FA) helps in examination of the retino-choroidal circulation. Photographs of the retina are taken by a fundus camera after intravenous injection of sodium fluorescein dye with mol wt 376 daltons. Fluorescein dye fluoresces at wavelength of 520–530 nm (green) after excitation by a light with wavelength 465–490 nm (blue). 80% of the dye is protein bound. The remaining 20% unbound fluorescein circulates in the vasculature of the retina and choroid, where it can be visualized.

Indocyanine green angiography (ICGA-Flower and Hochheimer, 1973) is fast emerging as useful adjunct to the traditional FA. ICG is a tricarbocyanine dye with mol wt 775 daltons. ICG angiography uses near-infrared portion of spectrum with absorption at 805 nm and emission at 835 nm. It is almost completely protein bound (98%) with limited diffusion through the small fenestrations of the choriocapillaris. The retention of ICG in the choroidal circulation makes it ideal for imaging choroidal circulation.

21.1.7 Electrophysiological Tests

Electrophysiological tests involve assessing the function of the photorecptor system and proximal visual pathway. Electroretinogram (ERG), Electrooculogram (EOG), and Visual-evoked potential (VEP) are the tests commonly performed.

The electroretinogram (ERG) measures the electrical responses generated in the retina. The pattern electroretinogram (PERG) is the retinal response to a structured stimulus, such as a reversing checkerboard or grating. It helps in both the objective clinical evaluation of macular function (P50) and a direct assessment of retinal ganglion cell function (N95). Pattern ERG is affected by diseases confined to the macula. Multifocal electroretinography (mfERG) can measure multiple electroretinographic responses simultaneously by cross-correlation. It allows mapping of retinal function in the central 40–50°.

The EOG is a measure of the function of the retinal pigment epithelium (RPE) and the interaction between the RPE and the photoreceptor. Arden ratio represents ratio between the light and dark troughs and peaks in the EOG. The Arden ratio above 1.8 is normal and below 1.6 is abnormal. Between 1.8 and 1.6, it is suspicious.

VEP is a cortical response that is time-locked to a visual stimulus event, such as the contrast-reversal of a checkerboard pattern or a flash of light. The amplitude is typically 4–15 μV, and the latency is 90–100 mS. Pattern VEP is used in patients who can detect a pattern stimulus. It is helpful to study optic nerve function. A delay in the latency is suggestive of optic nerve dysfunction, whereas a reduction in the amplitude is usually suggestive of visual disturbance proximal to the optic nerve or neuronal tissue. Flash VEP helps to rule out the presence or absence of visual response from the optic nerve in uncooperative patient or in case of dense media opacity.

Bright-light flash ERG and VEP are useful for evaluation of visual potential in severely traumatized eye. However, these tests may be affected by media haze and may not be confirmatory for loss of visual potential in such cases.

21.1.8 Radiographic Imaging

21.1.8.1 Plain x-Ray

In current day practice, plain x-rays have a limited role in ophthalmic trauma. Prior to the advent of high-resolution CT scans, it was the imaging of choice for the diagnosis of orbital and orbito facial fractures and retained radio-opaque foreign bodies. However, owing to less reliability indices in comparison to CT scan, they are no longer utilized as first-line choice.

21.1.8.2 Computerized Tomography (CT Scan)

Computed tomography scan (CT or CAT scan) uses computer-processed combinations of multiple radiographic projections (X-ray) taken from different angles to produce cross-sectional images (virtual "slices") of specific areas. The relative attenuation of X-ray beam is expressed as Hounsfield units (HU), named in honor of the inventor of CT scanning—Godfrey N. Hounsfield. Water has a value of 0 HU, air a value of −1000 HU, and dense bone has a value of +1000 HU. Although, originally, the images generated were in the axial or transverse plane, modern scanners allow digital processing of images to generate 3-D volume of an object from series of images taken around a single axis. A typical CT can involve 10–20 mGy for specific organs, and can go up to 80 mGy for certain specialized scans. Contrary to this, a typical plain X-ray involves radiation dose of 0.01–0.15 mGy [9].

21.1.8.3 Magnetic Resonance Imaging (MRI)

Magnetic Resonance Imaging (MRI) produces three-dimensional detailed anatomical images. Developed with pioneering work of Paul Lauterbur and Peter Mansfield (1971), MRI scanners use strong magnetic radio waves to generate images of the organs in the body. A strong oscillating magnetic field forces protons in the body to align with the field. A radiofrequency (RF) current is then pulsed to stimulate the protons and spin out of equilibrium, straining against the pull of the magnetic field. When the RF field is turned off, the MRI sensors detect the energy released as the protons realign with the magnetic field. The time taken by the protons to realign with the magnetic field, as well as the amount of energy released, changes depending on the environment and the nature of the tissue. Through manipulation of the RF pulses and measurements of the resulting emitted energy, different images can be constructed. Each tissue returns to its equilibrium state after excitation by the independent relaxation processes of T1 (magnetization in the same direction as the static magnetic field) and T2 (transverse to the static magnetic field). To create a T1-weighted image, magnetization is allowed to "recover" before measuring the MR signal by changing the "repetition time" (RT), whereas to create a T2-weighted image, signal is recorded by changing the "echo- time" (ET) after magnetization is allowed to "decay." Fat-suppression protocols have been developed to decrease the signal intensity of orbital fat, which, in combination with contrast agents (often containing Gadolinium), can improve visualization of the optic nerve and vascular lesions. Contrast agents help to increase the speed at which protons realign with the magnetic field, resulting in brighter image quality.

21.2 Imaging in Specific Conditions

- Anterior segment trauma
- Posterior segment trauma
- Globe integrity
- Posterior segment Foreign body
- Orbital fracture
- Extraocular muscle injury
- Optic nerve trauma
- Carotid cavernous fistula

21.2.1 Anterior Segment Trauma

21.2.1.1 Ultrasound Evaluation of the Anterior Segment

Ocular trauma with hyphema and corneal opacities may obscure visualization of anterior segment structures. However, conventional B-scan is not good enough to scan the anterior segment structures. Immersion technique may be used, provided any open wound is repaired or has healed. Standard B -Scan can be accomplished with the use of a scleral shell filled with coupling fluid (e.g., methylcellulose or balanced salt solution) avoiding air bubbles within the shell. The probe is placed on top of the shell [10]. With contact B-scan, to adequately center a lesion, the patient needs to look toward the direction of the lesion, while the probe is held opposite to it. With immersion technique, the patient needs to look in opposite direction of the lesion to center the area of interest. Using transverse scanning along the nonaxial plane of the eyeball, B-scan USG helps in localization of IOFBs in the anterior segment [11]. Examination through the lids with a soft standoff technique may also be of help if the immersion technique cannot be performed. Ultrasound may reveal the status of the anterior chamber, angle recession, ciliary body detachment, integrity of the lens, and retained IOFB. Hyphema may be presented with multiple echoes in the anterior chamber. Angle recession should be suspected if the anterior chamber is abnormally deep with wide angles. Now, ultrasound biomicroscopy (UBM) is used more effectively for imaging anterior segment.

21.2.1.2 Ultrasound Biomicroscopy (UBM)

UBM is helpful in precise evaluation of anterior segment and can demonstrate disruption of the intraocular structures as seen in iridodialysis, angle recession, cyclodialysis, zonular dehiscence, scleral laceration, foreign body, and epithelial ingrowth, irrespective of the opaque media. The scleral spur is the only constant morphological landmark, allowing to interpret UBM images of the status of anterior chamber angle. UBM can be performed over a soft contact lens in a micro-open wound.

With the help of UBM, angle recession can be differentiated from cyclodialysis. In angle recession, the ciliary body is torn between its circular and longitudinal fibers, creating in a wide-angle appearance with no disruption of the interface between the sclera and ciliary body. In contrast, in cyclodialysis, there is detachment of the ciliary body from the scleral spur, creating a communication from the anterior chamber to the suprachoroidal space (Fig. 21.1).

UBM can identify the exact location, size, and nature of a foreign body in the anterior segment along with the appearance of surrounding tissue better than conventional ultrasound or CT scan [12, 13].

Foreign bodies generate various artifact patterns based on their acoustic characteristics. In general, hard and dense materials (e.g., metal or glass) generate "comet tail" appearance by reflecting ultrasound back and forth. In contrast, softer materials that contain air (e.g., wood) create "shadowing artifact" by absorbing most of the ultrasound.

UBM can be used to accurately assess the presence, position, and integrity of the lens capsule and zonular defects associated with traumatic cataract: this allows the surgeon to plan preoperatively to prevent complications like vitreous loss or nucleus drop (Figs. 21.2 and 21.3).

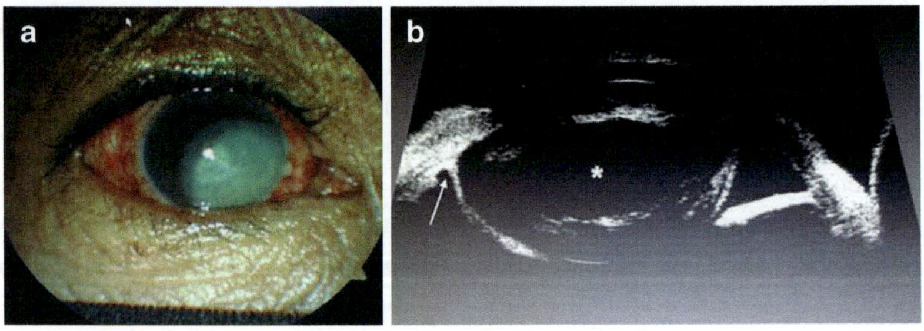

Fig. 21.1 A case of traumatic anterior dislocation of lens with cyclodialysis. (**a**) Clinical appearance shows anterior dislocation of cataractous lens. (**b**) Ultrasound biomicroscopy shows anterior displacement of the lens (asterisk) along with a cyclodialysis cleft (arrow)

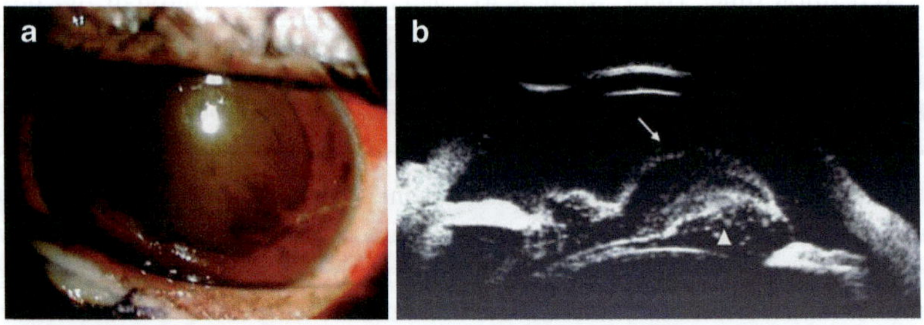

Fig. 21.2 A case of traumatic zonular dialysis with vitreous prolapse. (**a**) Clinical appearance shows prolapsed vitreous with blood staining. (**b**) Ultrasound biomicroscopy shows vitreous prolapsed (arrow) into the anterior chamber through the area of zonular dialysis with layering of blood (arrowhead)

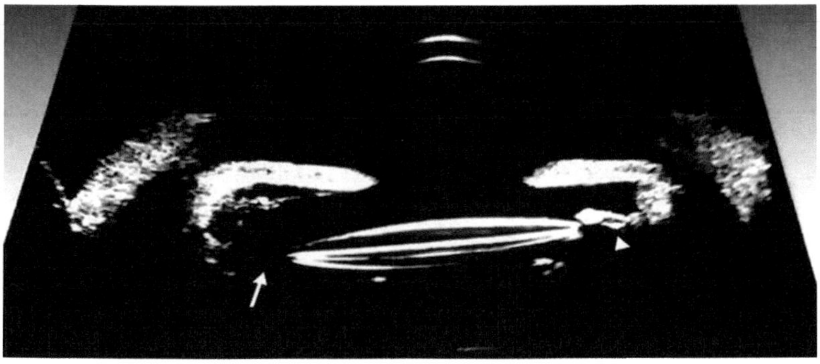

Fig. 21.3 UBM image of an eye with a subluxated IOL. Note the arrowhead showing intact zonular support. The zonular dehiscence is marked with arrow. The tilt of the IOL is evident from the difference in vertical distance from the posterior iris surface to the anterior surface of the IOL

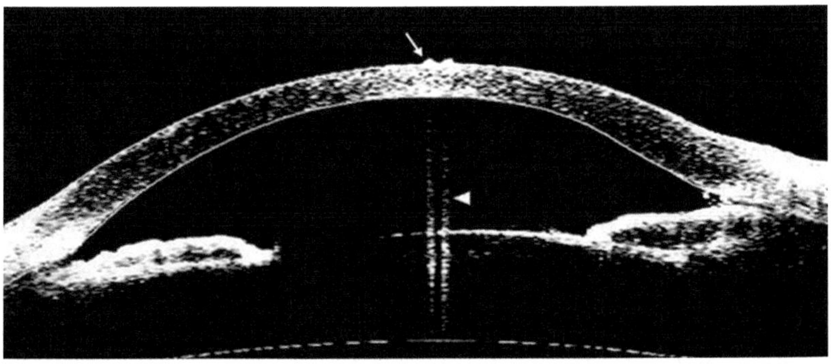

Fig. 21.4 Anterior segment optical coherence tomography shows superficial corneal foreign body (arrow) with corresponding back shadowing (arrowhead)

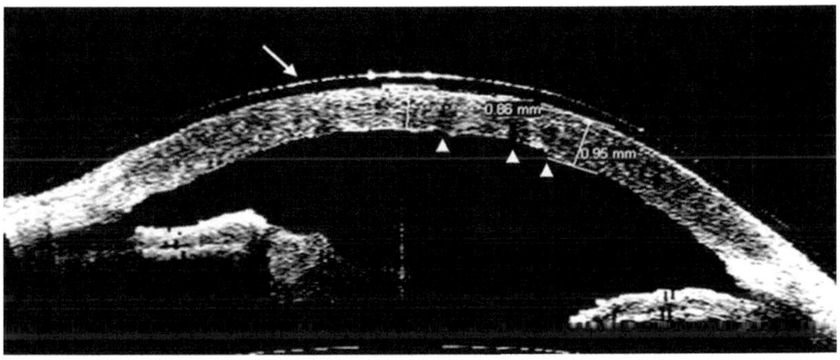

Fig. 21.5 A case of blast injury. Anterior segment optical coherence tomography shows multiple corneal foreign bodies (arrowheads), corneal edema with overlying bandage contact lens (arrow)

21.2.1.3 Anterior Segment Optical Coherence Tomography (ASOCT)

ASOCT helps to evaluate ocular surface injuries and anterior segment lesions. It helps to detect subtle lesion or small FB that are difficult to recognize on routine slit-lamp examination and in monitoring the healing process [14]. It can be performed in open-globe injuries or in a soft globe due to its noncontact approach. It has advantages of accuracy and repeatability (Figs. 21.4 and 21.5).

ASOCT allows rapid imaging of depths up to 6 mm into ocular tissue and provides accurate measurements of foreign body location, number, and dimensions. Different reflectivity is appreciable depending on the nature of foreign body. Metal and stone foreign bodies show high anterior reflectivity with shadowing. Wood foreign body shows moderate reflectivity, while glass

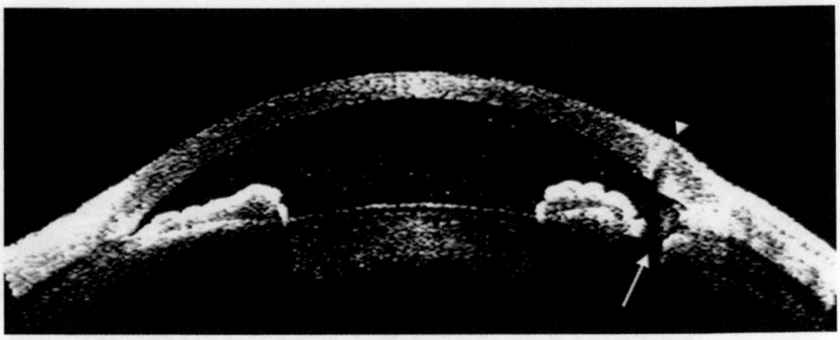

Fig. 21.6 A case of penetrating injury with foreign body. Anterior segment optical coherence tomography shows sealed corneal perforation (arrowhead) with traumatic iridotomy caused by foreign body (arrow)

foreign body is well delineated without reflectivity. It can provide vital details about status of DM integrity and site of entry of foreign body (Fig. 21.6).

Other conditions that may be diagnosed with ASOCT include damage to the iris, angle structures, cyclodialysis cleft, and status of lens capsule.

Limitations of ASOCT, however, include inability to penetrate pigmented tissue and, thus, inability to image past the posterior pigmented epithelium of the iris.

Anterior Segment Optical Coherence Tomography (ASOCT) Versus Ultrasound Biomicroscopy

	ASOCT	UBM
Principle	Optical	Ultrasound
Resolution	15 μm	50 μm
Scan dimensions	16 × 6 mm	5 × 5 mm
Scan depth	6 mm	5 mm
Contact with eye	No	Requires immersion bath
Imaging posterior to iris	No	Yes
Real-time imaging	Yes	Yes
Quantitative measurement	Yes	Yes

21.2.1.4 Scheimpflug Imaging

Scheimpflug Imaging may calculate pachymetry and topography of the anterior and posterior surfaces of the cornea. It helps in quantification of opacity in cornea and lens. It also provides an objective way to document and quantify the PC tear; it also helps to quantify the density of the associated traumatic cataract and monitor its progression over time.

However, scheimpflug system is affected by clarity of the refractive media and pupillary size [15].

21.2.2 Posterior Segment Trauma

21.2.2.1 Ultrasound of the Posterior Segment

Vitreo-retinal abnormalities have been reported to be associated with traumatic cataract as high as 20–30% cases [16]. Posterior segment structures that may be imaged in the presence of anterior segment opacity include the vitreous, retina, choroid, and the optic nerve head.

Vitreous hemorrhage: Vitreous hemorrhage is one of the commonest findings in patients with trauma. The echographic pattern of a vitreous hemorrhage depends upon its duration and severity. Fresh and mild hemorrhages appear as small dots or linear areas of low reflective mobile vitreous opacities in B Scan and as chain of low amplitude spikes on A-scan. In more severe and older hemorrhages, blood organizes and forms membranes, giving rise to increased and mixed pattern of ecogenicity on B-scan and higher reflectivity on A-scan. Old vitreous hemorrhages may also layer inferiorly (Figs. 21.7 and 21.8).

Acute vitreous hemorrhage
• Scattered, ill-defined collections of slightly echogenic opacities
• Often requires considerable increase in gain to visualize
• Demonstrates mobility in kinetic echography
Subacute/chronic vitreous hemorrhage
• Organization into more echogenic membranous structures

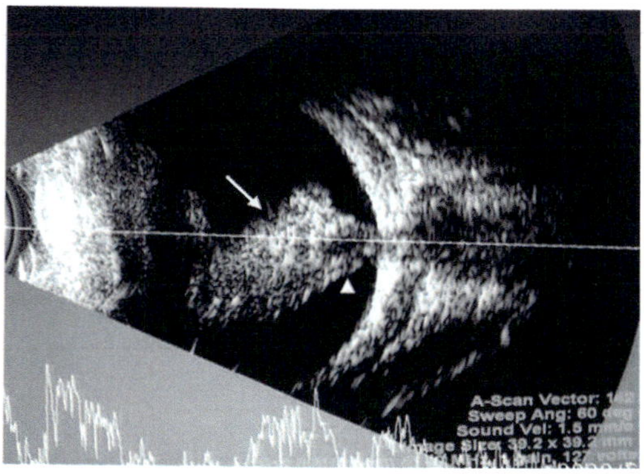

Fig. 21.7 A case of blunt ocular trauma. Ultrasound B scan shows moderate reflective dot-like echoes (arrow) along with a low reflective membrane (arrowhead) attached to the optic disc suggestive of vitreous hemorrhage with incomplete posterior vitreous detachment. The retinochoroidal thickness is increased

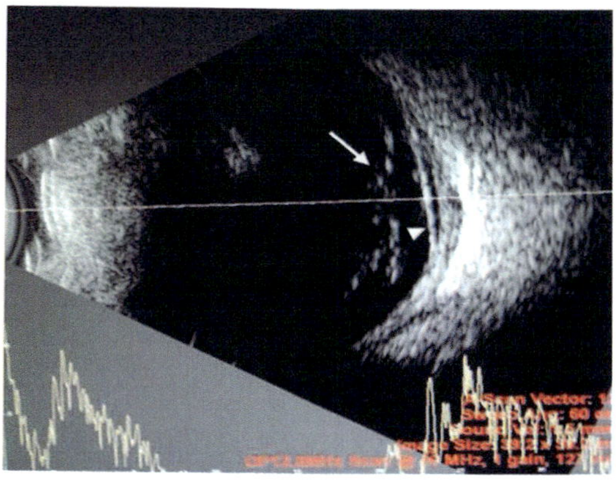

Fig. 21.8 Ultrasound B scan shows moderate reflective dot-like echoes (arrow) dispersed in vitreous cavity suggestive of vitreous hemorrhage. Note the high reflective membrane echo with limited after movement (arrowhead) and underlying moderate reflective dot-like echoes suggestive of localized retinal detachment with subretinal hemorrhage

• When severe, may obliterate vitreous body as a confluent, echogenic hematoma
• Retains mobility, but declines with age of hemorrhage

Posterior Vitreous Detachment (PVD)

Posterior vitreous detachment (PVD) is usually smooth but may be thick when blood is layered along its surface (*Ochre membrane*). Reflectivity may vary from low (in the normal eyes), to high (in dense hemorrhage). It may be attached to ONH (incomplete PVD) or separated from the ONH (complete PVD). Kinetic B-scan shows an undulating after-movement, which normally allows the PVD to differentiate from less mobile retinal detachments. On A-scan, horizontal and vertical spikes with after movement are seen.

Vitreous Traction Band and Track

Vitreous traction bands extending to an area of external wound demonstrated ultrasonically may be sign of vitreous incarceration within the wound. These bands may sometimes help identify sites of occult scleral rupture. There may be tractional retinal breaks and retinal detachment opposite to the site (Fig. 21.9). A hemorrhagic track can be seen along the path of a foreign body or a perforation. This information helps in planning further management [17].

Vitreous Base Avulsion

During blunt trauma, there is antero-posterior compression and rapid equatorial expansion. This may avulse the vitreous base from the retina and pars plana due to differences in their elasticity. Vitreous base avulsion is a sign of ocular blunt trauma ("bucket handle" sign). Vitreous base avulsion may be associated with retinal tear, retinal dialysis, or vitreous hemorrhage. Vitreous base avulsion is often difficult to capture using conventional imaging due to its peripheral location. A thorough peripheral retinal examination is helpful to diagnose in presence of clear media that may be documented with ultra-wide-field imaging techniques (e.g., Optos). Careful ultrasound B scan in suspected cases with media opacity may be helpful.

Retina and Choroid

Traumatic retinal detachment (RD) accounts for 10–40% of all retinal detachments and has been reported to occur in up to 30% of open-globe injuries and 6–36% of those with posterior segment IOFBs [18, 19]. Traumatic RD is usually rhegmatogenous or tractional. Rhegmatogenous RD typically appears as a high reflective, continuous, smooth, and somewhat folded membrane within the vitreous and attached to the disc, showing mobility on real-time ultrasonog-

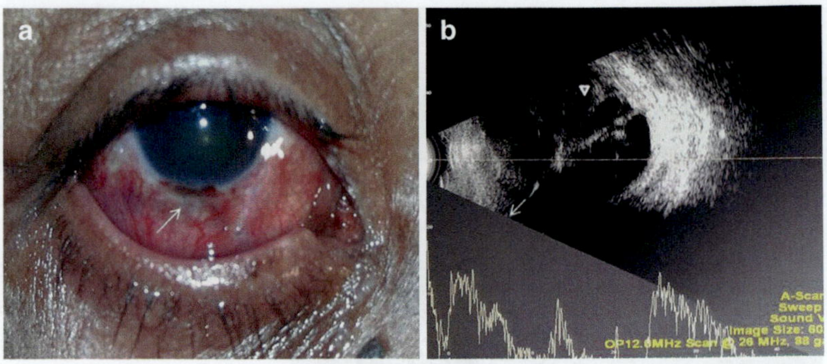

Fig. 21.9 (**a**) Case of open-globe injury (status post repair) with scleral laceration inferior to limbus (arrow). (**b**) US B scan shows vitreous tract extending anteriorly to the wound (arrow). Localized retinal traction noted posteriorly (arrowhead)

raphy. Detachment may be total, partial, or focal, depending on its extension. In cases of total or extensive retinal detachment, the detached retina appears as a "V" shape with insertion into the optic disc posteriorly and ora serrata anteriorly. On A-scan, a 100% tall spike is produced when the sound beam is directed perpendicular to the detached retina. In partial detachment, a linear echogenic membrane can be seen, usually extending to the optic nerve head, but not across it. The point of fixation at the optic nerve head is a useful feature for differentiating between retinal detachment and vitreous membrane (Fig. 21.10).

The tractional RD appears as a tented or table-top configuration with the vitreous or membranous band connected to the anterior surface. Tractional retinal detachments have limited after-movements. Traction can occur within the vitreous base either near the injury site or more commonly at the opposite quadrant.

Chronic detachment is often seen as a rigid "triangle sign." A narrow or close funnel configuration, limited after movement, with or without evidence of multiple membranous echoes and cystic changes, are signs of chronicity (Fig. 21.11).

Peripheral retinal tears and retinal dialysis may also occur in blunt trauma. Disinsertion of the peripheral retina from the ora serrata can be detected in B scan. Giant Retinal Tear may show a classical "double linear echo" sign with two high-amplitude linear echoes, one extending from the optic disc and the other almost parallel to it corresponding to the inverted posterior flap (Fig. 21.12). Echoes from PVD and inverted

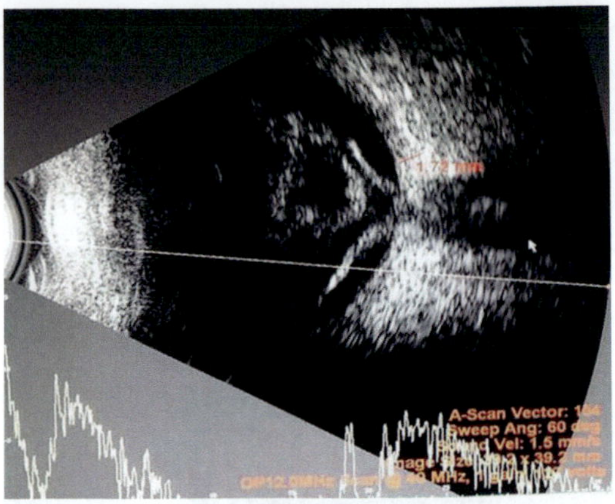

Fig. 21.10 Case of retinal detachment with vitreous hemorrhage. Note "v"-shaped high reflective membranous echo attached to disc with multiple low to moderately reflective dot echoes in vitreous cavity

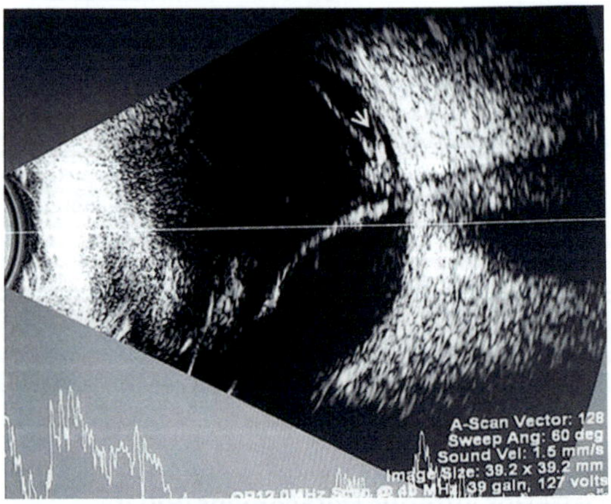

Fig. 21.11 Ultrasound B scan shows moderate reflective membranous echo (with limited after movement) and attachment to the disc suggestive of chronic retinal detachment. A subretinal gliotic band noted near the ONH suggesting chronicity (arrow)

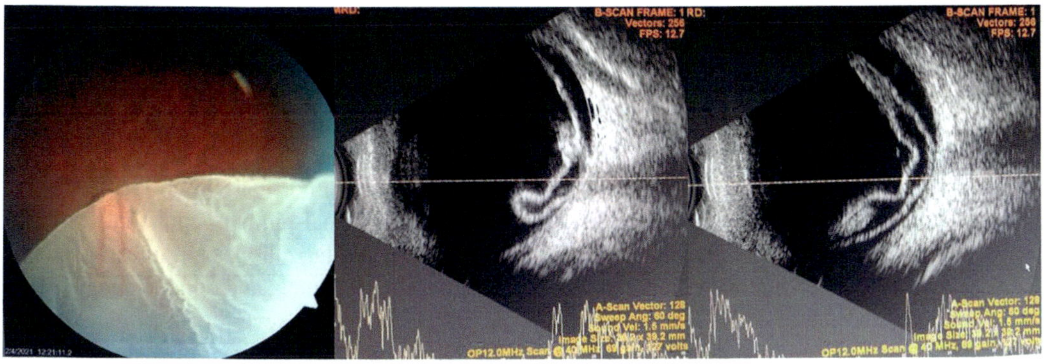

Fig. 21.12 A case of Giant Retinal tear. Note A "double linear echo" sign in B scan USG with two high-amplitude linear echoes, one extending from the optic disc and continuous with the globe contour and the other (inverted posterior flap) lying almost parallel to it and discontinuous with the globe contour

posterior flap help in differentiating it from a giant retinal dialysis.

Sometimes, RD may be associated with subretinal haemorrhage, which produces echoes in the subretinal space on B and A-scans.

Retinal Detachment (RD) Versus Posterior Vitreous Detachment (PVD)

	Retinal detachment	Posterior vitreous detachment (PVD)
• Attachment to optic disc	Attached to the optic disc	In incomplete PVD, PVD may be attached to optic disc margin. In complete PVD, it is not attached to the optic disc
• Shape	Triangular, thick folded membrane May be smooth	Usually fine, smooth/folded membrane. May be thick especially in cases with vitreous hemorrhage or fibrovascular proliferation of disc
• Character of Echo	100% amplitude compared to choroid-sclera. Persists in low gain (40–50 dB)	Usually less than 100% amplitude. Disappears at low gain (40–50 dB)
• After-movement	Limited	Good
• Associated features	May have associated vitreous or subretinal echoes s/o hemorrhage, cystic changes, subretinal or peripheral membrane with 100% amplitude or choroidal detachment	May be associated with intragel echoes, s/o hemorrhage and attachment at multiple points of retina at areas other than disc. Peripheral or anterior part of the membrane usually has <100% spike

Choroidal Detachment (CD)

CD is less common than retinal detachment. On B-scan, CD typically appears as smooth, thick, dome-shaped membranous echo in the periphery with little or no after-movement, which is limited posteriorly by the uveoscleral attachments (Fig. 21.13). They do not extend to the optic disc. On A-scan, at tissue sensitivity, thick, steeply rising 100% high spike is produced, which, on low sensitivity, shows "M" (double peak) shape. Slight vertical after-movement may be appreciated. When 360° choroidal detachment is present, transverse B-scan reveals multiple bullae, producing a scalloped appearance ("kissing choroidals") [20].

Traumatic choroidal detachments are often hemorrhagic, rather than serous. Hemorrhagic CD may be represented by low- or medium-level echoes between the choroid and the sclera. In cases of massive suprachoroidal haemorrhages, ultrasound follow-up is important in evaluating clot size and clot lysis. As the blood liquifies, the density of clot changes from high irregular internal reflectivity to a low, regular reflectivity. This helps to determine the timing for surgical intervention and the area of drainage.

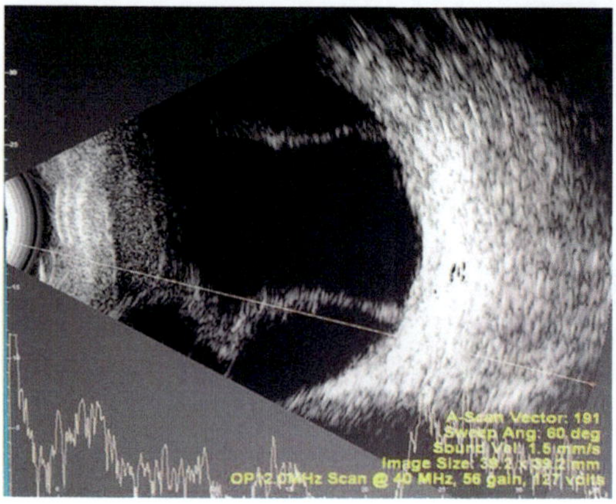

Fig. 21.13 Ultrasound B-Scan showing coroidal detachment characterized by paired, convex echogenic bands extending posteriorly from the ciliary body. Posterior extension does not reach optic disc due to the insertion of the vortex veins, to which the sclera and choroid are tightly adherent

21.2.2.2 OCT in Posterior Segment Trauma

In ocular trauma, posterior segment OCT aids in diagnosis and evaluation of Berlin's edema (commotio retinae), traumatic macular hole, preretinal or submacular hemorrhage, choroidal rupture or detachment, retinal pigment epithelial tear, subretinal neovascularization, or traumatic retinoschisis. It is easy, quick, and reliable imaging tool.

Depending on the severity of the blunt trauma, SD-OCT can reveal different optical densities of intraretinal spaces in traumatic macular edema. There may be transient hyper-reflectivity of the outer retina [21]. Mild lesions have shown transient hyper-reflectivity of the outer retina with disappearance of the hypo-reflective optical spaces, often associated with good visual prognosis. More severe trauma is accompanied by actual disruption of the IS/OS junction along with hyper-reflectivity of the overlying retina, pigment disturbance, and retinal atrophy, leading to poor visual prognosis [22] (Figs. 21.14 and 21.15).

OCT-based studies on traumatic macular hole have shown that these are more eccentric and horizontally oval, in comparison to idiopathic macular holes. This eccentricity is consistent with the tangential traction theory of development of such hole. As the equatorial horizontal diameter of the globe is longer than its vertical diameter, a stronger shearing force is more likely applied at the macula in the horizontal meridian, resulting in the greater horizontal hole diameter. Significant differences in the average size of trau-

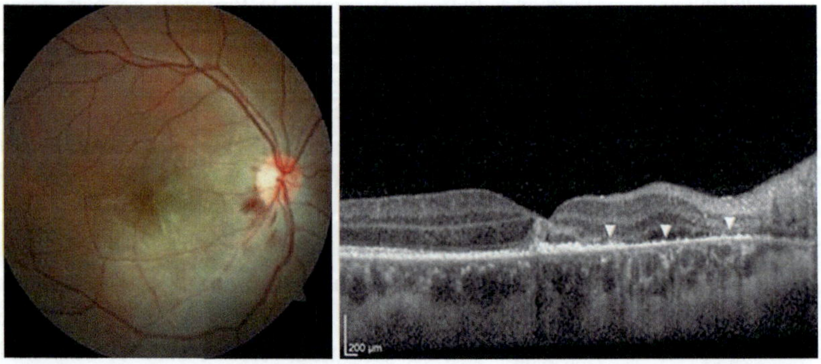

Fig. 21.14 A case of commotio retinae following blunt trauma. Color fundus photograph shows retinal whitening inferotemporal to the disc with few flame-shaped hemorrhages. Optical coherence tomography shows discontinuity of the inner segment/outer segment junction (arrowheads) at the corresponding area

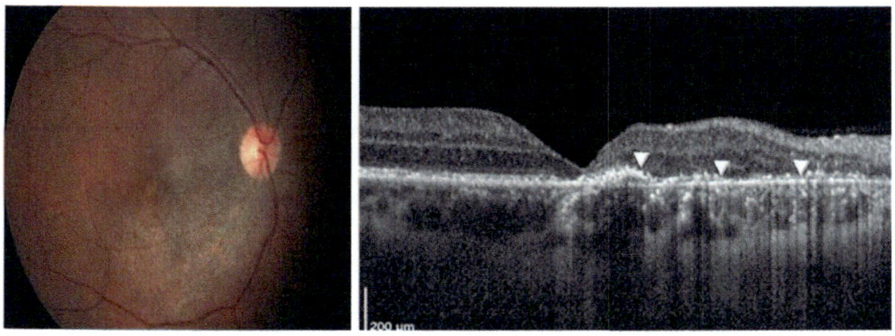

Fig. 21.15 Follow-up case of commotio retinae. Color fundus photograph shows resolution of retinal whitening and hemorrhages. Optical coherence tomography shows discontinuity of the inner segment/outer segment (IS/OS) junction (arrowheads) at the corresponding area of the commotio retinae

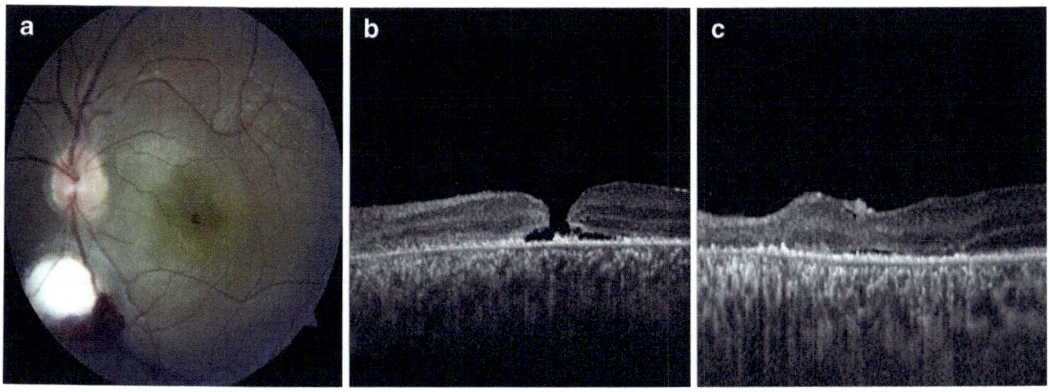

Fig. 21.16 (**a**) Color fundus photo and (**b**) Optical coherence tomography (OCT) showing traumatic macular hole, grade V retinochoroidal coloboma with adjacent hemorrhage in a young adult. (**c**) OCT shows spontaneous closure of the hole after 2 weeks

matic versus idiopathic MHs have been noted. A larger basal diameter and basal area of 1338.45 μm and 176.85 μm^2 versus 958.57 μm and 77.92 μm^2, respectively, with retinal thickness much lower at 248.4 μm compared to 408.8 μm at the edge have been reported. However, in contrast to idiopathic MHs, no correlation has been noted between visual acuity (VA) and size of the hole in cases of trauma. There may be no PVD or operculae in traumatic macular hole [23, 24]. They may close spontaneously (Fig. 21.16).

Indirect choroidal ruptures (ICRs) are characterized by discontinuities in the choroid, Bruch's membrane, and the retinal pigment epithelium (RPE). It results from concussional force in blunt trauma that transmits through the wall of the globe. Approximately 5–10% of patients with such injury may develop choroidal rupture [25]. Two patterns of choroidal ruptures on SD-OCT have been described. The first pattern (Type 1 ICR) is characterized by a forward protrusion of the retinal pigment epithelium-choriocapillaris (RPE-CC) complex associated with small discontinuity of the RPE layer or a break in the wall of the elevated RPE-CC complex. Reflectivity under the dome is variable. The second type (Type 2 ICR) is more extensive and comprises a posteriorly concave area of disruption of the RPE-CC complex. This is associated with loss of photoreceptor inner segment/outer segment and external limiting membrane reflectivity [26].

Fig. 21.17 (**a**) Right eye color fundus photo shows nonresolving retinal detachment after surgery following open-globe injury. (**b**) Left eye fundus photo showing disc hyperemia and multiple pockets of exudative detachment of the neurosensory retina suggestive of sympathetic ophthalmia

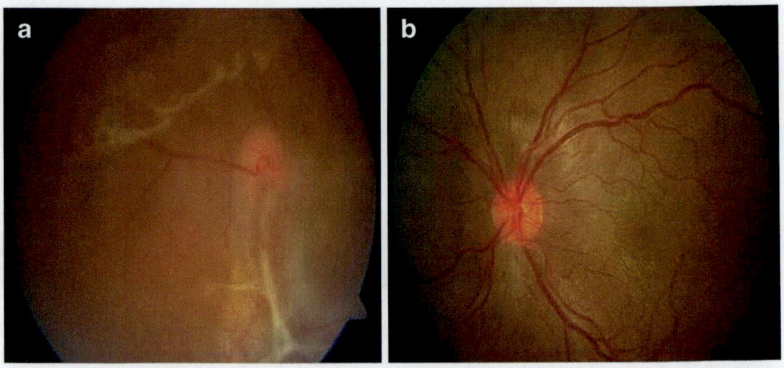

Fig. 21.18 Left eye fluorescein angiogram (**a**) early venous phase showing multiple pinpoint leaks and optic nerve head leakage, (**b**–**d**) the late phase showing dye pooling in subretinal space suggestive of sympathetic ophthalmia

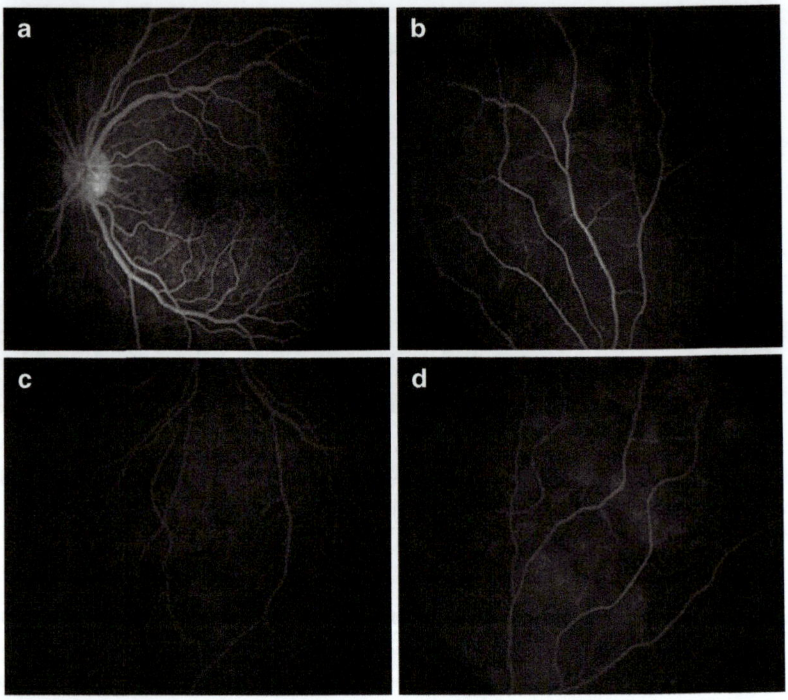

21.2.2.3 Angiography in Posterior Segment Trauma

Angiographic findings in trauma may vary depending on the severity and pattern of injury. In mild cases of blunt trauma, there may be no breakdown of the blood–retinal barrier representing normal fluorescence, while in cases of severe trauma, fluorescein leakage is observed, denoting disruption of the RPE outer blood–retinal barrier. Areas of retinal opacity with fluorescein leakage following trauma may develop a salt-and-pepper appearance, which correlate with focal loss of retinal function. In late cases of severe trauma, RPE atrophy presenting as window defects has been noted. Fluorescein angiography is highly suggestive in cases of sympathetic ophthalmia, where it presents characteristic feature of starry, pin point leakages pattern in the sympathizing eye [27, 28] (Figs. 21.17 and 21.18).

Indocyanine Green Angiography (ICG), on the other hand, helps in assessing disturbance of choroidal circulation that is vital to the outer retinal layer. Local delayed filling of choroidal vessels in the event of blunt trauma indicates choroidal insult. There might be intrachoroidal ICG leakage indicating damage to the veins

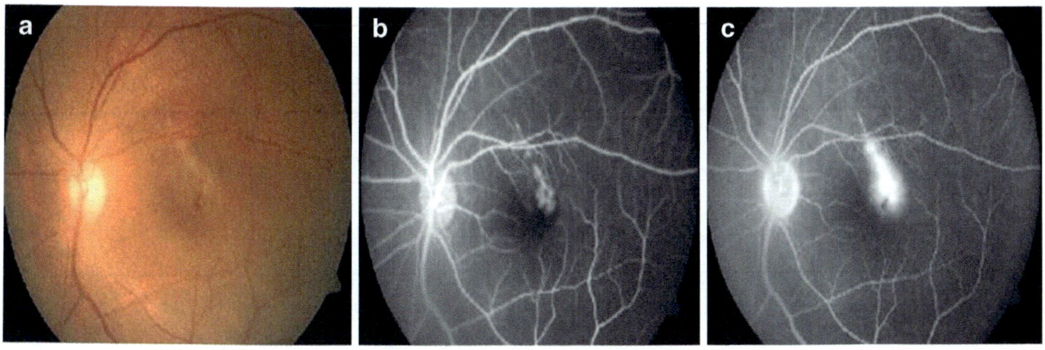

Fig. 21.19 (**a**) Color fundus photo showing choroidal rupture involving fovea, (**b**, **c**) Fluorescein angiography showing leakage of dye in the area of choroidal rupture suggesting underlying neovascularization

draining the choroid [29]. Dilation of small choroidal vessels and narrowing and irregular diameters of choriocapillaris can also be observed at leakage site, which often coincides with the fluorescein leakage.

Purtscher retinopathy has been described as a chorioretinopathy secondary to indirect trauma as in case of compression trauma. It is represented by a constellation of retinal findings including cotton-wool spots, retinal hemorrhages, optic disc edema, and Purtscher flecken. FA shows blocked choroidal fluorescence due to retinal whitening or blood, occluded retinal arterioles, capillary nonperfusion, and late leakage from the retinal vessels in areas of ischemia and optic disc edema. Acute changes (within 2 h) show masking of choroidal fluorescence in the affected area with subsequent arteriolar leakage, which may persist up to 5 months after diagnosis. Leakage from the optic nerve head is also seen. Areas of hypofluorescence have also been noted on ICGA, implying that the choroidal vasculature is also involved [30, 31].

FFA along with OCT and OCT angiography (OCT-A) are useful adjunct in follow-up cases of choroidal ruptures, which may lead to secondary CNVM (Figs. 21.19 and 21.20).

21.2.2.4 Fundus Autofluorescence in Posterior Segment Trauma

Most of the patients with closed-globe injury present with commotio retinae, which may result in posttraumatic pigment epitheliopathy (TPE) represented by areas of patchy discoloration due to RPE atrophy along with pigment clumping. In these cases, FAF imaging shows a hypoautofluorescence alternating with punctiform hyperautofluorescent lesions. If the macular region is involved, TPE may lead to poor visual prognosis [32].

FAF images also help to delineate ambiguous choroidal ruptures as hypoautofluorescent line. Healed choroidal rupture represents as hypoautofluorescent area surrounded by a hyperautofluorescent ring corresponding to RPE hyperplasia, that occurs as the rupture heals [32].

Recent subretinal or intraretinal hemorrhage presents as hypoautofluorescent lesion on FAF images and helps to define the extension of hemorrhage. As blood cells are degraded, the FAF images become hyperautofluorescent. Devitalized blood cells are considered harmful to photoreceptors in the long run and may be associated with a poor visual prognosis [32].

In Purtcher's retinopathy, FAF shows hypoautofluorescence in the areas corresponding to Purtscher's flecken, hyperautofluorescence in area affected by ischemia during the acute phase, whereas a granular pattern of hyperautofluorescence and hypoautofluorescence in the region previously affected by the Purtscher's spots after the retinopathy had been resolved [33].

Fundus autofluorescence (AF) also shows characteristic pattern in macular holes. Relative hypoautofluorescence is seen at the fovea due to the lutein and zeaxanthin pigments. However, in eyes with MH, lack of these pigments results in hyperautofluorescence. This disappears with suc-

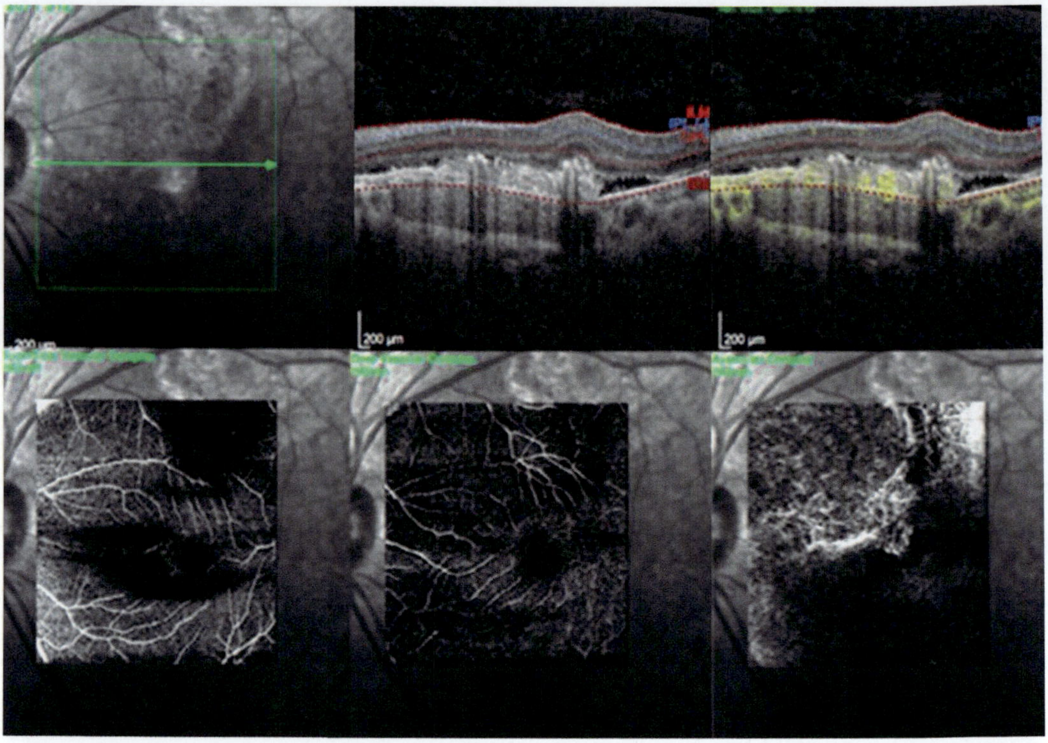

Fig. 21.20 Optical coherence tomogram angiography (OCT-A) images of choroidal neovascular membrane. The superficial and deep retinal complexes are depicted along with the avascular complex. Note the presence of CNVM in avascular complex showing loops and anastomoses. Subretinal fluid can be seen in the SD- OCT sections

cessful anatomic closure. Stellate hyperautofluorescence with striae may be noted with cysts in the outer plexiform layer and indicates better visual prognosis after surgical closure [34, 35].

21.2.3 Evaluation of Intraocular Foreign Body

Perforating injuries of the globe with retained intraocular foreign bodies most frequently result from occupational activities and hence predominantly involve males in third to fourth decade. 10–28% of blast injuries may be accompanied by ocular injuries. Open-globe injuries with intraocular or intraorbital foreign bodies are the commonest mode of presentations in such cases [36]. Intraorbital foreign bodies are present in approximately 10–17% of all ocular injuries, and as many as 41% of open-globe injuries [37]. Timely detection and management of retained foreign bodies is important, because they may lead to infection, retinal toxicity, retinal detachment, and permanent blindness, if not appropriately treated.

21.2.3.1 Ultrasound

While CT scanning is considered more sensitive in detection and localization of foreign bodies, US- B scan often complements it due to its advantages of ready availability, low cost, and nonionizing nature. Ultrasound has an edge over CT scan in precise localization of foreign bodies relative to the ocular coats and showing extent of damage to the surrounding tissues associated with an IOFB. The dynamic nature of ultrasound scores over other radiographic examination techniques [38].

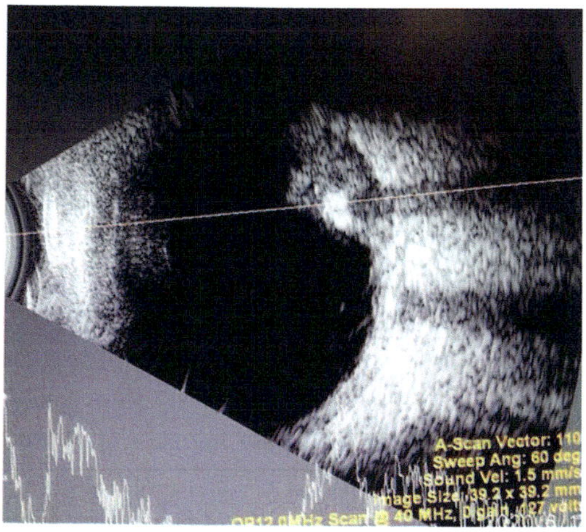

Fig. 21.21 Ultrasound B scan shows a high reflective echo (arrow) over retinal surface with back shadowing (arrowhead) suggestive of intraocular foreign body. Surrounding low-to-moderate reflective dot echoes suggestive of vitreous hemorrhage

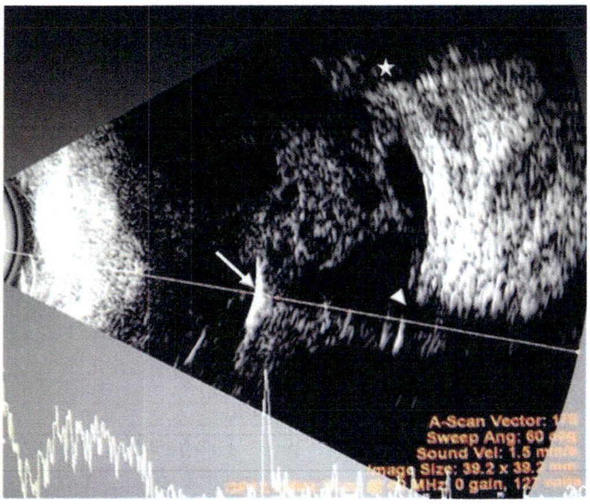

Fig. 21.22 Ultrasound B scan shows moderate reflective dot-like echoes suggestive of vitreous hemorrhage. A high reflective echo (arrow) in the vitreous cavity with back shadowing (arrowhead) suggestive of intraocular foreign body along with loss of ocular coat integrity and vitreous incarceration (star) in a case of blast injury

Metallic FBs produce steeply rising spikes with high (100%) reflectivity that persists at low gain settings even when the sensitivity is decreased by 20–30 db [20]. In addition, there is usually marked shadowing of the ocular and orbital structures posterior to the foreign body. FB <0.5 mm in diameter or very thin elongated FB, (like a metallic wire) though produces high reflective echoes, may not produce obvious shadowing. In case of a thin elongated FB cases, examination with the A-scan, using oblique sound beam, may help to confirm the foreign body. This technique is also useful in detecting foreign bodies located anteriorly, adjacent to, or within the ocular coats. Topographic and kinetic echography can show exact location and other details of a FB in relation with other intraocular structures. B-scan ultrasonography also helps to access associated intraocular pathologies like vitreous hemorrhage, retinal detachment, and choroidal detachment, to locate entry or exit wounds and status of lens (Figs. 21.21, 21.22, and 21.23).

Ultrasound can be used to differentiate a magnetic IOFB from a nonmagnetic IOFB by demonstrating movement of the IOFB in a magnetic field [39]. Standardized echography, as described

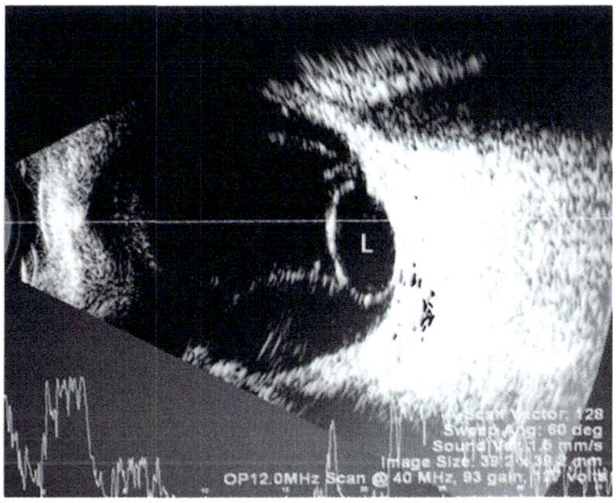

Fig. 21.23 Case of blunt ocular trauma with crystalline lens dislocation into vitreous cavity. Ultrasound B scan shows dislocated clear lens (L). Note the biconvex structure with clear-cut margins and no internal echoes

by Ossoinig, may be used to monitor the magnetic response of a foreign body to a pulsed magnet using standardized A-scan [40]. The technique of extraction of nonmagnetic foreign bodies under ultrasound guidance was described by Bronson N.R [41]. However, these techniques are rarely used in current practice.

Spherical FBs like a gunshot pellet produce echographic feature characterized by "reduplication signals." When sound waves pass through a spherical, metallic body, a portion of the sound waves reverberates within the object. When each time reverberation occurs, some of the sound energy passes back to the transducer, producing a series of echoes of decreasing amplitudes (reduplication signals). On A-scan, a long chain of spikes of decreasing amplitude is produced, whereas on B-scan, multiple, short, bright echoes appear in decreasing brightness immediately following the foreign body signal.

Glass FB usually has a smooth surface. Usually, glass enters the eye as a sliver. In such cases, when ultrasonic wave strikes the smooth surface of the FB at an oblique angle, most of the sound gets reflected away from the probe. As a result, a relatively large piece of FB may be missed or mistaken for a small FB. Therefore, when glass FB is suspected, a thorough screening with scanning perpendicular to the long flat surface of the FB should be performed.

Wood or other types of vegetative material may produce varying echographic findings. Initially, they may be highly reflectile, which decreases with time due to change in consistency and may even be difficult to detect over a period of time. Similarly, small particles lodged at or near the orbital apex may be difficult to detect due to highly reflectile surrounding tissues. In such cases, reducing and adjusting the gain against surrounding tissues may help to confirm the diagnosis.

Small air bubbles may enter the vitreous cavity as a result of penetrating ocular injury. These are highly reflective and the echographic pattern may be confusing with true foreign bodies. Air bubbles are spherical and smooth and produce echoes of similar appearance when evaluated from different probe orientations. In the vitreous cavity, they tend to float opposite to the direction of head tilt. If the diagnosis is still uncertain, follow-up examination in a day or two may be of help, as small air bubbles usually disappear with time.

21.2.3.2 Radioimaging for Foreign Body

CT scanning is the most reliable method for identification of intraocular foreign bodies. CT scan can determine location of IOFB and its relationship to the surrounding ocular structures. Both coronal and axial scans are required for exact localization. Metal foreign bodies up to 0.5 mm can be detected with CT scan, whereas stone, plastic, or wood <1.5 mm sizes are usually difficult to be visualized (Fig. 21.24).

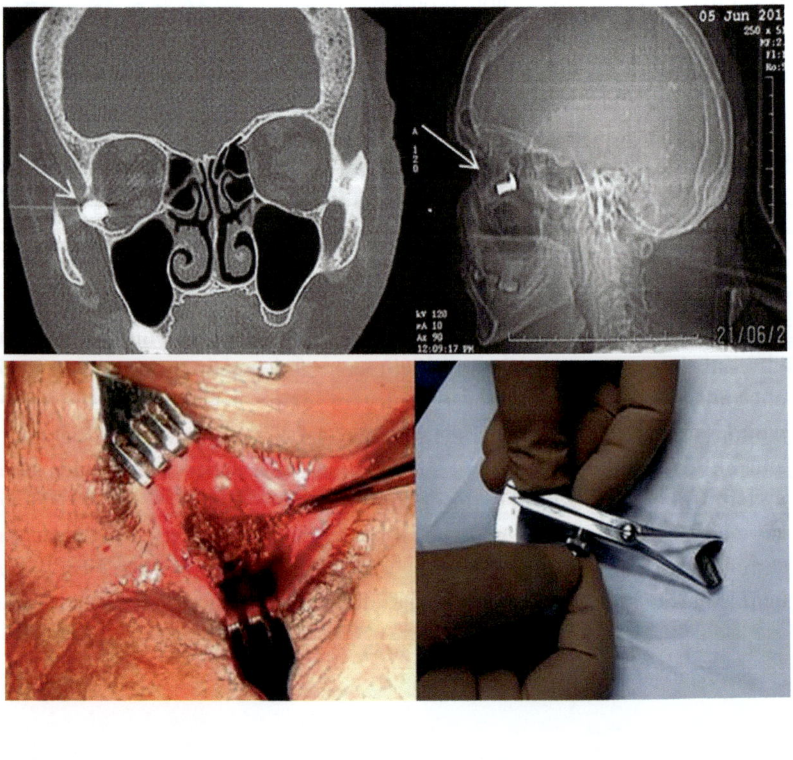

Fig. 21.24 CT scan of the radiodense foreign body in the right posterolateral part of the orbit leading to beam hardening due to metal artifact (bullet). Foreign body removed by surgical approach through the inferolateral fornix of eye (Courtesy: Dr. J K Das)

CT scan is also more sensitive in comparison to US-B scan or MRI in detecting intraocular glass fragments. Glass has attenuation coefficient of 1400–2800 HU. Studies have shown that CT can detect intraocular glass foreign bodies of 1.5-mm diameter in 96% cases, whereas glass fragments of 0.5-mm size can be detected in 48% cases. Not only the size, but also the type of glass and its location can affect detection rates [42]. Unlike metallic and glass foreign bodies, small wooden or organic foreign bodies are often missed in CT scan, which appear hypoattenuating and may be confused with air There is a wide range of attenuation of wood on CT ranging from air density (−1000 HU) to soft tissue/fluid density (+23 HU), depending upon the type of wood and amount of fluid content in it. In such situations, FB should be suspected if the low-attenuation collection displays a specific geometric margin [43].

MR imaging may be helpful in case of wooden or organic foreign bodies. On MRI, dry wood is typically hypointense to fat on both T1- and T2-weighted studies because of its high air content and presents geometric shape depending on the plane of section. On the other hand, greenwood (recently harvested) is typically hypo- or isointense on T1-weighted studies depending on the amount of hydration. Sometimes, the inflammation and edema surrounding the foreign bodies can give clue to their existence. T2-weighted or contrast-enhanced MR imaging performed with fat suppression can demonstrate an intraorbital foreign body by enhancing the inflammatory response seen surrounding the foreign body.

In cases where foreign body is associated with a hematoma, MRI can better delineate the hematoma (Fig. 21.25). Hemorrhage <7 days old is usually isointense to the cerebral white matter on T1- and T2-weighted sequences. During organization of the hemorrhage, the image becomes bright both on T1- and T2-weighted sequences. Eventually, when the hematoma is fully organized with production of hemosiderin, it becomes hypointense compared to cerebral white matter on both T1- and T2-weighted scans [44].

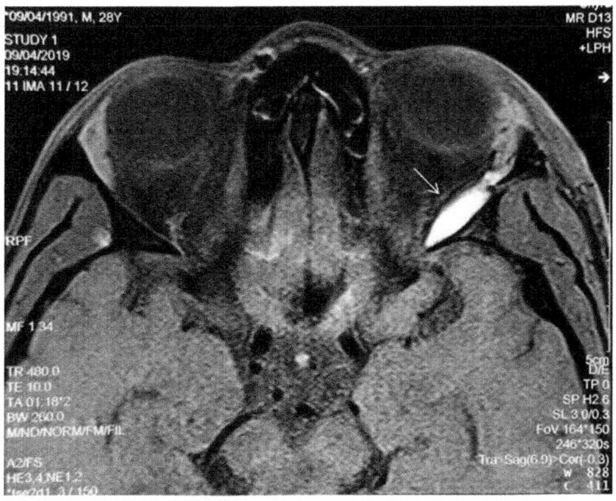

Fig. 21.25 Axial MRI (T1) image showing well-defined biconvex hyperintense lesion along left orbital wall suggestive of hematoma in the subperiosteal space

21.2.3.3 Electrophysiological Tests

ERG has specific role in follow-up and prognostic evaluation of cases with iron or copper foreign body injury to rule out metallosis.

Siderosis bulbi is caused by retention and oxidation of an iron-containing intraocular foreign body, while *Chalcosis bulbi* refers to chronic ocular inflammation due to intraocular foreign body containing copper between about 70–85%. These may develop within weeks, but the course is variable depending on the metal content in the foreign body and its location.

Iron retinotoxicity leads to a dysfunction of all the layers of the retina with more severe damage occurring in the inner retina than in the outer retina [45]. Rod-dominated responses are predominantly affected. Full-field ERG is the most common means for detecting siderosis [46]. ERG changes in the early phase (1–2 weeks) of siderosis include an increased a-wave and normal or high b-wave amplitude, followed by both diminishing b-wave and a-wave amplitude, causing the b-wave/a-wave ratio to fall as the disease progresses (1–2 year period). Eventually, the ERG becomes extinguished (Figs. 21.26 and 21.27). Serial ERGs can be helpful for following eyes with small retained foreign bodies or when diagnosis is not confirmed.

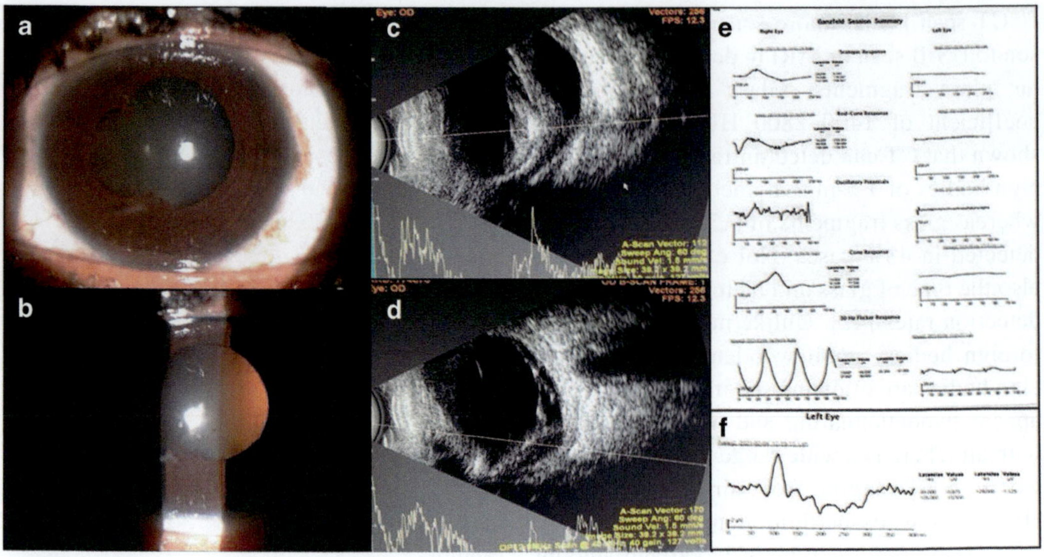

Fig. 21.26 Case with retained intraocular metallic foreign body (Left eye) showing siderotic change. Image **a** and **b** shows healed corneal wound, evidence of anterior segment inflammation with rusty pigmentation over iris and lens. US B-Scan (Image **c** and **d**) shows evidence of intraocular foreign body with vitreous hemorrhage, TRD, shallow choroidale. ERG (Image **e**) shows normal wave pattern in right eye and extinguished response in left eye suggestive of siderotic change in left eye. VEP of the same eye (Image **f**) shows normal amplitude and latency, indicating intact optic nerve function

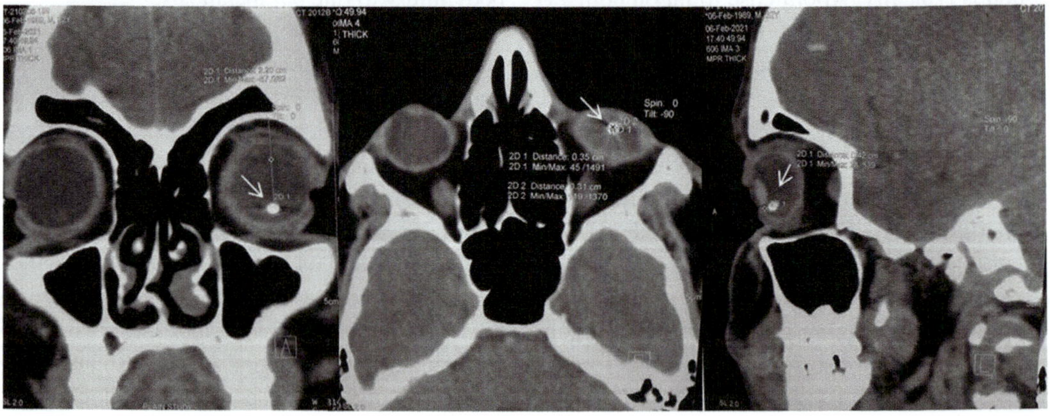

Fig. 21.27 CT Scan reveals a foreign body (3.5 × 3.1 mm) in a siderotic eye (Fig. 21.26). Left eyeball is slightly smaller with possible vitreous hemorrhage. Retrobulbar space including optic nerve is normal

Early changes in b-wave amplitude are indication for exploration and removal of the foreign body. Increased latency in mfERG may serve as an early predictor of retinal damage from siderosis when full-field ERG is normal [47].

EOG changes does not occur in eyes with metallic intraocular foreign bodies presumably because of sparing of the outer segments of the rod and the retinal pigment epithelium. EOG abnormalities indicate severe metallosis and poor visual prognosis.

Small, intraocular copper foreign bodies can be tolerated for long periods of time without significant retinal toxicity. Thus, ERG changes observed in chronic chalcosis are less severe than those seen in siderosis: very few patients with chalcosis experience more than 50% reduction in b-wave amplitude. Moreover, after the ERG amplitudes fall to a certain level, they usually remain stable without further deterioration for many years [48].

21.2.4 Globe Integrity

21.2.4.1 Ultrasound

Blunt trauma can lead to posterior scleral rupture that may sometime be difficult to detect clinically. While obvious globe rupture is a contraindication to ocular ultrasonography, less obvious cases may be incidentally detected with ultrasonography after ocular trauma. AC depth is decreased or even collapsed. AC may contain layering, homogenous echogenic debris consistent with hyphema. Globe volume is reduced with loss of spherical contour and areas of decreased reflectivity. Posterior scleral buckling associated with vitreous hemorrhage can be a sign of globe rupture. Perforating injuries often produce vitreous hemorrhage. When caused by sharp objects or FB, it usually produces a hemorrhagic track that may lead to the exit wound. A careful search should be made for a hemorrhagic track to confirm scleral integrity or an impacted IOFB. There may be traction bands or folds extending in the direction of suspected rupture. RD or CD with irregular thickening of ocular coats, intraocular or periocular air with scattered echogenicities and shadowing are other indirect signs of globe rupture (Fig. 21.28).

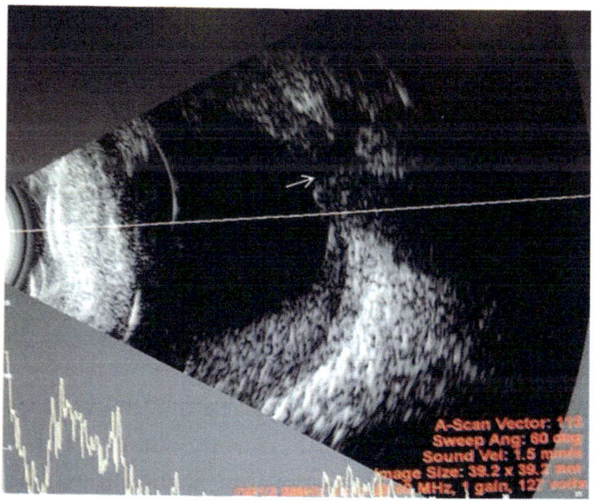

Fig. 21.28 Ultrasound B scan shows discontinuity of ocular coats suggestive of globe rupture (arrow). Also there are dot-like echoes inside the eye suggestive of vitreous hemorrhage

21.2.4.2 Radioimaging

Sensitivity of CT in detecting open-globe injuries has been reported to be approximately 71–75%, whereas specificity is approximately 93%. However, the sensitivity of CT for detecting clinically occult open-globe injuries varied from 56% to 68%, depending on the observer [49, 50].

CT findings suggestive of globe rupture include an obvious scleral discontinuity, altered anterior chamber depth (ACD), change in globe contour and globe volume (the "flat tyre" sign), and the presence of intraocular air, hemorrhage, or foreign body.

The ACD may be reduced after full-thickness corneal laceration due to extrusion of aqueous humor. Alternatively, in case of posterior scleral rupture, there is extrusion of vitreous humor causing retropulsion of the lens and resulting increase in ACD. A deep anterior chamber can be useful clue to diagnose ruptured globe on CT images. A difference in ACD of 0.4 mm or greater between the two eyes has been found to be 73% sensitive and 100% specific for the identification of globe rupture [51].

Certain nontraumatic causes (e.g., optic nerve head coloboma or posterior staphyloma) causing altered globe contour may occasionally mimic an open-globe injury. A posttraumatic orbital hematoma may also deform the globe.

MR imaging is found to be superior to CT scan in providing information about the globe outline (Fig. 21.29). However, presence of fer-

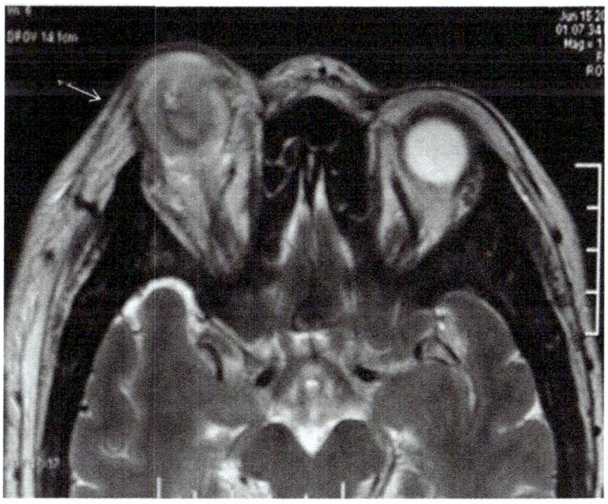

Fig. 21.29 Axial MRI (T2) scan showing distorted right globe with hematoma suggestive of globe rupture

romagnetic foreign bodies must be ruled out prior to MRI due to risk for the worsening the injury.

21.2.5 Optic Nerve Injury

21.2.5.1 Optic Nerve Avulsion

Optic nerve avulsion may occur due to sudden extreme rotation of the globe causing extreme pull on optic nerve. It is a rare presentation of ocular injury and typically results from concussion of the globe, blunt injury to the orbit, or severe facial trauma. The diagnosis in most of the cases is clinical with typical appearance of excavated optic nerve head surrounded by hemorrhage and engorged retinal vasculature [52]. However, the clinical diagnosis may be obscured by the presence of concomitant vitreous hemorrhage.

USG B scan, though not confirmatory in all cases, yet can play important role in the diagnosis. US B scan demonstrates vitreous hemorrhage overlying the site of optic nerve insertion. The optic nerve is not seen to reach the optic disc and an area of hypolucency may be seen just posterior to the optic nerve head indicating retraction of the nerve into its sheath posterior to the lamina cribrosa. A "retinal step sign," representing the transition from an edematous retina to a bare choroid, may be displayed in US B scan.

CT scan may reveal disruption of the optic nerve at its attachment to the globe. MRI may show hypointensities in the posterior globe consistent with optic nerve avulsion (ONA). However, optic nerve dural sheath usually remains attached to the globe, making diagnosis difficult [53, 54].

21.2.5.2 Traumatic Optic Neuropathy (TON)

Traumatic optic neuropathy (TON) can be classified according to the mode of injury (direct or indirect) or depending on the site of injury (optic nerve head, intraorbital, intracanalicular, or intracranial) [55, 56].

Direct TON may be caused by a projectile penetrating the orbit or as a result of optic nerve avulsion. It is associated with significant anatomical disruption to the optic nerve. Indirect TON is caused by the transmission of forces to the skull in cases of blunt trauma. The intracanalicular segment of the optic nerve is more vulnerable to this form of injury [57]. Indirect TON is the more common occurrence and is associated with 0.5–5% of all closed head trauma cases, and in 2.5% of those with midfacial fractures [58].

VEP in TON

Flash visual-evoked potentials (FVEPs) are not only helpful in diagnosis of traumatic optic neuropathy, but also highly predictive of the degree of visual function in TON. The amplitude in TON is found to be significantly lower in comparison to those with other causes of ON [59]. FVEP amplitudes that are at least 50% of the normal eye in unilateral TON appear to be critical in anticipating good, long-term visual outcome [60]. Automated visual field testing such as Humphrey (HVF) can be used to characterize visual field defects/scotomas in patients with TON over time.

Radioimaging in TON

When traumatic optic neuropathy is suspected, special attention should be paid to the intraorbital and intracanalicular segments of the optic nerve. A displaced bone fragment or compression due to associated intracanalicular hematoma from a fracture in the canal may lead to optic nerve injury. Orbital CT scan allows assessment of the integrity of the optic nerve, presence of an optic nerve sheath hematoma, intraconal emphysema, and optic canal injury. CT of the orbit with coronal and axial thin sections [0.6–1 mm] through the optic canal is crucial to visualize the optic nerve as well as the optic canal for evidence of a hematoma or bony fragments impinging on the optic nerve. CT may also show orbital fat-stranding around the nerve with a linear hypodensity near its attachment to the globe [61].

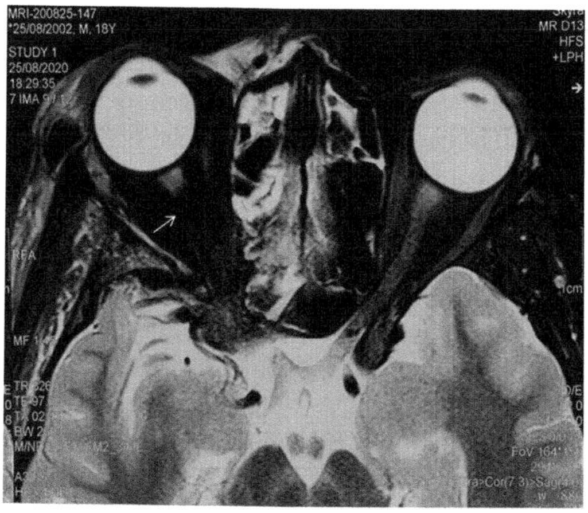

Fig. 21.30 Axial MRI Orbit (T2) shows discontinuity of optic nerve on the right with hyperintensity in the region of optic nerve canal suggestive of optic nerve edema

MRI in TON demonstrates hyperintense T2 signal along with diffusion restriction within the affected optic nerve. However, these findings are nonspecific and should be correlated clinically [62, 63] (Fig. 21.30).

There are some other distinctive conditions related to optic nerve injury that may be recognized by neuro-imaging using CT or MRI scanning [64].

Optic nerve transection may occur as a rare complication of orbital fracture and midfacial trauma. CT scanning may detect a bone fragment transecting the optic nerve, while MRI may help to locate the defect in the Optic nerve.

Optic nerve sheath hemorrhage may cause potentially reversible vision loss and may be difficult to recognize clinically. An expanded nerve sheath with shaggy irregularity and adjacent fat stranding detected on CT or MRI imaging helps in diagnosing hematoma in the optic nerve sheath.

21.2.6 Orbital Imaging

21.2.6.1 Orbital Hemorrhage

Orbital hemorrhage may be diffuse or localized to the orbit. There is usually associated proptosis and ophthalmoplegia. On contrast-enhanced CT, there may be heterogeneous density depending upon its location in the orbit. The hematomas represent variable density compared to the enhancing extraocular muscles. On MRI, hematomas represent variable signal intensity depending upon its duration. On T1- weighted images, a hyperacute hematoma may have low signal, and high signal in the subacute (3–7 days) phase. Conversely, on T2-weighted images, the hematoma commonly presents high signal in the hyperacute phase, and low signal in the subacute phase [65].

21.2.6.2 Orbital Fracture

CT is the primary method for the identification of facial and orbital fractures. CT scan can often be helpful in demonstrating entrapped extraocular muscles in the fracture site. CT typically demonstrates linear floor fractures with minimal displacement and little or no soft tissue displacement into the maxillary antrum. However, associated soft tissue swelling, muscle hematoma, or fat stranding can make radiographic interpretation difficult. This emphasizes the importance of clinical correlation. Finally, CT can also be used to estimate the fracture area, which can be utilized as criterion for operative repair [66].

Orbital floor fractures are common in the relatively thinner posterior part of the floor. Orbital blowout fractures refer to the fractures of orbital floor that do not involve the orbital rim. The CT findings demonstrate a downward curvature of the orbital floor with bony discontinuity and displacement of fragments into the maxillary sinus. Prolapse of orbital fat, entrapment of inferior rectus muscle, opacification of the maxillary sinus with or without fluid level may be associated finding. Trapdoor fractures in children may not be easily noticed in CT scans. In such cases, “teardrop sign,” “missing rectus sign,” movement restriction, forced duction test, and oculocardiac reflex can be clue to diagnosing the fractures.

In medial wall fractures, “orbital emphysema” may be seen in addition to bony discontinuity.

Optic canal fractures should be suspected in cases of head injuries associated with impaired vision. Soft-tissue density within ethmoid sinus detected on the CT scan due to presence of blood can be helpful clue to detect optic canal fracture. Thin-sections in CT scan of the orbital apex and anterior clinoid process may demonstrate fractures at the optic canal [67].

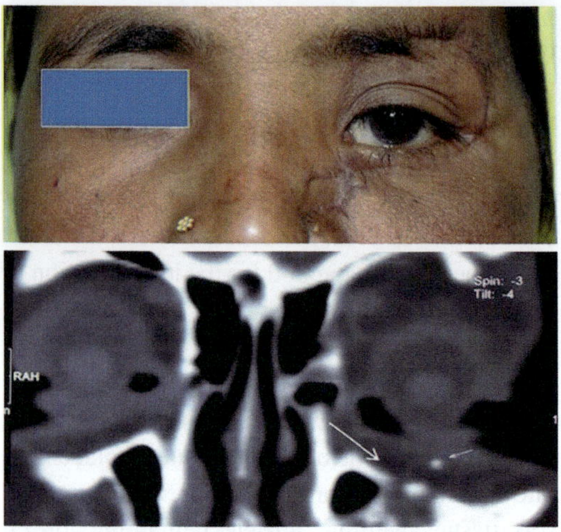

Fig. 21.31 External photograph of the patient showing scar along the injury site. Coronal CT scan of brain and orbit showing orbital floor fracture, hypoglobus, and radiodense fracture fragments

CT scan can also be employed for intraoperative navigation in cases of orbitofacial fractures with 3-D modeling, in which images are acquired in the 0.6–1 mm formats. 3D reconstructions also help in patient information and treatment planning (Figs. 21.31 and 21.32).

21.2.6.3 Orbital Emphysema

Orbital emphysema is a clinical entity in the setting of injury involving the paranasal sinuses. A hair-line fracture of the thin bony wall may produce a "ball-valve" effect leading to accumulation of air in the orbit. CT is effective in identifying the fracture as well presence and location of air when orbital emphysema is suspected. In true orbital emphysema, air is located behind an intact orbital septum, which occurs following fracture of an orbital wall and tearing of the sinus mucosa. Palpebral emphysema, where subcutaneous air remains restricted to the eyelid, is a rare event arising from disruption of the lacrimal sac and bone. Occasionally, wooden foreign body can mimic the presence of orbital emphysema in CT scan [68]. In such cases, a

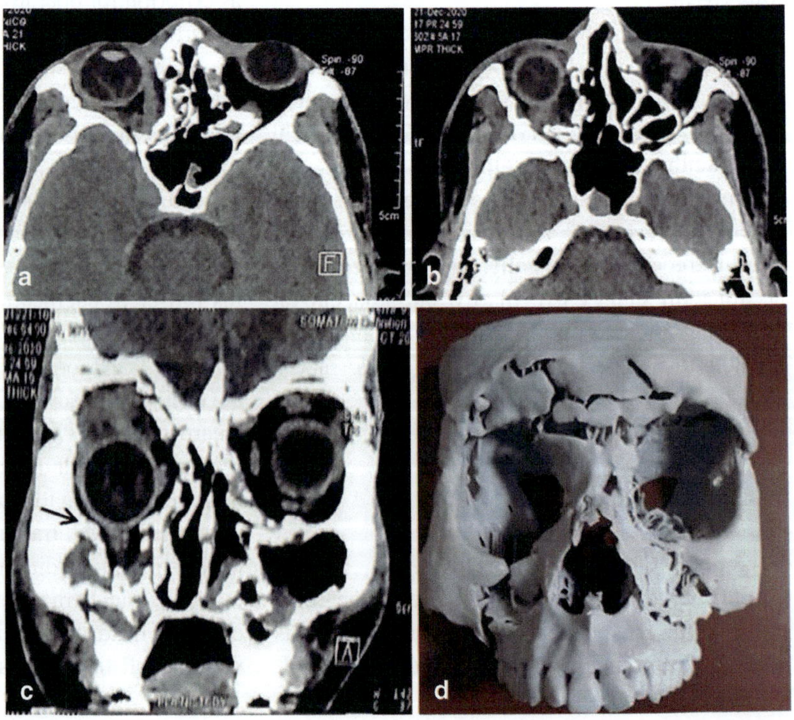

Fig. 21.32 Image **a–c**: CT scan (axial and coronal) showing comminuted fracture involving walls of both orbit, maxillary, frontal, and ethmoidal sinuses. There is herniation of orbital contents into maxillary antrum through fractured floor of right orbit (**c**, black arrow). There is evidence of vitreous hemorrhage in right eye. (**d**) 3-D printed model of CT scan showing fractures for planning surgical management

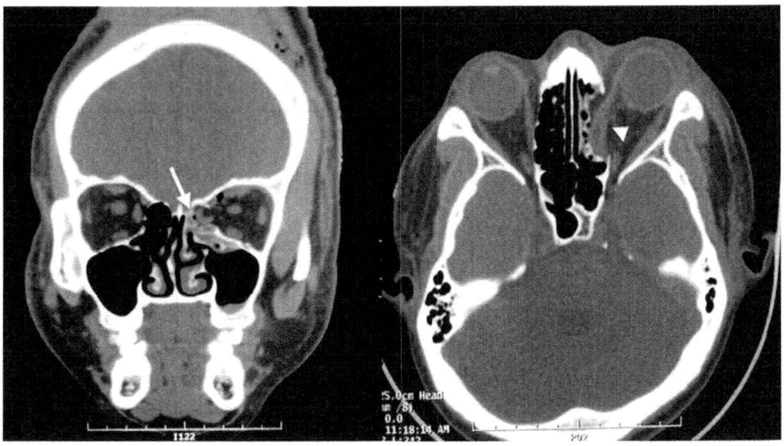

Fig. 21.33 Coronal and Axial CT images showing medial orbital wall fracture with herniation of the medial rectus and orbital soft tissue (arrow and arrowhead) into the fracture site

careful history and MRI scanning is helpful in making the correct diagnosis.

21.2.6.4 Orbital Compartment Syndrome

Orbital compartment syndrome results from a rise in pressure within a tight anatomical space leading to damage to the vital structure contained therein. Normal intraorbital pressure has been measured at 3–6 mmHg [69]. In traumatic setting, this tissue pressure can elevate above arterial pressure. Irreversible visual loss can occur after 60–100 min of raised orbital pressure due to obstruction in blood flow [70]. The initial management of orbital compartment syndrome is usually clinical. Imaging may be indicated when initial decompressive measures fail. CT is the preferred modality. Imaging may reveal large subperiosteal hematoma and tenting of the posterior globe. A posterior globe contour angle of less than 120° with proptosis has been shown to carry a poorer prognosis of visual recovery [71]. CT can also identify a retrobulbar hemorrhage, foreign body, or emphysema. MRI is rarely indicated in the acute case of compartment syndrome. If used, it may provide additional clues regarding the age of a hematoma.

21.2.6.5 Extraocular Muscle Injury

Extraocular muscles can be entrapped, avulsed, or lacerated from trauma. The muscle injuries are often located at or near their tendon insertion. A lacerated or avulsed muscle typically presents with weakness or loss of movement in the cardinal direction of the involved muscle. MRI is superior in detecting muscle contour irregularity in case of a lacerated muscle. While CT has high sensitivity (>70%), in detecting muscle entrapment, its sensitivity in detecting muscle laceration or intramuscular injury is much lower in comparison to MRI (Fig. 21.33).

21.2.6.6 Carotid Cavernous Fistula

Carotid cavernous fistulas consist of abnormal communication between the internal carotid arterial system and the cavernous sinus. Carotid cavernous fistulas can be classified etiologically as traumatic or spontaneous, hemodynamically as high flow or low flow, and anatomically as direct or dural [72].

High-flow, direct "Type A" carotid cavernous fistulas are classically seen following head trauma, and they represent 70–90% of all carotid cavernous fistulas. They often present days or weeks after head injury with a triad of pulsating exophthalmos, conjunctival chemosis with arterialization, and orbital bruit. If not treated, progressive visual loss may ensue [73]. The diagnosis of direct carotid cavernous fistula can be made with orbital US–B Scan, CT, or MRI. Findings of a dilated superior ophthalmic vein along with diffuse enlargement of the extraocular muscles are suggestive of a carotid cavernous fistula in the

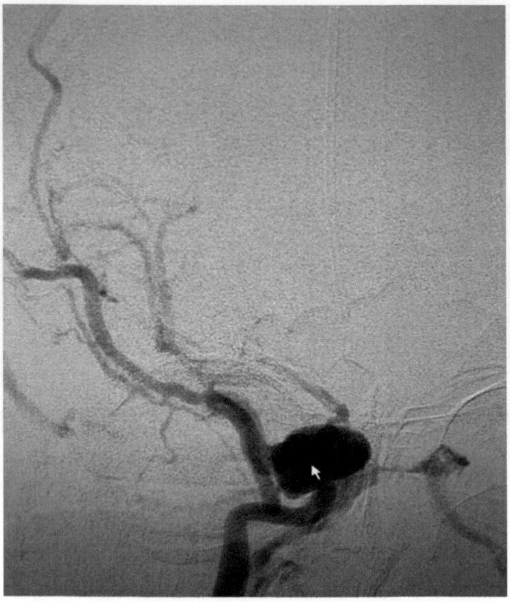

Fig. 21.34 Digital subtraction angiography (DSA) scan showing dilated cavernous sinus due to backflow from the intra-cavernous internal carotid artery segment suggestive of a carotico-cavernous fistula (direct type) following blunt trauma to head (Courtesy: Dr. Aditi M Grewal)

context of trauma. However, isolated dilatation of the superior ophthalmic vein may also be seen in some other conditions, including cavernous sinus thrombosis, Graves disease, venous varix, and occasionally as a normal variant. CT angiography or, more definitively, conventional angiography are confirmatory tests for diagnosis of carotid cavernous fistula (Fig. 21.34).

21.3 Conclusion

Vision loss in the setting of trauma is common and can result from a multiple mechanisms. A comprehensive knowledge of various imaging techniques, their relative and absolute contraindications, and interpretation, coupled with their judicious and appropriate use, aids in developing a holistic diagnosis of severity of trauma. This in turn aids in planning most appropriate treatment, prognostication, and patient counseling that helps deliver the most appropriate care for the patient.

References

1. Koo L, Kapadia MK, Singh RP, Sheridan R, Hatton MP. Gender differences in etiology and outcome of open globe injuries. J Trauma. 2005;59(1):175–8.
2. Guly CM, Guly HR, Bouamra O, Gray RH, Lecky FE. Ocular injuries in patients with major trauma. Emerg Med J. 2006;23(12):915–7.
3. Mundt GH, Hughes WF. Ultrasonics in ocular diagnosis. Am J Ophthalmol. 1956;42:488–98.
4. Baum G, Greenwood I. The application of ultrasonic locating techniques to ophthalmology. II. Ultrasonic slit-lamp in the ultrasonic visualization of soft tissues. Arch Ophthalmol. 1958;60:263–79.
5. Anvari A, Forsberg F, Samir AE. A primer on the physical principles of tissue harmonic imaging. Radiographics. 2015;35(7):1955–64.
6. Pavlin CJ, Harasiewicz K, Sherar MD, Foster FS. Clinical use of ultrasound biomicroscopy. Ophthalmology. 1991;98:287–95.
7. Izatt JA, Hee MR, Swanson EA, et al. Micrometer-scale resolution imaging of the anterior eye in vivo with optical coherence tomography. Arch Ophthalmol. 1994;112:1584–9.
8. Brunk UT, Wihlmark U, Wrigstad A, et al. Accumulation of lipofuscin within retinal pigment epithelial cells results in enhanced sensitivity to photo-oxidation. Gerontology. 1995;41(Suppl 2):201–12.
9. Hall EJ, Brenner DJ. Cancer risks from diagnostic radiology. Br J Radiol. 2008;81(965):362–78. https://doi.org/10.1259/bjr/01948454.
10. Vodapalli H, Murthy SI, Jalali S, Ali MJ, Rani PK. Comparison of immersion ultrasonography, ultrasound biomicroscopy and anterior segment optical coherence tomography in the evaluation of traumatic phacoceles. Indian J Ophthalmol. 2012;60(1):63–5.
11. Wang K, Liu J, Chen M. Role of B-scan ultrasonography in the localization of intraocular foreign bodies in the anterior segment: a report of three cases. BMC Ophthalmol. 2015;15:102; Published 2015 Aug 14. https://doi.org/10.1186/s12886-015-0076-1.
12. Nouby Mahmoud G, Silverman RH, Coleman DJ. Using high-frequency ultrasound to characterize intraocular foreign bodies. Ophthalmic Surg. 1993;24:94–9.
13. Deramo VA, Shah GK, Baumal CR, Fineman MS, Corrêa ZM, et al. Ultrasound biomicroscopy as a tool for detecting and localizing occult foreign bodies after ocular trauma. Ophthalmology. 1999;106:301–5.
14. McGwin G, Owsley C. Incidence of emergency department-treated eye in the United States. Arch Ophthalmol. 2005;123:662–6.
15. Magalhaes FP, Costa EF, Cariello AJ, Rodrigues EB, Hofling-Lima AL. Comparative analysis of the nuclear lens opalescence by the lens opacities classification system III with nuclear density values provided by oculus Pentacam: a cross-section study using Pentacam nucleus staging software. Arq Bras Oftalmol. 2011;74:110–3.

16. Kaskalogu M. US findings in eyes with traumatic cataracts. Am J Ophthalmol. 1985;9:496.
17. Susheel, Chugh JP, Verma M. Role of ultrasonography in ocular trauma. Indian J Radiol Imaging. 2001;11(2):75–9.
18. Balles MW. Traumatic retinopathy. In: Albert DM, Jakobiec FA, editors. Principles and practice of ophthalmology, vol. 2. Philadelphia, PA: WB Saunders; 1994. p. 1029–31.
19. Wickham L, Xing W, Bunce C, Sullivan P. Outcomes of surgery for posterior segment intraocular foreign bodies—a retrospective review of 17 years of clinical experience. Graefes Arch Clin Exp Ophthalmol. 2006;244(12):1620–6.
20. Kaur I, Kaur P, Handa A, Agrawal P. Diagnostic and therapeutic role of B scan ultrasonography in traumatized eyes. J Evol Med Dent Sci. 2014;3:3543–50.
21. Saleh M, Letsch J, Bourcier T, Munsch C, Speeg-Schatz C, Gaucher D. Long-term outcomes of acute traumatic maculopathy. Retina. 2011;31(10):2037–43.
22. Souza-Santos F, Lavinsky D, Moraes NS, Castro AR, Cardillo JA, Farah ME. Spectral-domain optical coherence tomography in patients with commotio retinae. Retina. 2012;32(4):711–8.
23. Huang J, Liu X, Wu Z, Sadda S. Comparison of full-thickness traumatic macular holes and idiopathic macular holes by optical coherence tomography. Graefes Arch Clin Exp Ophthalmol. 2010;248(8):1071–5.
24. Bekerman I, Gottlieb P, Vaiman M. Variations in eyeball diameters of the healthy adults. J Ophthalmol. 2014;2014:503645, 5 pages
25. Bressler NM, Bressler SB, Gragoudas ES. Clinical characteristics of choroidal neovascular membranes. Arch Ophthalmol. 1987;105(2):209–13.
26. Nair U, Soman M, Ganekal S, Batmanabane V, Nair K. Morphological patterns of indirect choroidal rupture on spectral domain optical coherence tomography. Clin Ophthalmol. 2013;7:1503–9. https://doi.org/10.2147/OPTH.S46223.
27. Duke-Elder S, MacFaul PA. Contusion effects on the choroid: contusion effects on the retina. In: Duke-Elder S, editor. System of ophthalmology, vol. 14, Part 1. London: Henry Kimpton; 1972. p. 150–87.
28. Yamana T. Retinochoroidal lesions in concussional injuries of the eyes: an experimental study. Acta Soc Ophthalmol Jpn. 1981;90:1049–66.
29. Yannuzzi LA, Slakter JS, Sorenson JA, Guyer DR, Orlock DA. Digital indocyanine green videoangiography and choroidal neovascularization. Retina. 1992;12:191–223.
30. Beckingsale AB, Rosenthal AR. Early fundus fluorescein angiographic findings and sequelae in traumatic retinopathy: case report. Br J Ophthalmol. 1983;67(2):119–23.
31. Gomez-Ulla FB, Torreiro MG, Salorio MSGF. Choroidal vascular abnormality in Purtscher's retinopathy shown by indocyanine green angiography. Am J Ophthalmol. 1996;122(2):261–3.
32. Lavinsky D, Martins EN, Cardillo JA, Farah ME. Fundus autofluorescence in patients with blunt ocular trauma. Acta Ophthalmol. 2011;89:e89–94.
33. Guerra RL, Silva IS, Marback EF, Maia Ode O Jr, Marback RL. Fundus autofluorescence in blunt ocular trauma. Arq Bras Oftalmol. 2014;77:139–42.
34. Wakabayashi T, Ikuno Y, Sayanagi K, Soga K, Oshima Y, Tano Y. Fundus autofluorescence related to retinal morphological and functional changes in idiopathic macular holes. Acta Ophthalmol. 2008;86(8):897–901.
35. Ciardella AP, Lee GC, Langton K, Sparrow J, Chang S. Autofluorescence as a novel approach to diagnosing macular holes. Am J Ophthalmol. 2004;137(5):956–9.
36. Morley MG, Nguyen JK, Heier JS, Shingleton BJ, Pasternak JF, Bower KS. Blast eye injuries: a review for first responders. Disaster Med Public Health Prep. 2010;4(2):154–60.
37. Pinto A, Brunese L, Daniele S, et al. Role of computed tomography in the assessment of intraorbital foreign bodies. Semin Ultrasound CT MR. 2012;33(5):392–5.
38. Zacks DN, Hart L, Young LH. Ultrasonography in the traumatized eye: intraocular foreign body versus artifact. Int Ophthalmol Clin. 2002;42(3):121–34.
39. Coleman DJ, Trokel SL. A protocol for B-scan and radiographic foreign body localization. Am J Ophthalmol. 1971;71(1):84–9.
40. Ossoinig KC. The evaluation of kinetic properties ofecho signals. In: Oksala A, Gernet H, editors. Ultrasonics in ophthalmology. Basel: Karger; 1967. p. 88–96.
41. Bronson NR. Managementof intraocular foreign bodies. Am J Opthalmol. 1968;66(2):279–84.
42. Gor DM, Kirsch CF, Leen J, et al. Radiologic differentiation of intraocular glass: evaluation of imaging techniques, glass types, size, and effect of intraocular hemorrhage. AJR Am J Roentgenol. 2001;177:1199–203.
43. Go JL, Vu VN, Lee KJ, Becker TS. Orbital trauma. Neuroimaging Clin N Am. 2002;12:311–24.
44. Gomori JM, Grossman RI, Goldberg HI, Zimmerman RA, Bilaniuk LT. Intracranial hematomas: imaging by high-field MR. Radiology. 1985;157:87–93.
45. Imaizumi M, Matsumoto CS, Yamada K, Nanba Y, Takaki Y, Nakatsuka K. Electroretinographic assessment of early changes in ocular siderosis. Ophthalmologica. 2000;214(5):354–9.
46. Faure C, Gocho K, Le Mer Y, Sahel JA, Paques M, Audo I. Functional and high resolution retinal imaging assessment in a case of ocular siderosis. Doc Ophthalmol. 2014;128(1):69–75.
47. Gupta S, Midha N, Gogia V, Sahay P, Pandey V, Venkatesh P. Sensitivity of multifocal electroretinography (mfERG) in detecting siderosis. Can J Ophthalmol. 2015;50(6):485–90. https://doi.org/10.1016/j.jcjo.2015.08.011.
48. Rosenthal AR, Marmor MF, Leuenberger P. Chalcosis: a study of natural history. Ophthalmology. 1979;86:1956–72.

49. Joseph DP, Pieramici DJ, Beauchamp NJ. Computed tomography in the diagnosis and prognosis of open globe injuries. Ophthalmology. 2000;107:1899–906.
50. Arey ML, Mootha VV, Whittemore AR, et al. Computed tomography in the diagnosis of occult open globe injuries. Ophthalmology. 2007;114:1448–52.
51. Lee HJ, Jilani M, Frohman L, Baker S. CT of orbital trauma. Emerg Radiol. 2004;10:168–72.
52. Roth DB, Warman R. Optic nerve avulsion from a golfing injury. Am J Ophthalmol. 1999;128:657–8.
53. Williams DF, Williams GA, Abrams GW, et al. Evulsion of the retina associated with optic nerve evulsion. AMJ Ophthalmol. 1987;104:5–9.
54. Foster BS, March GA, Lucarelli MJ, et al. Optic nerve avulsion. Arch Ophthalmol. 1997;115:623–30.
55. Sarkies N. Traumatic optic neuropathy. Eye. 2004;18:1122–5.
56. Steinsapir KD, Goldberg RA. Traumatic optic neuropathy. Surv Ophthalmol. 1994;38:487–518.
57. Anderson RL, Panje WR, Gross CE. Optic-nerve blindness following blunt forehead trauma. Ophthalmology. 1982;89:445–55.
58. Carta A, Ferrigno L, Salvo M, Bianchi-Marzoli S, Boschi A, Carta F. Visual prognosis after indirect traumatic optic neuropathy. J Neurol Neurosurg Psychiatry. 2003;74(2):246–8. https://doi.org/10.1136/jnnp.74.2.246.
59. Ikejiri M, Adachi-Usami E, Mizota A, Tsuyama Y, Miyauchi O, Suehiro S. Pattern visual evoked potentials in traumatic optic neuropathy. Ophthalmologica. 2002;216(6):415–9.
60. Holmes MD, Sires BS. Flash visual evoked potentials predict visual outcome in traumatic optic neuropathy. Ophthalmic Plast Reconstr Surg. 2004;20(5):342–6. https://doi.org/10.1097/01.IOP.0000134272.55294.4C.
61. Bodanapally UK, Van der Byl G, Shanmuganathan K, Katzman L, Geraymovych E, Saksobhavivat N, Mirvis SE, Sudini KR, Krejza J, Shin RK. Traumatic optic neuropathy prediction after blunt facial trauma: derivation of a risk score based on facial CT findings at admission. Radiology. 2014;272(3):824–31. https://doi.org/10.1148/radiol.14131873.
62. Nguyen VD, Singh AK, Altmeyer WB, Tantiwongkosi B. Demystifying orbital emergencies: a pictorial review. Radiographics. 2017;37(3):947–62. https://doi.org/10.1148/rg.2017160119.
63. Bodanapally UK, Shanmuganathan K, Shin RK, Dreizin D, Katzman L, Reddy RP, Mascarenhas D. Hyperintense optic nerve due to diffusion restriction: diffusion-weighted imaging in traumatic optic neuropathy. AJNR Am J Neuroradiol. 2015;36(8):1536–41. https://doi.org/10.3174/ajnr.A4290.
64. Sarkies NJC. Neuro-ophthalmological aspects of head injury. In: Macfarlane R, Hardy D, editors. Outcome after head neck and spinal trauma. Oxford: Butterworth Heinemann; 1977. p. 163–77.
65. Atalla ML, McNab AA, Sullivan TJ, et al. Nontraumatic subperiosteal orbital hemorrhage. Ophthalmology. 2001;108(1):183–9.
66. Borstedt KJ, Alinasab B. The measurement of orbital blowout fractures cannot be made with geometric estimations. Otorhinolaryngol Head Neck Surg. 2019;4:1–6. https://doi.org/10.15761/OHNS.1000220.
67. American Academy of Ophthalmology. Section 7: Orbit, eyelid and lacrimal system. In: Levine LM, editor. Basic and clinical science course. San Francisco: American Academy of Ophthalmology; 2016–2017. p. 94–101.
68. Birrer RB, Robinson T, Papachristos P. Orbital emphysema: how common, how significant? Ann Emerg Med. 1994;24(6):1115–8.
69. Kratky V, Hurwitz JJ, Avram DR. Orbital compartment syndrome. Direct measurement of orbital tissue pressure. Can J Ophthalmol. 1990;25:293–7.
70. Hayreh SS, Kolder WE, Weingeist TA. Central retinal artery occlusion and retinal tolerance time. Ophthalmology. 1980;87:75–8.
71. Dalley RW, Robertson WD, Rootman J. Globe tenting: a sign of increased orbital tension. AJNR Am J Neuroradiol. 1989;10:181–6.
72. Barrow DL, Spector RH, Braun IF, et al. Classification and treatment of spontaneous carotid-cavernous sinus fistulas. J Neurosurg. 1985;62:248–56.
73. Biousse V, Mendicino ME, Simon DJ, et al. The ophthalmology of intracranial vascular abnormalities. Am J Ophthalmol. 1998;125:527–44.

22 Prevention of Ocular Injuries in the Armed Forces and Rehabilitation of the Visually Impaired

Supriya Phadke, Parikshit Gogate, Muskan Shaikh, Amruta Chavan, Siddharth Gogate, and O. K. Radhakrishnan

Eyes occupy only 0.1% of the total and 0.27% of the anterior body surface area; however, ocular trauma is far more commonly seen than what these small figures might indicate. Loss of vision in one or both eyes is so significant that it has been classified as a 24% of whole-person impairment and 85% of whole-person disability, respectively. Approximately 19 million people worldwide are unilaterally blind and 1.6 million are bilaterally blind due to ocular trauma [1]. Ocular injuries constitute a major cause of visual morbidity, with a significant socioeconomic impact. They are also considered an important, preventable, public health problem the world over. These injuries are far more commonly seen in males (the male to female ratio being 4:1) and, in them, it occurs at a much younger age (average age, 36 years) than in women (average age, 73 years) [2]. Out of all types of ocular emergencies, ocular trauma is by far the commonest, constituting nearly 75% of all ocular emergencies. According to the World Health Organization, there are approximately 55 million eye injuries that restrict all activities for 1 or more days occurring each year. Approximately 200,000 open globe injuries occur every year. Ocular trauma is the most frequent cause of eye-related emergency department visits [3].

Eye injuries have a bimodal age distribution, with the first peak in young adults under the age of 30 years. Armed forces have majority of its personnel in this age group. A second peak occurs in the elderly individuals above 70 years of age associated with falls and war veterans belong to this group [2]. Majority of ocular injuries occur in either the workplace or home environment. When occupational injuries do occur, the majority of individuals are not wearing devices to protect the eye. This highlights the importance of improving safety standards and education regarding ocular trauma.

Eye trauma has a devastating impact on both the individual and society at large. Beyond the direct cost of medical care, indirect costs such workdays lost, long-term disability, and loss of trained manpower are huge. Prevention of ocular trauma should be a major health goal for all eye care professionals. Ocular trauma not only results in significant visual loss but can also have a tremendous psychological impact. Depression

S. Phadke · M. Shaikh · A. Chavan
Community Eye Care Foundation, Dr. Gogate's Eye Clinic, Pune, Maharashtra, India

P. Gogate (✉)
Community Eye Care Foundation, Dr. Gogate's Eye Clinic, Pune, Maharashtra, India

Department of Ophthalmology, Dr. D.Y.Patil Medical College, Pune, Maharashtra, India

S. Gogate
Armed Forces Medical College, Pune, Maharashtra, India

O. K. Radhakrishnan
Department of Ophthalmology, Dr. D.Y.Patil Medical College, Pune, Maharashtra, India

S. Waikar (ed.), *Ocular Trauma in Armed Conflicts*, https://doi.org/10.1007/978-981-19-4021-7_22

and anxiety can occur after significant ocular trauma. Psychological support is often required in helping patients to overcome these obstacles. Patients with significant monocular visual loss require assistance in adjusting to a new life. Low vision services and rehabilitation therapy are often required for these individuals to carry on with life [4, 5].

Military ocular injuries cannot be directly compared with the experience of civilian trauma. Armed Forces personnel are more vulnerable to ocular trauma due to their outdoor activities and need to be in violent surroundings as compared to other professions. Injury to the eye constitutes a grievous injury. It has serious implications for armed forces personnel's fitness for duty. A person with below par vision is deemed unfit for service.

The vast majority of military patients are male (98%). High-energy explosive blast injuries are sustained in 83% compared with 3% in civilians. Military injuries cause greater ocular damage, with an initial VA of ≤6/60 recorded in 71% compared with 27% among civilians. Military ocular injuries are often associated with severe polytrauma in 75% of cases; this is rare in the civilian setting [6].

Armed forces personnel are predisposed to all types of trauma that a noncombatant is exposed to in their civilian life including injury at workplace, home environment, sports and recreational activities, assault, and fireworks. He is however predisposed to trauma that are peculiar to combat duties involving a knife, bayonet, various types of gunshots injuries, IED blasts, bow and arrow injuries, anti-aircraft guns, aircraft crashes, blast injuries, chemical warfare, or radiation. Soldiers serving in high altitude areas and sea are prone to snow and sea blindness. In 1998, approximately 1% of all members of the US Armed Forces were treated for eye injuries [7].

Ocular injury and significant visual loss have significant implications on the future of the patient as well as the family. It has effect on employment, and emotional and social well-being of an individual. So, it is important to give a critical support to minimize the handicap.

22.1 Prevention of Ocular Injuries

Eye injuries range from minor bruises and scratches to serious lacerations, fractures, and burns. Wearing of protective eyewear by personnel of Armed Forces during combat and noncombat duties is important. Consistent use of eye protection could significantly prevent a high proportion of all eye injuries among the Armed Forces personnel [7].

Various types of protective eyewear are available. Use of polycarbonate eyewear should be prescribed and encouraged. There are protective goggles and face shields for protection against knife wounds, bullet injury, and chemical burns. There are special sun goggles for UV protection for soldiers in high altitude and high seas.

There are special aviator glasses for use of pilots and airmen. The professions that use high impact protection in eyewear include not just armed forces personnel but also welders, carpenters, plumbers, people working with moving machines, mill workers, and some construction workers. The National Institute for Occupational Safety and Health (NIOSH) recommends safety goggles for protection against splashes splatter and spray of blood, other body fluids, or chemicals for health-care personnel [8].

22.2 Classification of Ocular Protective Devices

Safety lenses are of two types: basic and high impact. The "drop ball" test is used to ascertain the basic impact safety classification for lenses [9]. In this test, a one-inch diameter steel ball is dropped onto the lens from a height of 50 inches. The lens must not crack, chip, or break to pass the test. Polycarbonate material and its variants are widely used. For high impact testing, a special high velocity test is performed. In this, a quarter-inch diameter steel ball is shot at the lens at a speed of 150 feet per second from a distance of 10 inches. For high mass impact, a 1-in. diameter steel ball weighing 17.6 ounces is dropped through a tube at the height of 50 in. onto the safety lens mounted in a frame. The lens must not crack, chip, or break to pass this test, and it must not become dislodged from the lens holder. A plus (+) mark indicates its approval at high impact. A "V" mark indicates that the lens is photo chromatic, while "S" mark denotes a special tint [10].

22.3 Low Vision Assessment

The purpose of low vision assessment is to assess the residual vision of the patient, correlate it with the individual's social and emotional needs, and identify the ways and means to enhance the residual vision. Functional vision is the residual vision resulting from some pathological conditions that cannot be corrected or treated, which results in situations such as insufficient visual resolution, inadequate field of vision, and reduced contrast sensitivity [11].

According to WHO, blindness is defined as having visual acuity less than 3/60 in the better eye, after best possible correction or visual field less than 10° from the point of fixation.

Categories of visual disabilities that are currently in use are defined in Table 22.1 [12]:

22.4 Low Vision Assessment

The low vision assessment has three goals:

1. To quantify the patient's vision
2. To improve the residual vision
3. To recommend vision rehabilitation interventions

22.5 Examination

Observation: Patient should be observed for mobility, posture, ocular fixation, and psychological well-being

22.5.1 History

General history: Demographic information, marital status, orientation and mobility.

Ocular history: Diagnosis, onset of symptoms, previous treatments or surgeries, and LVAs and possible outcomes.

History of systemic diseases: General health, current medications, and psychological status.

Table 22.1 Categories of blindness

Better eye Best corrected	Worst eye Best corrected	Percentage impairment	Disability category
6/6 to 6/18	6/6 to 6/18 6/24 to 6/60 Less than 6/60 to 3/60 Less than 3/60 to light perception	0% 10% 20% 30%	0 0 I II (one eyed person)
6/24 to 6/60 or visual field less than 40 up to 20° around centre of fixation or hemianopia involving macula	6/24 to 6/60 Less than 3/60 to 6/60 Less than 3/60 to no light perception	40% 50% 60%	III a (low vision) III b (low vision) III c (low vision)
Less than 6/60 to 3/60 Or Visual field less than 20 up to 10° around centre of fixation	Less than 6/60 to 3/60 Less than 3/60 to no light perception	70% 80%	III d (low vision) III e (low vision)
Less than 3/60 to 1/60 Or Visual filed less than 10° around centre of fixation	Less than 3/60 to no light perception	90%	IV a (blindness)
Only HMCF Only light perception No light perception	Only HMCF Only light perception No light perception	100%	IV a (blindness)

Financial status: Affordability of low vision aids (LVA).

22.5.2 Visual Acuity

Distance vision assessment: Chart should be handheld or movable. ETDRS is the preferred chart and testing distance should be 4 m.

Near acuity assessment: Allow the patient at their preferred distance. Measure the near vision for each eye separately. The eye with better vision should be given the low vision aid.

Functional visual acuity should be measured at 40 cm.

Refraction: Should be over—corrected for near and distance vision. 6/12 is taken as reference acuity to be achieved.

Visual field analysis: Humphrey perimetry and Amsler grid testing to find out field of vision, peripheral and central scotomas.

Other tests that need to be done are pinhole test, color vision and glare sensitivity.

22.6 Treatment

Different low vision devices are given based on principles of magnification listed below:

1. Relative distance magnification. e.g., holding a book close to the eye
2. Relative size magnification., larger print
3. Angular magnification, e.g., Telescopes
4. Electronic magnification, e.g., CCTV

The following treatment options are available for the patients:

22.6.1 Optical Devices

22.6.1.1 Low Vision Devices for Distance

- Spectacles
- Contact Lenses
- Telescopes

Telescopes are based on the principle of angular magnification.

They can be

1. Monocular: They are cheap, handy, and can be used for the dominant eye (Fig. 22.1).
2. Binocular: They are more effective in cases of nystagmus (Fig. 22.2).

22.6.1.2 Low Vision Devices for Near Vision

1. Spectacle magnifiers: They are hands-free and provide large field of vision but provide lot of distortions, aberrations, and poor illumination.
   (a) Full field spectacle magnifiers (Fig. 22.3)
   (b) Half field spectacle magnifiers (Fig. 22.4)
   (c) Bifocal spectacles (Fig. 22.5)
   (d) Prismatic spectacles (Fig. 22.6)
2. Hand magnifiers: They have good working distance. Accommodation is also not required.

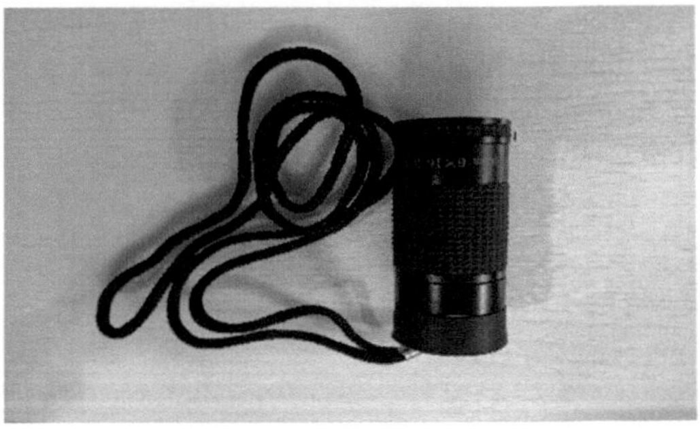

Fig. 22.1 Monocular Telescope

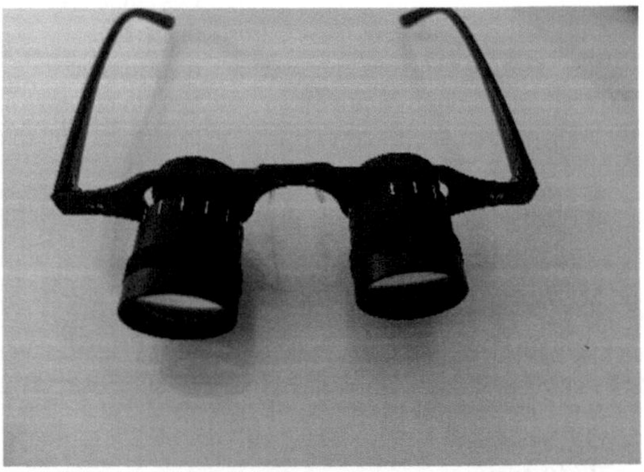

Fig. 22.2 Binocular Telescope

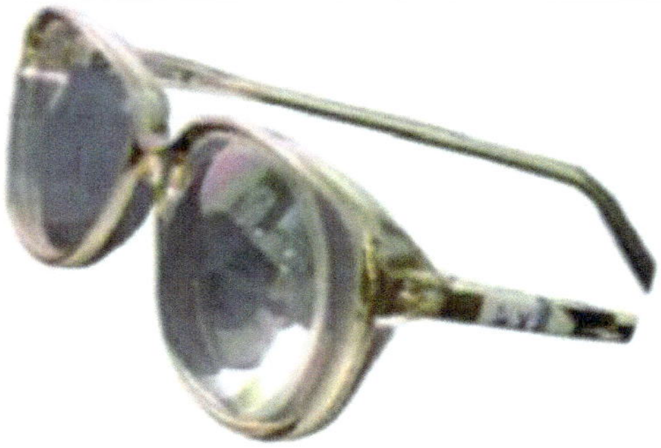

Fig. 22.3 Full field spectacle magnifier

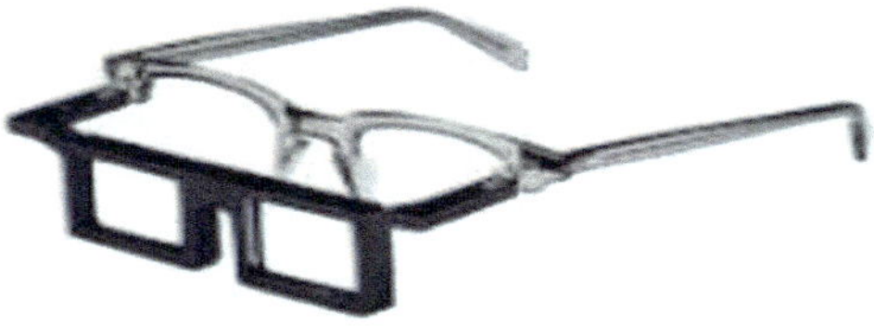

Fig. 22.4 Half field spectacle magnifier

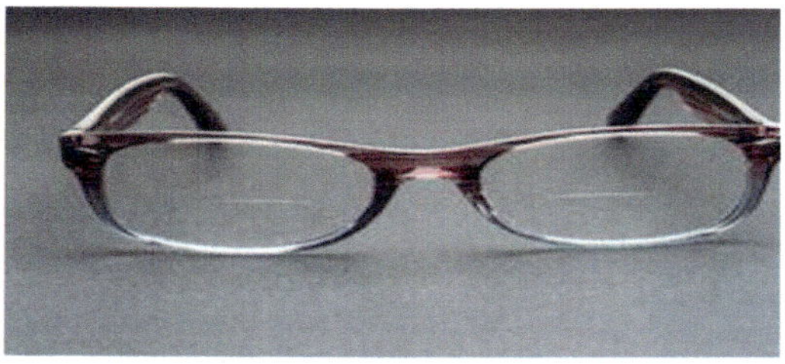

Fig. 22.5 Bifocal Spectacles

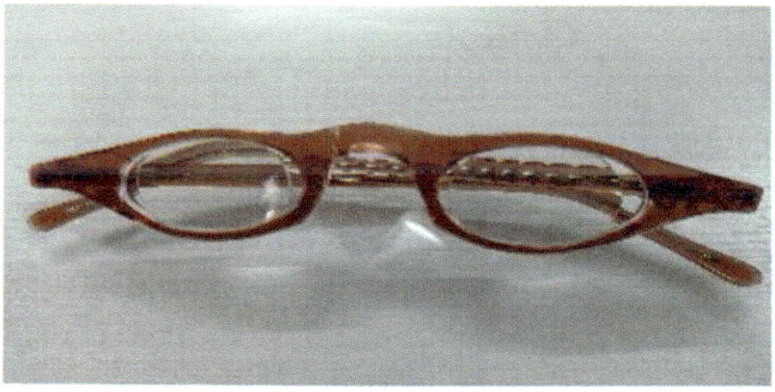

Fig. 22.6 Prismatic Spectacle

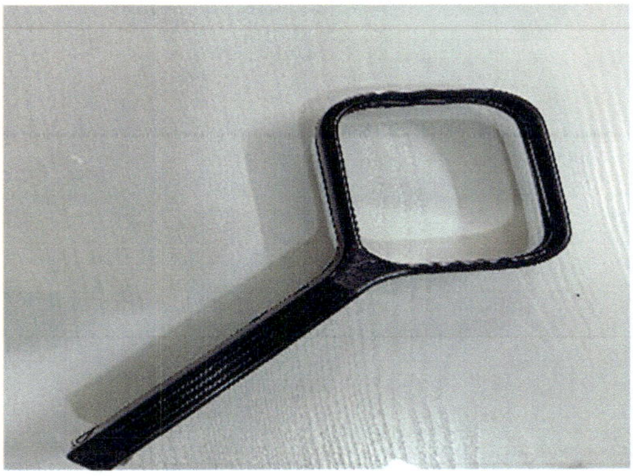

Fig. 22.7 Hand Magnifier

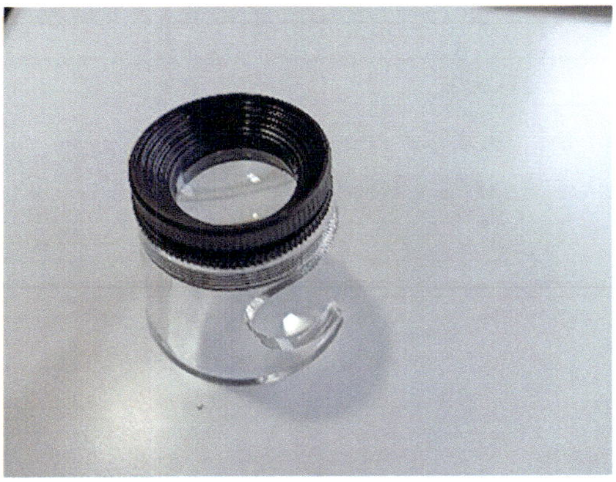

Fig. 22.8 Stand Magnifier

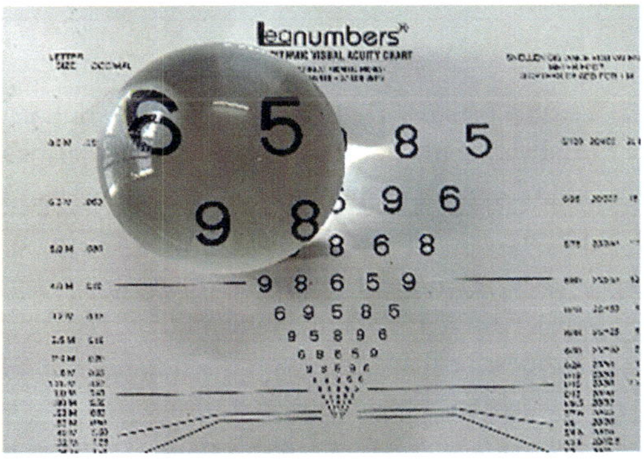

Fig. 22.9 Dome Magnifier

However, it is not hand-free and has smaller field of vision (Fig. 22.7).

3. Stand magnifiers: While stand magnifiers are hand-free and are helpful in cases with tremors, they have small visual field and the reading distance is too small, resulting in bad posture (Fig. 22.8).
4. Dome magnifiers: Fig. 22.9

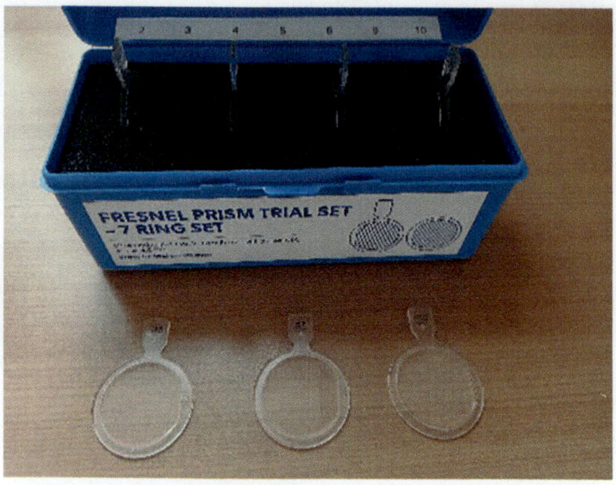

Fig. 22.10 Fresnel Prism Set

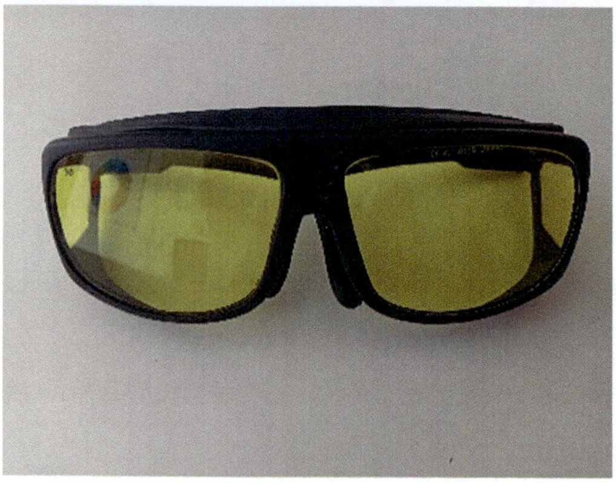

Fig. 22.11 Glare Control glass

5. Fresnel prisms: They are lightweight, stick-on prisms that are helpful in patients with peripheral, central and hemianopic or sectoral field detects.

   The prism will shift the image from the nonseeing to the seeing area (Fig. 22.10).
6. Devices for glare and photophobia.

   Coating, tints, polarized filters or photo chromatic lenses are used to decrease the glare (Fig. 22.11).

22.6.2 Nonoptical Devices

Nonoptical devices can be prescribed with or without optical visual aids.

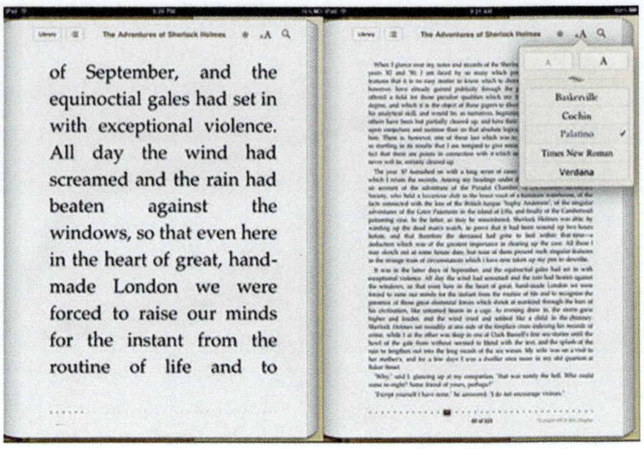

Fig. 22.12 Large Print Book

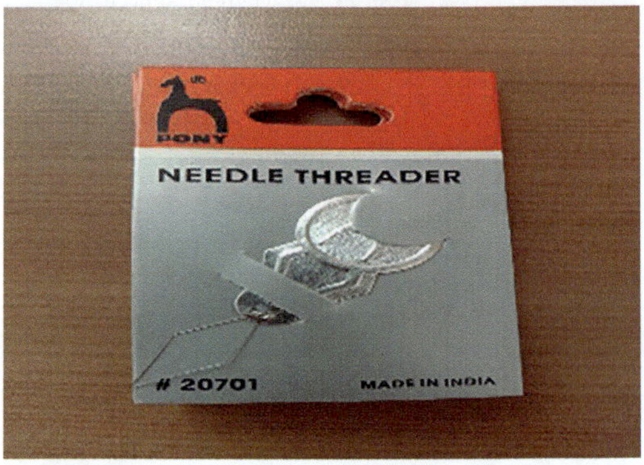

Fig. 22.13 Needle Threaders

22.6.2.1 Relative Size Devices

Large objects are used, e.g., large print books, needle threaders, etc. (Figs. 22.12 and 22.13).

22.6.2.2 Light and Illumination Controls

Patients can have better vision with extra illumination (Fig. 22.14).

22.6.2.3 Writing and Communication Devices

Writing and communication devices: help a visually impaired person to read and write print.E.g., typoscope, writing guide, etc. (Figs. 22.15 and 22.16).

22.6.2.4 Mobility Devices

Mobility devices help the patient in moving independently, e.g., foldable and nonfoldable canes.

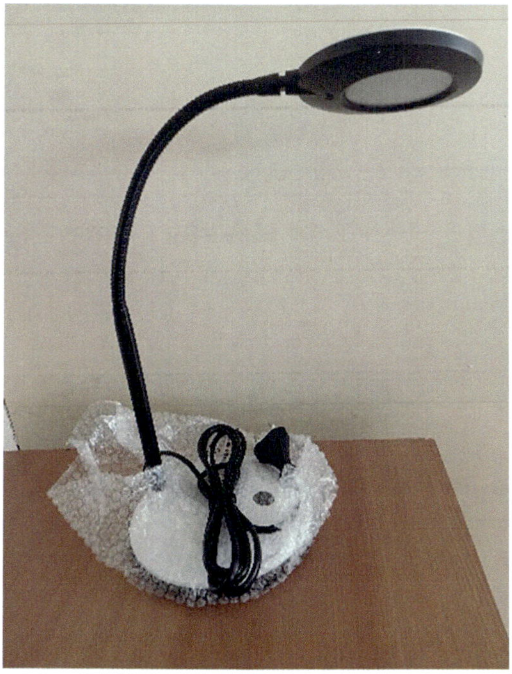

Fig. 22.14 LED Table Lamp

Fig. 22.15 Typoscope

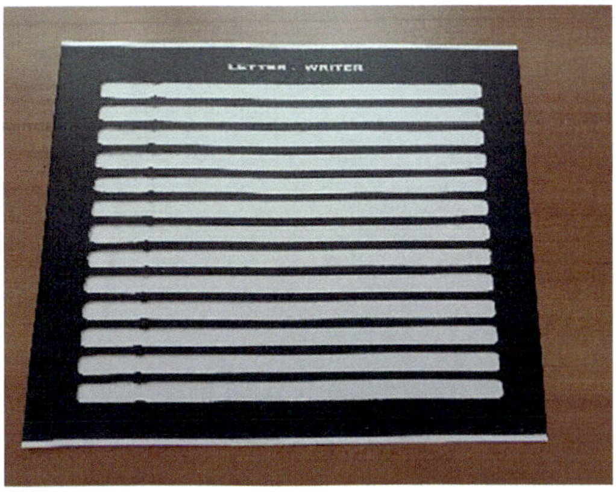

Fig. 22.16 Writing Guide

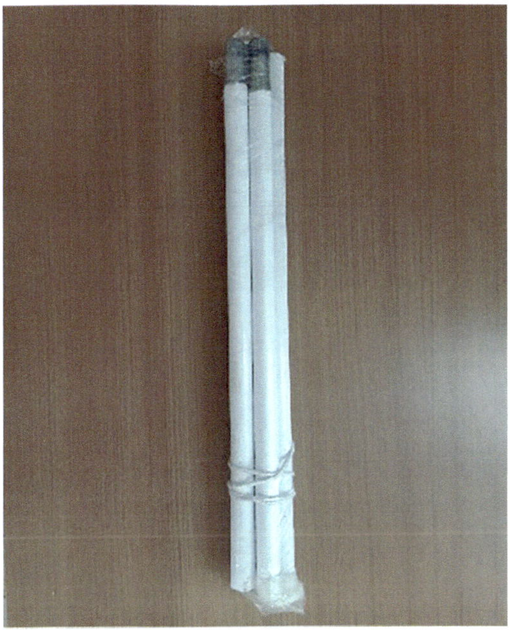

Fig. 22.17 Mobility Cane

Dog guides are used in many European countries (Fig. 22.17).

22.6.2.5 Sensory Substitution Devices

Sense of seeing is substituted with tactile or auditory senses, e.g., talking clocks and calculators, Notex (Figs. 22.18 and 22.19).

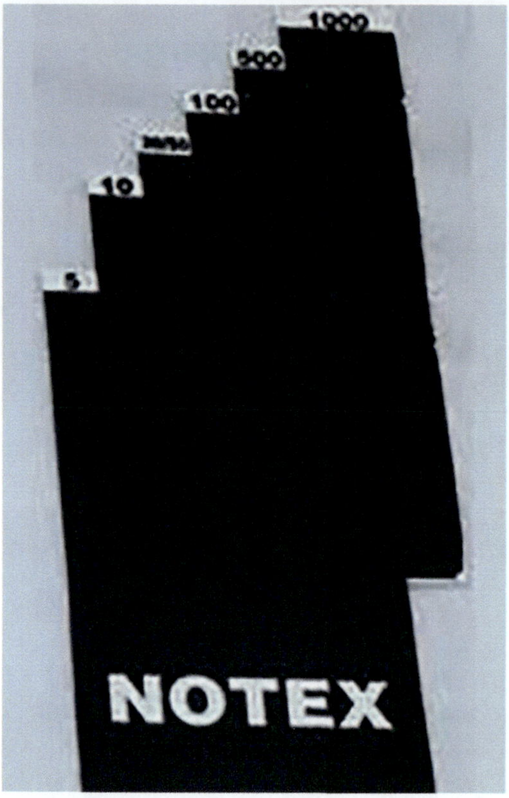

Fig. 22.18 Notex

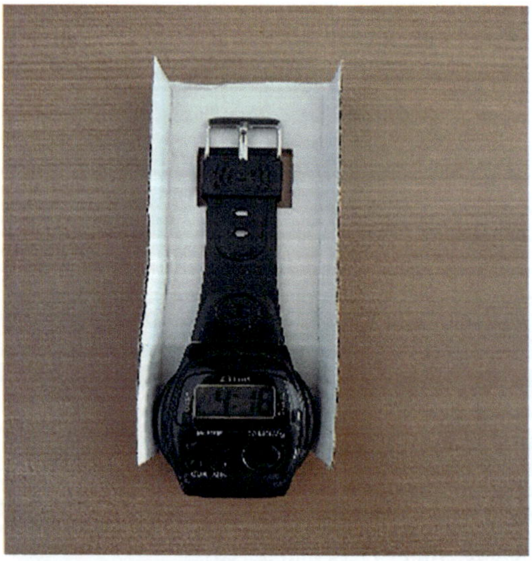

Fig. 22.19 Talking Watch

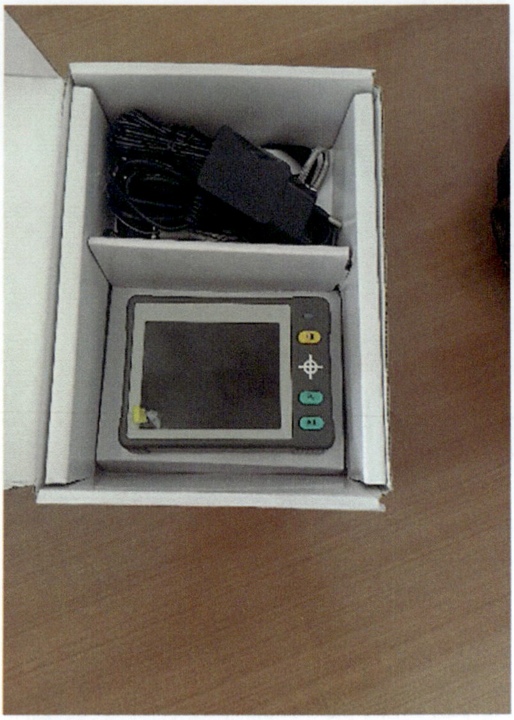

Fig. 22.20 Video Magnifier

22.6.2.6 Electronic Devices

Electronic devices assist in moderate-to-severe visual impairment patients who are not benefitted by other devices, e.g., video magnification systems and CCTV systems (Fig. 22.20).

22.7 Rehabilitation

Rehabilitation is aimed at giving psychological counseling, career guidance, independence in daily activities, and teaching orientation and mobility. It also aims at providing skilled training such as computers, Braille, training in writing and English-speaking skills, and home management.

Treatment of patients with low vision is not the job of a single specialty; it is a joint effort between ophthalmologists, optometrists, low vision aid specialists and rehabilitation experts, and, most importantly, the patient and his family.

Most people have problems coping with vision loss and some may need psychological counseling. They go through the five stages of coping, denial, anger, barter, depression, and acceptance. Those in the working age group may need career counseling to adjust in their respective professions or choose an entirely different one. People of all age groups may need mobility training in the form of "white cane training," guide dogs, and mobile phone applications to retain their independence of movement. The Royal National Institute for the Blind was established in London in 1868 by Thomas Armitage, a doctor with problems with his eyesight [13]. It focused on rehabilitation of the blind. The Royal Normal College and Academy for the Blind was founded in 1872 for the education of the blind and visually impaired and is now the Royal National College for the Blind [14].

Most serving uniformed personnel are retired on losing vision and may need help in coping with a new world. The First World War was the starting point for having special centers for rehabilitation of blinded soldiers in Italy (*Comitatofiorentino per iciechi di Guerra*, the Florentine Committee for the War Blinded, established in 1915) and its Director Aurelio Nicolodi, from Austro-Italian border, was a visually impaired war veteran [15]. The prolonged use of artillery and explosives with numerous projectiles ensured numerous eye wounds and injuries. The eyes were the least protected part of the body in trench warfare as the helmets protected only the head and goggles were irregularly supplied and used even less.

In the United States of America, Russell C. Williams, World War II veteran who was blinded in the war, was selected to be the first chief of the Hines Blind Rehabilitation Centre [16]. He ensured that the center won the respect of both the military and medical bureaucracies. President Franklin D. Roosevelt signed an executive order declaring: "No blinded servicemen from WW II would be returned to their homes without adequate training to meet the problems of necessity imposed upon them by their blindness." The Hines center in 1949 helped more than five hundred US armed personnel blinded in the Korean War. They accounted for nearly 5% of all casualties demonstrating how risky modern warfare was, not just to limb and life, but also to eyes and vision.

Recreational activities for the visually impaired: There are numerous indoor games that have been modified for the visually impaired. Chess, carom, playing cards, Uno, and board games like Monopoly, Bananagrams, Checkers, and Scrabble have all been adapted for the visual impaired as have been numerous computer games. Outdoor games like cricket and basketball have visually impaired teams and tournaments.

With proper low vision assessment and dispensing of optical and nonoptical aids, many visually impaired can lead near-normal life, albeit out of the uniform. Rehabilitation helps them to cope with the disability better, and markedly improves psychological well-being and quality of life.

References

1. Scott R. The injured eye. Philos Trans R Soc Lond B Biol Sci. 2011;366(1562):251–60.
2. Mishra A, Verma AK, Baranwal VK, Aggarwal S, Bhargava N, Parihar JKS. The pattern and visual outcomes of ocular trauma in a large zonal hospital in a non-operational role: a 36 months retrospective analysis. J Clin Ophthalmol Res. 2014;2:141–4.
3. Negrel AD, Thylefors B. The global impact of eye injuries. Ophthalmic Epidemiol. 1998;5(3):143–69.
4. Do AT, Ilango K, Ramasamy D, Kalidasan S, Balakrishnan V, Chang RT. Effectiveness of low vision services in improving quality of life at Aravind eye hospital. Indian J Ophthalmol. 2014;62(12):1125–31.
5. Williams DR. Non-optical aids. J Am Optom Assoc. 1986;57(8):608–15.
6. Blanch RJ, Bindra MS, Jacks AS, Scott RAH. Ophthalmic injuries in British armed forces in Iraq and Afghanistan. Eye. 2010;25:218–23.
7. Andreotti G, Lange JL, Brundage JF. The nature, incidence, and impact of eye injuries among US military personnel: implications for prevention. Arch Ophthalmol. 2001;119(11):1693–7.
8. National Institute of Occupational Safety & Health. https://www.cdc.gov/niosh. Accessed 20 Feb 2021.
9. McMahon JM, Beckerman S. Testing safety eyewear: how frame and lens design affect lens retention. Optometry. 2007;78(2):78–87.
10. Safety glasses and protective wear. https://www.allaboutvision.com/safety/safety-glasses.htm. Accessed 20 Feb 2021.

11. Kavitha V, Manumali MS, Praveen K, Heralgi MM. Low vision aid- a ray of hope for irreversible visual loss in the pediatric age group. Taiwan J Ophthalmol. 2015;5:63–7.
12. Gazette of India. Extraordinary Part II-Section 3- Subsection (ii) New Delhi, January 5, 2018/PAUSHA 15,1939, Ministry of social justice and empowerment [Department of Empowerment of Persons with Disabilities (Divyangjan).
13. Royal National Institute for the Blind, London, UK. www.rnib.org.uk. Accessed 20 Feb 2021.
14. Royal National College for the Blind. www.rnc.ac.uk. Accessed 20 Feb 2021.
15. Salvante M. 'Thanks to the great war the blind gets the recognition of his ability to act': the rehabilitation of blinded servicemen in Florence. First World War Stud. 2015;6(1):21–35.
16. Edward Hines, Jr VA Hospital, Central Blind Rehabilitation Centre. www.hines.va.gov. Accessed 20 Feb 2021.